Springer Series on Geriatric Nursing

Mathy D. Mezey, RN, EdD, FAAN, Series Editor
New York University, The Steinhardt School of Education, Division of Nursing

Advisory Board: Margaret Diamond, PhD, RN, FAAN; Steven H. Ferris, PhD; Terry Fulmer, RN, PhD, FAAN; Linda Kaeser, PhD, RN, ACSW, FAAN; Virgene Kayser-Jones, PhD, RN, FAAN; Eugenia Siegler, MD; Neville Strumpf, PhD, RN, FAAN; May Wykle, PhD, RN, FAAN; Mary Walker, PhD, RN, FAAN

Mathy Doval Mezey, EdD, RN, FAAN, received her undergraduate and graduate education at Columbia University. Dr. Mezey taught at Lehman College of the City University of New York. For 10 years she was a professor at the University of Pennsylvania School of Nursing, where she directed the geriatric nurse practitioner program and was director of the Robert Wood Johnson Foundation Teaching Nursing Home Program. Since 1991 she has been the Independence Foundation Professor of Nursing at New York University, and, since 1996, director of the John A. Hartford Foundation Institute for Geriatric Nursing Practice, the only nurse-led institute in the country. Dr. Mezey has authored 5 books and has over 60 publications that focus on the preparation of advanced practice nurses to care for older adults and bioethical issues that effect end of life decisions. She is Editor for the Springer Series in Geriatric Nursing and of the Springer publication *The Encyclopedia of Elder Care.* Dr. Mezey is a Fellow of the Gerontological Society of America, sits on the board of the Visiting Nurse Service of New York, and is Trustee Emeritus of Columbia University.

Terry Fulmer, RN, PhD, FAAN is the Division head for New York University. She is also a Professor of Nursing and Director of the Muriel and Virginia Center for Nursing Research at NYU, Co-Director for the John A. Hartford Foundation Institute for the Advancement of Geriatric Nursing Practice, and Director of the Consortium of New York Geriatric Education Centers. Dr. Fulmer's program of research focuses on acute care of the elderly and specifically on the subject of elder abuse and neglect. She has written extensively and has published over 90 articles and 40 chapters. Two of her nine books have received the American Journal of Nursing Book of the Year Awards.

Ivo Abraham, PhD, FAAN is the president and CEO of the Epsilon Group, an international healthcare research and consulting company and Clinical Professor of Nursing at the University of Virginia. Over the past two decades, Ivo's clinical research and development efforts have focused on aging, mental health nursing, and the integration of quantitative methods in nursing research. Previously, Dr. Abraham was on the faculty in the Schools of Nursing and Medicine at the University of Virginia and founding Director of the Center of Aging and Health and the NIMH Rural Mental Health Research Center.

DeAnne Zwicker, MS, APRN, BC is an ANCC certified adult and geriatric nurse practitioner and a senior advisor for Special Projects at The Hartford Foundation Institute of Geriatric Nursing in the NYU Division of Nursing. Most recently she was project editor for the NYU on-line Geriatric Nursing Review Course. Additionally, she is a primary care provider in a nursing home. She previously worked as a clinical services manager, an NP in primary care and long term care, and has taught in the Master's level nurse practitioner program at NYU.

Geriatric Nursing Protocols for Best Practice
Second Edition

Mathy Mezey, *EdD, RN, FAAN*
Terry Fulmer, *PhD, RN, FAAN*
Ivo Abraham, *PhD, FAAN*
Editors

DeAnne Zwicker, *MS, APRN, BC*
Managing Editor

 Springer Publishing Company

The protocols presented in this book have been selected by the National Guideline Clearinghouse (www.guideline.gov) for inclusion in their Internet database of clinical practice guidelines.

The National Guideline Clearinghouse (NGC) is a comprehensive database of evidence-based clinical practice guidelines and related documents sponsored by the U.S. Agency for Healthcare Research and Quality (AHRQ) (formerly the Agency for Health Care Policy and Research [AHCPR]), in partnership with the American Medical Association (AMA) and the American Association of Health Plans (AAHP).

Copyright © 2003 by Springer Publishing Company, Inc.

Springer Publishing Company, Inc.
536 Broadway
New York, NY 10012-3955

Acquisitions Editor: Ruth Chasek
Production Editor: Pamela Lankas
Cover design by Joanne Honigman

03 04 05 06 07 / 5 4 3 2

Library of Congress Cataloging-in-Publication Data

Geriatric nursing protocols for best practice / Mathy Mezey . . . [et al.], editors — 2nd ed.
      p. ; cm. — (Springer series on geriatric nursing)
Includes bibliographical references and index.
ISBN 0-8261-1834-8
1. Geriatric nursing. 2. Nursing care plans.
   [DNLM: 1. Geriatric Nursing—methods. 2. Nursing Care—Aged.
3. Hospitalization—Aged. 4. Nursing Assessment—Aged. WY 152
G3698 2003] I. Mezey, Mathy Doval. II. Series.
RC954 .G465 2003
610.73'65—dc21

                                                        2003054363

Printed in the United States of America by Maple-Vail Book Manufacturing Group.

The Geriatric Nursing Protocols for Best Practice, Second Edition is dedicated to all hospitals participating in Nurses Improving Care for Health System Elders (NICHE). The John A. Hartford Foundation Institute for Geriatric Nursing and the NICHE faculty recognize the commitment of "geriatric-friendly hospitals" to provide quality care for older adults. The support and activity of NICHE hospitals are instrumental in driving geriatric nursing to the forefront of health care for the elderly. The following is a list of the hospitals participating in NICHE.

Arizona
Tucson Medical Center, Tucson

California
Tulare Local Healthcare District (TDH), Tulare
University of California, San Francisco, San Francisco

Connecticut
Stamford Hospital, Stamford

Delaware
Christiana Care Health System at Newark, Newark
Christiana Care Health System at Riverside Long Term & Transitional Care, Bloomington
Christiana Care Health System at Wilmington Hospital, Wilmington

Florida
Florida Hospital Medical Center, Orlando
Morton Plant Mease Health Care, Morton Plant Hospital, Clearwater
Morton Plant Mease, Mease Dunedin Hospital, Clearwater
Sarasota Memorial Hospital, Sarasota

Hawaii
Kaiser Permanente, Honolulu

Iowa
Mercy Medical Center North Iowa, Marson City
University of Iowa Hospitals and Clinics, Iowa City

Idaho
Kootenai Medical Services, Coeur d'Alene

Illinois
Memorial Medical Center, Springfield
OSF Saint Anthony Medical Center, Rockford
OSF Saint Francis Medical Center, Peoria
Rush North Shore Medical Center, Skokie

Indiana
Wishard Hospital, Indianapolis

Louisiana
Ochsner Clinic Foundation, Nursing Executive Office, New Orleans
St. Charles General Hospital, New Orleans
Tenet Health Center, Memorial Medical Center, New Orleans

Massachusetts
Jewish Geriatric Services, Longmeadow
Massachusetts General Hospital, Boston
Spaulding Rehabilitation Hospital, Boston

Michigan
Bronson Methodist Hospital, Kalamazoo
Oakwood Healthcare System, Dearborn
Spectrum Health, Grand Rapids, Grand Rapids
St. John's Hospital and Medical Center, Detroit
St. Joseph Mercy–Oakland, Pontiac
W. A. Foote Memorial Hospital, Jackson
William Beaumont Hospital, Royal Oak

Minnesota
Fairview University Medical Center, Minneapolis
Mayo Clinic, Rochester
Mayo Clinic, St. Mary's Hospital, Rochester
North Memorial Medical Center, Robbinsdale

North Carolina
Mission St. Joseph's Healthcare System, Asheville
Moses Cone Health System, Greensboro
University of North Carolina Hospitals, Chapel Hill

New Hampshire
Frisbie Memorial Hospital, Rochester

New Jersey
Meridian Health System, Ann May Center for Nursing, Neptune
Meridian Health System, Jersey Shore Medical Center, Neptune
Meridian Health System, Medical Center of Ocean County, Brick

New Jersey *(continued)*
Meridian Health System, Riverview
Medical Center, Red Bank
Trinitas Hospital, Elizabeth

New York
Benedictine Hospital, Kingston
Kaledia Health, Buffalo General Hospital
Site, Buffalo
Long Island Jewish (LIJ) Medical Center,
New Hyde Park
Mount Sinai Medical Center, New York
New York Presbyterian Hospital—The Allen
Pavilion, New York
North Shore LIH: Huntington Hospital,
Huntington
North Shore University Hospital (NSUH) at
Manhasset, Manhasset
NYU Downtown Hospital, New York
NYU Medical Center, Tisch Hospital,
New York

Ohio
Premiere Health Partners, Good Samaritan
Hospital, Dayton
Premiere Health Partners, Miami Valley
Hospital, Dayton
The Cleveland Clinic Foundation,
Cleveland
The Cleveland Clinic Health System,
Euclid Hospital, Euclid
University Hospitals of Cleveland,
Cleveland

Oregon
Peace Health, Sacred Heart Medical
Center, Eugene
Providence Milwaukie Hospital, Milwaukie
Providence Portland Medical Center,
Portland
Providence St. Vincent Medical Center,
Portland

Pennsylvania
Community Medical Center, Scranton
Crozer Keystone Health System, Crozer
Chester, Upland
Crozer Keystone Health System, Delaware
County, Drexel Hill
Crozer Keystone Health System, Taylor
Hospital, Ridley
Moses Taylor Hospital, Scranton
Suburban General Hospital, Pittsburgh

Tennessee
Covenant Health: Fort Sanders Loudon
Medical Center, Loudon
Covenant Health: Fort Sanders Regional
Medical Center, Knoxville
Covenant Health: Fort Sanders Regional
Parkwest Hospitals, Knoxville

Texas
Rolling Plains Memorial Hospital,
Sweetwater
St. Luke's Episcopal Hospital, Houston
University of Texas Medical Branch,
Galveston

Virginia
Bon Secours DePaul Medical Center,
Norfolk
Inova Fairfax Hospital, Falls Church
University of Virginia Health System,
Charlottesville

Washington
Virginia Mason Medical Center, Seattle

Wisconsin
Aurora Health Care, St. Luke's South Shore
Hospital, Cudahy
Covenant Healthcare, Marian Franciscan
Center, Milwaukee
Covenant Healthcare, St. Francis Hospital,
Brown Deer
Covenant Healthcare, St. Michael Hospital,
Milwaukee
Meriter Health Services, Madison
Waukesha Memorial Hospital, Waukesha

West Virginia
Charleston Area Medical Center, Charleston
General Hospital, Charleston

Canada
St. Boniface General Hospital, Winnipeg

CONTENTS

FOREWORD

Older patients present a challenge to hospitals in a time of nursing shortage and cost containment. The decreased length of stay, complexity of medical regimens, and multiple co-morbid conditions increase the risk of adverse health outcomes in older patients. Although the hospital is often an ideal place for patients requiring "high tech" acute care, the environment poses a threat to many older persons, particularly the frail elderly. The hospital has been viewed as a culprit for adverse outcomes for the elderly (Kohn, Corrigan, & Donaldson, 2000). Older patients frequently experience cognitive decline (usually delirium with an underlying cause), functional decline, falls, fractures, pressure ulcers, urinary incontinence, fecal impaction, dehydration, and urinary infection while hospitalized or soon after discharge. Additionally, hospitalization poses risks to older patients due to exposure to drugs, diagnostic testing, and treatments. Complications that result from these risks add to older patients already slowed convalescence period.

For many older people, hospitalization is a "sentinel event," triggering a downward trajectory in health and function that is all too often permanent. The negative consequences of a hospitalization are particularly noticeable in the already frail older persons: those who already have compromised function, multiple chronic illnesses, cognitive impairment, or complex medications regimens. Because of cost constraints many older patients are being discharged home much earlier and much sicker, further increasing the risk of complications after discharge and the need for re-admission to the hospital.

Nurses are at the forefront of care in the hospital setting and must be looked to for help in reducing adverse consequences of hospitalization. All nurses need to be knowledgeable as to the unique needs of their older patients in order to improve outcomes and quality of life. Additionally nurses, who are the primary advocates for patient care, have to meet the increasing demands of cost containment while maintaining safety and quality outcomes. Nurses will need to take a proactive role instituting preventive measures to avoid common iatrogenic conditions that occur in the hospital.

We know quite a lot about the events that can turn a routine hospitalization into a cascade of negative outcomes for older people. We also know quite a lot about what triggers these events, including excessive use of physical restraints; less than optimal drugs, dosages and duration of medications; inappropriate treatment of pain; and failure to address nutritional needs of older people.

Geriatric nurses and geriatricians have long recognized that negative outcomes are not inevitable consequences of a hospitalization. Quite the contrary, careful assessment and planning can avert or minimize many complications (Cohen, Feussner, Weinberger, Carnes, Hamdy, Hsieh, et al., 2002). Over the past 18 years, many demonstration projects have taught us much about how to provide optimum care for the elderly in hospitals. One of the most prominent of these efforts, funded by The John A. Hartford Foundation, was The Hospital Outcomes Program for the Elderly (HOPE). HOPE projects were instrumental in demonstrating the benefits of such service reconfigurations as units specialized in the care of older people (Acute Care of the Elderly [ACE] units) (Francis, Fletcher, & Simon; 1998; Fulmer et al., 2002; Landfeld et al., 1995), and of unit-based Geriatric Resource Nurses (GRN) working with geriatric nurse specialists and geriatricians (Francis et al., 1998; Lee & Fletcher, 2002). Many other programs have emerged from the original HOPE program, GRN model, and ACE units; including the NICHE (Nurses Improving Care for Health System Elders) program, which focuses on nursing practice to improve care of elders (Fulmer et al., 2001; Francis et al., 1998; Lee & Fletcher, 2002).

Yet despite these and other projects, the infusion of knowledge as to how to create a safer hospital environment for older people has been slow to take hold. It is to address this need that the editors have prepared this book of protocols. The nursing protocols are specifically designed for the in-patient setting. Each represents a distillation of what constitutes "best practice" for 14 clinical syndromes that are commonly experienced by older people in hospitals. Originally tested by nurses in eight hospitals, we are confident that these protocols address many of the needs of the practicing nurse at the bedside. One protocol from the first edition, Eating and Feeding Difficulties, has also been tested in the long-term care setting (chapter 1). The protocols that appear in this book reflect the efforts of many nurse experts in the field. We hope that they will prove useful in your setting and that they will directly benefit the older people who come under your care. We are confident that your use of these approaches and feedback to the authors will lead to new "best practice" in geriatric nursing. These in turn will improve the quality, outcomes, and cost-effectiveness of inpatient care. Today and tomorrow's patients, their families or other caregivers, and their health practitioners will all be the beneficiaries of such changes.

DONNA REGENSTREIF, PhD
Senior Program Officer
The John A. Hartford Foundation of New York City

REFERENCES

Cohen, H., Feussner, J., Weinberger, M., Carnes, M., Hamdy, R., Hsieh, F., et al. (2002). A controlled trial of inpatient and outpatient geriatric evaluation and management. *New England Journal of Medicine, 346,* 905–912.

Francis, D., Fletcher, K., & Simon, L. (1998). The geriatric resource nurse model of care: A vision for the future. *Nursing Clinics of North America, 33,* 481–496.

Fulmer, T., Mezey, M., Bottrell, M., Abraham, I., Sazant, J., Grossman, S., & Grisham, E. (2002). Nurses Improving Care for Healthsystem Elders (NICHE: Using outcomes and benchmarks for evidenced-based practice). *Geriatric Nursing, 23,* 120–127.

Kohn, L. T., Corrigan, J. M., Donaldson, M. S. (Eds.). (2000). *To err is human: Building a safer health system.* Washington, DC: Institute of Medicine.

Landfeld, C. S., Palmer, R. M., Kresevic, D. M., et al. (1995). A randomized trial of care in a hospital medical unit especially designed to improve the functional outcomes of acutely ill older patients. *New England Journal of Medicine, 332,* 1338–1344.

Lee, V., & Fletcher, K. (2002). Sustaining the geriatric resource nurse model at the University of Virginia. *Geriatric Nursing, 23,* 128–1132.

PREFACE

The delivery of quality care during acute, ever-shortening episodes of care for the hospitalized elderly has become a major concern to families, staff nurses, nursing leadership, the chief nursing executive, medical staff, risk managers, and finance leaders alike. The percentage of the population that is aging is steadily rising, and the average age of members of this group is similarly rising. The multiplicity of problems imposed by each episode of hospitalization for the older patient proliferates. Their care needs are posing more complex challenges to nursing staff in particular, because frequently the problems requiring superb application of the nursing process are not disease specific, and are not generally amenable to standard medical regimes.

Although most organizations and health care systems have at least the rudiments of standards of practice for care, which focus on the process of care for specific patient groups, the development of such standards is a daunting project for the nursing staff. These nurses must be supported in their quest for methods and means of improving care delivery. Therefore, the focus of practice protocols is the staff nurse, the key critical element in the older person's survival in the institutional setting, or in the provider-supported program at home, as many elderly are supported in varying forms of home care services.

The purpose of this text is to present geriatric nursing protocols that have been developed as part of the NICHE Project, or Nurses Improving Care for Health System Elders. The 14 care problems commonly presented by sick elders to challenge staff nurses serve as the topic headings. The practice protocols each follow the conceptual framework of the professional nursing process: assessment, specialized tools specific to the problem area, nursing care strategies, and evaluation of expected outcomes. Each protocol is research or evidence-based, thus providing the critical foundation of knowledge that has been tested.

This text serves many audiences, each of whom may be invested in some aspect of geriatric care: For the staff nurse at the bedside, these ready-to-use protocols provide a sound and sophisticated basis for the delivery and improvement of care. For resource nurses, nursing leadership, clinical specialists, case managers, and staff development instructors, these protocols provide substance and resources for either the development or modification of whatever standards model the organization has established. Administrators and educators in health care organizations seeking ideas and a rationale for age-specific features, now a critical element in Joint Commission on Accreditation of Health Care Organizations standards, will find that the basis for competency assessment tailored to the care of the elderly in this volume. Patient-care-quality-and-improvement experts will find that the content and tools provide clinically appropriate avenues for designing or enhancing programs, establishing baseline parameters, and desired outcomes to be achieved.

For students, this volume provides a role model for the breadth of thinking and application of knowledge required for advanced nursing practice. For the very educated public, these protocols pose the means by which to evaluate the practice level of the institution in which family members or significant others are actual or potential patients. For administrators of insurance plans, these protocols provide a professional nursing care-based means of determining the level of service that optimally should be provided.

The reader must be cautioned that the presentation of such process standards does not ensure their implementation. This collection serves, however, as a substantive foundation for the identification of the problems posed, research-based assessment and interventions, and evaluation of outcomes.

SUSAN BOWER-FERRES, PhD, RN, CNAA
Vice President for Nursing Senior Administrator
New York University Medical Center

CONTRIBUTORS

Elaine J. Amella, PhD, APRN, BC, GNP
Assistant Professor
College of Nursing, Medical
    University of South Carolina
Charleston, SC

Elizabeth A. Ayello, PhD, RN, CS, CWOCN
Clinical Associate Professor and
    Senior Advisor
John A. Hartford Institute for
    Geriatric Nursing
Division of Nursing, The Steinhardt
    School of Education, New York
    University
New York, NY

Melissa M. Bottrell, MPH, PhD
Project Director
VHA National Center for Ethics
    in Health Care
VA Puget Sound Health Care
    System
Seattle, WA

Christine Wanich Bradway, MSN, RN, CS
Gerontologic Nurse Practitioner
    and Doctoral Candidate
University of Pennsylvania School
    of Nursing
Philadelphia, PA

Eileen R. Chasens, DSN, RN
Postdoctoral Fellow in Sleep
    Research
School of Nursing
University of Pennsylvania
Philadelphia, PA

Annemarie Dowling-Castronovo, APRN-BC
Gerontolgical Nurse Practitioner,
    New York University
The Steinhardt School of
    Education's Division of Nursing
New York, NY

Kathleen Fletcher, RN, MSN, APRN, BC
Administrator of Senior Services
University of Virginia Health
    Systems
Charlottesville, VA

Marquis D. Foreman, PhD, RN, FAAN
Associate Professor
University of Illinois at Chicago,
    College of Nursing
Chicago, IL

Deborah C. Francis, APRN, BC
Geriatric Clinical Nurse Specialist
Kaiser Permanente Medical
    Center
Sacramento, CA

Ann L. Horgas, PhD, RN
Associate Professor
University of Florida, College of
  Nursing and Institute on Aging
Gainesville, FL

**Denise M. Kresevic, RN, PhD, CS,
  GNP-C**
Nurse Researcher, Clinical Nurse
  Specialist
Cleveland VAMC
University Hospitals of Cleveland
Cleveland, OH

**Lenore H. Kurlowicz, PhD,
  RN, CS**
Assistant Professor of
  Geropsychiatric Nursing
School of Nursing, University of
  Pennsylvania
Philadelphia, PA

Judith A. Lucas EdD, RN, CS
Assistant Research Professor
Rutgers University
Institute for Health, Health Care
  Policy, and Aging Research
New Brunswick, NJ

Sue M. McLennon, MSN, ARNP
Doctoral Student, Research
  Assistant
University of Florida, College of
  Nursing
Gainesville, FL

Lorraine C. Mion, PhD, RN
Director, Geriatric Nursing
  Program
Division of Nursing
The Cleveland Clinic Foundation
Cleveland, OH

Ethel L. Mitty, EdD, RN
Adjunct Clinical Professor of
  Nursing
The John A. Hartford Foundation
  Institute for Geriatric Nursing
New York University,
  The Steinhardt School
  of Education
Division of Nursing
New York, NY

**Deborah M. Nadzam, PhD,
  FAAN**
The Quality Institute and Office of
  Quality Management
The Cleveland Clinic Foundation
Cleveland, OH

Anne O'Connell, MSN, RN
Clinical Nurse Specialist in
  Internal Medicine: Geriatrics
Cleveland Clinic Foundation-M13
Cleveland, OH

Gloria Picariello, APRN, BC
Director, Geriatric Case
  Management
HIP Health Plan of New York
New York, NY

Gloria Ramsey, RN, JD
Division of Nursing, The
  Steinhardt School of Education
New York University
New York, NY

**Barbara Resnick, PhD, CRNP,
  FAAN,**
Associate Professor, AHN
School of Nursing
University of Maryland
Baltimore, MD

Lark Trygstad, MA, ARNP-C
Geriatric Nurse Practitioner
Internal Medicine Geriatrics
Mason City, IA

Mary Grace Umlauf, PhD, RN
Professor, Graduate Program
University of Alabama School of
  Nursing
215 Nursing Building
Birmingham, AL

Terri E. Weaver, RN, PhD, CS,
  FAAN
Associate Professor
Chairperson, Division of
  Foundational Sciences and
  Health Systems
University of Pennsylvania School
  of Nursing
Nursing Education Building
Philadelphia, PA

INTRODUCTION

Mathy Mezey and DeAnne Zwicker

This book was written for acute care nurses working with the elderly. Although several models of acute care have been successful in improving care to the elderly, it is the bedside nurse who can ultimately make a difference in the outcome of elderly patients. Such a realization places a huge responsibility on the bedside nurse, but it can also be viewed as empowering for the bedside nurse as he or she is in a position of really making a difference in an elderly person's quality of life. Those patients with multiple comorbidities, multiple medications, and functional or mental impairment are particularly vulnerable to adverse outcomes. This is the population in which acute care nurses may significantly influence outcomes.

Nurses are well equipped to look at the geriatric patient in a preventive, holistic fashion because they have been developing care plans with a preventive focus since the onset of nursing diagnoses. Additionally, nurses have been in the forefront in communicating with patients and their families and understand how psychosocial issues impact patient outcomes during an acute episode. Therefore, the preventive focus and unique position of acute care nurses provide them with the tools they need to deal with the complexities of the geriatric population and the unique opportunity to help improve the quality of life for this population.

In order to do this, however, the acute care nurse must be well informed on common geriatric syndromes [broad categories of signs and symptoms (syndromes) that are more prevalent in the geriatric population, e.g., falls, eating difficulties, urinary incontinence], and how to assess these syndromes and initiate effective care strategies. Additionally, nurses must be informed about potential adverse events (e.g., delirium, pressure sores, adverse drug reactions, and falls) that can occur during an acute episode and how to prevent them or at least reduce their likelihood.

The Nurses Improving Care for Health System Elders (NICHE) project is a national initiative that provides a wealth of information to institutions to promote research-based quality of care to the aging population. Among the NICHE tools developed to aid in improving the care of the elderly are geriatric "best practice" protocols, which were piloted at NICHE hospital sites and later published in the first edition of this book. For more information on NICHE projects, visit www.niche.program@nyu.edu.

A recent publication in the *Journal of the American Medical Association* (Shekelle et al., 2001) indicates that protocols have a "shelf life" of about 3.8 years. Therefore, it became apparent that an update of the protocols in the book was necessary in order to provide the most recent research to augment improvement of care for the hospitalized elderly, a primary goal of the NICHE project.

The chapters from the first edition of *Geriatric Nursing Protocols for Best Practice* have been reviewed and updated based on clinical information obtained from the literature. Many of the guidelines have been written by research experts in the topic area in collaboration with practicing clinical practitioners of geriatrics/gerontology. Each protocol is accompanied by a case presentation to demonstrate application of the guideline in a realistic geriatric-specific case.

To date, the focus of practice guidelines has been on their development, with little attention given to evaluating and measuring guidelines, their clinical relevance, whether they are truly "evidence-based," and their impact on improving outcomes of care. Studies verifying the extent such evidence-based guidelines improve outcomes in geriatric care are scant. Two new chapters in this book (chapters 1 and 2) will walk readers through the process of evaluating the quality of practice guidelines, in hopes that many will be encouraged to critically evaluate and test the protocols while implementing them in the practice setting.

Elderly patients account for around 40% of all admissions to acute care hospitals in the United States. Acute care nurses must be up to date on the unique needs of this vulnerable population. It is an enormous task for nurses to access and assimilate the immense amount of information in the literature and figure out what is relevant to their current practice and how to apply it. It is our hope that the guidelines will provide nurses in the acute care setting with a shortcut to this process by providing research-based guidelines that need only to be tailored to the setting. Each guideline provides readers with background information on the topic, assessment parameters, care strategies, and suggestions for evaluation of outcomes. We hope readers enjoy the book and find the guidelines "user-friendly" and practical for application in the acute care setting, and we welcome any and all feedback.

We would like to thank the following for their involvement and support during the production of this book:

- All of the expert contributors for this book
- The NICHE faculty members who have taken the lead in setting best geriatric nursing practice standards
- The institutions supporting the faculty and geriatric clinicians participating in writing the protocols
- The John A. Hartford Foundation Institute for Geriatric Nursing, providing ongoing support of initiatives to improve the care of the elderly
- The authors who provided a valuable contribution in the first edition and ongoing research in geriatrics
- Springer Publishing Company for its ongoing support of quality geriatric nursing publications

REFERENCE

Shekelle, P. G., Ortiz, E., Rhodes, S., Morton, S., Eccles, M. P., & Grimshaw, J. M. (2001). Validity of the AHRQ clinical practice guidelines: How quickly do guidelines become outdated? *Journal of the American Medical Association, 286,* 1461–1467.

Chapter 1

EVALUATING CLINICAL PRACTICE GUIDELINES: A BEST PRACTICE

Judith A. Lucas and Terry Fulmer

EDUCATIONAL OBJECTIVES

On completion of this chapter, the reader will be able to:

1. Discuss reasons why it is important to examine and test clinical protocols.
2. Describe several approaches for the assessment of clinical protocols.
3. Describe one example of empirically testing an elder-focused clinical protocol.

Over the past decade there has been great interest and considerable effort spent on the development and implementation of clinical practice guidelines among health care disciplines. It is generally believed that clinical practice guidelines and protocols can improve the quality, appropriateness, and cost effectiveness of health care, as well as promote patient satisfaction (Shaneyfelt, Mayo-Smith, & Rothwangl, 1999). However, the proliferation of clinical practice guidelines in addition to the dramatic increase in clinical research on patient problems and interventions may be overwhelming for the clinical nurse. How is the nurse to judge which guideline to implement?

Some clinical practice guidelines are multidisciplinary and consensus-based, some are research-based, and others use a combination of research and consensus. Some are disease-specific, and others, such as those in this book are developed to provide a synthesis of empirical evidence and expert knowledge for geriatric syndromes (e.g., acute confusion, falls, and pain) that nurses manage. Unlike traditional ritualized care, geriatric nursing practice is more likely to improve older patient care outcomes by using research-based protocols that guide clinical nursing practice (Conn, Burks, Rantz, & Knudsen, 2002; Titler, Mentes, Rakel, Abbott, & Baumler, 1999). Significant clinical evidence must underpin the guidelines that nurses use if they are to reach appropriate outcomes.

Clearly, best practice protocols and guidelines are not valuable for clinical decision making unless they are up-to-date (Shekelle et al., 2001) and provide current evidence from research, clinical expertise, and patient preferences (Conn et al., 2002; Shaneyfelt et al., 1999). They also need to be tailored to the clinical population and setting where they will be used (Titler & Mentes, 1999). The clinical research base that geriatric nurses use to solve older patients' problems is growing. The new challenge is to examine and assess the best clinical practice guidelines for use in daily practice.

The first objective of this chapter is to help clinicians and health care organizations recognize the need to examine and test guidelines as part of the process of accepting and implementing them into practice. The second objective is to highlight several approaches to assessment of protocols and specifically to describe one example of empirical testing of a Nurses Improving Care for Health System Elders (NICHE) elder-focused clinical protocol for use in the long-term care setting.

CLINICAL PRACTICE GUIDELINES: THE TOOLS TO GUIDE CLINICAL NURSING PRACTICE

Clinical practice guidelines (CPGs) are statements derived from the best available evidence for making decisions about the care of specified populations. CPGs have many names, such as protocols, practice standards, and algorithms, and are statements developed with evidence from clinical expertise, patient preferences, and research (Conn et al., 2002). Several methods are used to access and examine evidence, including synthesis of research findings (e.g., integrative reviews), meta-analyses (e.g., statistical methods), consensus panels, and expert opinion for guideline development (Conn et al., 2002; Titler & Mentes, 1999).

REASONS TO ASSESS PROTOCOLS
BEFORE IMPLEMENTING

Over time, clinical practice protocols have become the underpinning for performance improvement programs, emphasizing research-based interventions to improve patient outcomes. Clinical practice guidelines are not valuable to clinicians unless they are up-to-date and present current scientific knowledge. It is important to ascertain if the evidence on which the guidelines were developed is recent. Often the evidence is from studies conducted at least 2 years prior to guideline publication. In their survival analysis of national guidelines, Shekelle and colleagues (2001) reported that about half of the guidelines became obsolete at 5.8 years (or 3.8 years past publication). Some national guidelines use prescheduled review dates; however, these dates may be arbitrary. Guidelines less rigorously developed may become obsolete at a different rate. Shekelle's group recommended that guidelines require reassessment when new information on interventions, outcomes, or patient preferences is found during focused literature searches.

The process of how a clinical practice guideline was developed also needs examination prior to use. In their structured review of 279 guidelines published between 1985 and 1997, Shaneyfelt and associates (1999) reported that just over half of those guidelines reviewed met established standards for evaluation and synthesis of scientific evidence. Less than half specified outcomes or applicable patient populations. They noted that few of the guidelines specified methods used to identify evidence, to determine expert opinion, or to discuss the role of patient preferences in choosing options (see Conn et al., 2002; Lang, 1999; and Leipzig, 1998 for nursing and geriatric studies). In fact, the weaker the underlying evidence of a protocol, the stronger the argument for testing, so that patient outcomes will be improved when clinicians implement the clinical practice guideline. Research and evidence-based protocols are often general guidelines, so application for patient care requires individualization based on patient needs and preferences. Nurse researchers at the

University of Iowa recommend that best practice protocols need to be assessed and tailored to local needs at the specific clinical setting where they are to be used (Titler & Mentes, 1999). Integrated health care systems are challenged to ensure applicability of practice protocols as patient needs and preferences, practitioners, and resources all vary across the organizations within a health system. Evaluating general practice guidelines is critical prior to application.

A PARADIGM FOR EVALUATING CLINICAL PRACTICE GUIDELINES

Most literature on evidence-based practice and best practice guidelines is focused on search strategies, guideline development, and implementation. We integrated criteria for review of evidence and evaluation of methods for guideline development to identify a general paradigm for appraising clinical practice guidelines. Addressing these areas prior to implementation (Box 1.1) will help clinicians to recognize valid, appropriate, and applicable guidelines, as well as particular guideline limitations.

Questions can be asked to ascertain whether the guideline addresses a significant practice problem relevant to nursing. For example, was the protocol triggered by the identification of a clinically significant practice problem or scientific evidence? Do these guidelines address important health problems, provide evidence-based options for managing a problem, and cover outcomes for the particular population in the specific clinical setting? Are these made explicit? For example, are the benefits, harms, and costs specified or quantified? In geriatric nursing, nurses manage clinical phenomena and health problems commonly experienced by older patients that cross several types of health conditions. These common phenomena are more clinically relevant for guidelines than disease-specific protocols (Titler et al., 1999).

Once the problem is defined and the outcomes are specified, it is important to ask if appropriate sources of scientific evidence were systematically sought and reviewed. Different evidence is needed to address different clinical research questions. For example, if we are considering the experience of patients trying to resolve chronic pain, we want to review qualitative research. If we are identifying the best non-drug pain interventions, this requires quantitative research. If it is an interdisciplinary problem, appropriate evidence

---

BOX 1.1   A Paradigm for Evaluating Clinical Practice Guidelines*

Significant practice problem, relevant to nursing
Guideline triggered by a clinically significant practice problem or scientific evidence.
Provides evidence-based options for managing a problem, as well as outcomes for the population of interest.
Options and outcomes (e.g., benefits, harms, and costs) specified or quantified.

Evidence
Appropriate sources of scientific evidence systematically sought and reviewed.
High-quality evidence relevant to clinical decision making sought, including empirical evidence, expert opinion, physiologic principles, patient and family preferences, professional values, and system features for care provision.
Strength of the research-based evidence judged on statistical and clinical significance (effect size), the degree of certainty, and the reproducibility of findings with multiple studies.
Processes are made explicit.

Up-to-date
Guideline published within past 3 years. Studies supporting the guideline published less than 2 years prior to guideline publication date.
Focused literature search conducted, experts sought, and published guidelines on the same clinical problem reviewed.
All appropriate options considered in this guideline.
New options or outcomes since the guideline was developed are sufficient for a revision.

Guideline development
Explicit and sensible process used to identify, select, appraise, and integrate evidence. All elements are made explicit.

General clinical practice guidelines
The unique local practice circumstances, including practitioner and patient populations, resources, and institutional perspectives, considered.
Guideline and recommendations reviewed by local clinicians for their patient population.

---

* Recommendations from several sources were used in the development of the paradigm, including Friedland et al. (1998); Hayward, Wilson, Tunis, Bass, & Guyatt (1995); Shaneyfelt et al. (1999); Shekelle et al. (2001); and Titler & Mentes (1999).

of prevention and intervention should be sought from relevant disciplines. High-quality evidence relevant to clinical decision making should be sought, including empirical evidence (e.g., systematic reviews, meta-analyses, randomized clinical trials [RCTs], controlled experiments, and observational studies), expert opinion, physiologic principles, patient and family preferences, professional values, and system features (e.g., economic, legal, cultural, logistic, and facilitators/barriers) for care provision (Conn et al., 2002; Tonelli, 2001). The emphasis in judging the strength of the research-based evidence is on statistical and clinical significance (effect size), the degree of certainty of the findings (conclusiveness), and the reproducibility of findings with multiple studies.

Because of the time it takes to review evidence and achieve consensus, guidelines may be out-of-date by the time we see them. It is important to check the publication dates of the studies supporting the guideline. Shekelle and associates (2001) reviewed national guidelines and concluded that the lifetime validity of a clinical practice guideline is about 3 years. After that time period, they recommend reassessment with a focused literature search by the groups already familiar with the topics. Additionally, they recommend that automated searches be conducted at regular intervals and abstracts reviewed by expert panels. Smaller organizations might contact the original panel members to identify experts most qualified to assess current validity. Another strategy is to search the National Guideline Clearinghouse (www.guidelines.gov) and other Web sites for practice guidelines published on the same clinical problem under review to assess options that may have been excluded from this guideline. Also, look for new options, outcomes, intervention delivery systems, costs, or patient preferences since the guideline was developed.

The process used for guideline development is important to consider. Was an explicit and sensible process used to identify, select, and appraise and integrate evidence? How was consensus reached? These elements need to be made explicit. The identification and evaluation of scientific evidence is critical to ensuring validity of the guidelines. In their review of national guidelines, Shaneyfelt and associates (1999) reported that only a third of those reviewed follow standards for identification and summary of evidence. Many do not specify the methods used, the time period from which evidence was collected, or the formal methods used for integrating empirical evidence (e.g., meta-analysis) or determining expert opinion (e.g., delphi method). If developers have not included their methods for choosing options, outcomes, evidence, or values, then clinicians might suspect that these steps were not done systematically.

Many important clinical problems are technically, economically, or ethically difficult to address with RCTs. A variety of studies, as well as reports of expert and consumer experience, may be considered to fill in gaps in evidence. Assess if developers have candidly reported the type and quantity of evidence, as well as their appraisal of the strength of that evidence. When expert panels/consensus groups are used, it is important to know who the panel members are and who they represent (e.g., specialty groups/consumers), as well as the methods used to seek consensus (Hayward, Wilson, Tunis, Bass, & Guyatt, 1995). Frank reporting can help in the decision to adopt or adapt recommendations. Confidence in the validity of a protocol increases if external reviewers have judged the conclusions reasonable and clinicians have found the guidelines applicable in practice. Guidelines with weak underlying evidence need actual empirical testing to determine if a guideline's implementation improves patient outcomes or, at least, has no adverse effects (i.e., sensitivity testing, RCT).

Clinical practice guidelines may be general and need to be assessed before implementing in settings different from which they were originally developed. Titler and Mentes (1999) recommended that guidelines be assessed and tailored to local needs. Adoption of a guideline must consider unique local practice circumstances, including practitioner and patient populations, resources, and institutional perspectives. Evaluation and adaptation of a clinical practice guideline are regarded as steps along the final pathway through which the evidence must pass before being applied to practice (Haynes, Hayward, & Lomas, 1995). There will be little local impact, and adoption may not even take place, unless those who will be using the guidelines review and adapt them to their care practices. Local clinicians are professionally responsible for the review of clinical practice guidelines. They must assess if the guidelines are applicable to their patient population, their patients' preferences, and the institutional resources and culture that support the new practice guideline (Haynes et al., 1995).

Assessment and testing are particularly important when guidelines are developed locally (e.g., care maps) or are being adopted by an integrated health system. Many of these integrated health systems have a strategic goal to provide all levels of care within the system (i.e., acute, ambulatory, skilled, rehabilitation, long term, and home care). The challenge in adopting a clinical practice guideline will be to ensure validity and applicability for a patient population, particularly when patients' needs and preferences, as well as practitioners and resources, vary across different organizations within the health system (Goode & Titler, 1996).

AN EMPIRICAL TEST OF A NICHE PROTOCOL FOR BEST PRACTICE: USING THE PARADIGM

Our empirical test of the NICHE (Nurses Improving Care for Health System Elders) Eating and Feeding Best Practice Protocol (Amella, 1999) illustrates many of the areas from the paradigm for evaluating clinical practice guidelines depicted in Box 1.1. This was the first attempt to test a NICHE protocol for use in long-term care.

First, we considered the significance of the practice problem. Many independent eating functions may be lost, impaired, or misdiagnosed in nursing home residents. This may result in dehydration, malnutrition, significant weight loss, and feeding tube placement—all significant clinical and quality of life issues. Over 60% of nursing home residents need some nursing staff assistance for feeding (American Health Care Association, 1995). Yet nursing homes are often poorly staffed, with certified nursing assistants typically assisting 7 to 9 residents at daytime meals and 12–15 residents during the evening meal (Kayser-Jones & Schell, 1997). That means that even when oral supplements are ordered as a treatment for weight loss, they are often not served or actually consumed, so that many residents become frail and die having lost up to a third of their body weight (Kayser-Jones et al., 1998; Kayser-Jones & Schell, 1997).

The NICHE Eating and Feeding Best Practice Protocol (Amella, 1999) is evidence-based. Peer-reviewed clinical evidence, observational and experimental evidence, and the opinions of an expert panel were used to recommend assessment and intervention options. Some of the studies reviewed took place in long-term care. The actual processes used for judging the evidence for inclusion were not made explicit.

The evidence from nursing, medicine, nutrition, and sociology was recent—within 3 years of publication of the protocol. We contacted members of the original panel and conducted a focused search of studies for resident problems, values, interventions, and other nutrition guidelines specific to the nursing home setting as part of the evaluation. A panel of nationally recognized experts in geriatric nursing care developed the NICHE best practice protocols. How consensus was reached was not clearly delineated. The Eating and Feeding Difficulties Protocol is general in nature. Unique local practice and institutional circumstances of either the hospital or the nursing home are not presented. The focus is on the geriatric patient in general. Local clinicians are encouraged to review the guidelines for their particular patient populations.

Our initial examination of the NICHE Eating and Feeding Protocol (Amella, 1999) was planned in a nursing home similar to most in the United States. This also provided a crucial exploration of possible facilitators and barriers to the adoption and use of the protocol. We addressed three research questions: (1) What assessment, prevention, and management practices of the protocol are carried out and by whom in long-term care? (2) What parts are important to residents and to staff? (3) What are the circumstances that may affect use of the protocol in the context of long-term care nursing?

An eating problem was defined using the Resident Assessment Instrument /Minimum Data Set (RAI/MDS version 2.0) guidelines (U.S. Department of Health and Human Services, 1995). The research team interviewed residents, their primary certified nursing assistants (CNAs), and their licensed nurses (registered and licensed practical), for each of the 100+ items on the NICHE protocol. The context of mealtimes was observed. We also interviewed the two part-time dieticians, therapists (occupational and physical), and the assistant director of nursing (ADON) to review dietary and nursing policies and to discuss general processes used for managing eating and feeding problems.

For our analysis we identified the items with 100% consensus from all residents and all staff. Because the number of subjects was small, we conservatively defined this as 100% agreement on the question Does it matter? for each item. We then quantified how often these were reported as done and who carried out these steps. To identify divergence within nursing staff priorities, we conducted cross-tabulations and compared licensed nurse and CNA responses. We then reviewed the qualitative data from the interviews with other professionals (therapists, dieticians, assistant director of nursing) to help identify facilitators and barriers to implementing guidelines in nursing homes.

We only briefly summarize our findings here. A quarter of the assessment items (25.6%) achieved 100% consensus between residents and staff. Assessment for residents is all about nurses checking that "all is going alright" and for symptom relief. For nurses, height and weight are important to measure, but the basal metabolism index (BMI) is not calculated by these nursing home nurses. Signs of a swallowing disorder (neck position, slow eating, and coughing) are only grossly observed by the CNAs at meals "because we have the speech and language pathologist (SLP) do swallow assessment."

Only three intervention items received 100% consensus. Getting to choose foods and to set the pace of a meal is "a given" for residents. Using methods to remind or encourage residents to eat was important to staff. Only four evaluation items that focused on safety received 100% consensus. Overall, a picture of generalist nurses predominantly making resident assessments and evaluating outcomes, but referring to other professional team members for problem evaluation and treatment plans, emerged. The CNAs are the primary provider of the mealtime interventions. Several interventions were described as "doesn't matter," but they were carried out often "because they are required by regulation." Examples include examination of residents on antidepressants, documentation of drug side effects by the care team, diet history by the dietician and nurse on admission, advance directives for all residents, and alterations in weight and eating or feeding that require reassessment.

Several areas supported by recent analyses and clinical trials were not emphasized in the NICHE protocol (Amella et al., 1999) including

- Treating wounds, infections, and agitation/pacing that increase calorie needs
- Replenishing reserves posthospitalization
- Assessing and treating causes of unplanned weight loss (e.g., depression, cancer, cardiac and gastrointestinal disorders, medications, and polypharmacy)
- Performing a specific panel of tests for unintentional weight loss
- Utilizing recommendations from consultant pharmacists
- Recognizing the low activity level of residents in the nursing home setting and, whenever possible, encouraging exercise or physical therapy (Appetite and total energy intake have been shown to increase, and muscle weakness and frailty to decrease, when exercise is used concurrently with nutritional supplements.)

- Providing increased food choices, private areas, and groups for restorative programs, as well as teaching and involving the family at mealtimes
- Preventing and treating undernutrition: reducing restrictions (foods, diet, and precautions) and using regular/favorite foods as supplements (vs. commercially prepared foods); also, increasing the number of small-volume meals provided at the resident's preferred mealtime versus routine times; the last choice should be adding specific medications for weight gain (none are actually labeled by the U.S. Food and Drug Administration for this indication) and tube feedings—which have risks and benefits (they do not necessarily prevent aspiration or assure weight gain)
- Comfort care for terminally ill: administering food and fluids based on the advance directives/preferences.

Our examination of the protocol also identified five factors that may influence the adoption and continued use of clinical practice guidelines in nursing homes. These include

1. *Nursing roles.* The professional nurse in the nursing home site is valued by the team as the "first line for assessment," but even common geriatric problems were referred to other team members for evaluation. None of the nurses had training in gerontology or chronic disease management. Heavy workloads encourage routine care practices and shortcuts by nursing assistants. See eating and feeding chapter in this text.

2. *Regulation and staffing.* The nursing home industry is highly regulated, and regulations (e.g., staffing) are often minimum standards. Supervisors try to deliver "5-minute messages" as a way to keep busy staff up-to-date. Minimum staffing for efficiency and lack of continuing geriatric education are likely to act as barriers to protocol use.

3. *Team functioning.* Having many part-time members means there are rarely multidisciplinary rounds at which members can share their expertise, review new research, or discuss difficult geriatric issues such as end of life decisions and comfort care. Patterns of problems, such as prevalence of unplanned weight loss, are less likely to be addressed without an interdisciplinary effort for quality improvement.

4. *Availability of geriatric specialists.* We met no geriatric specialists at the particular nursing home in this study. As demonstrated in the NICHE project, the geriatric advanced practice nurse, who is particularly skilled at questioning care practices, seeking out evidence-based protocols, testing and championing protocol use, and empowering staff, could have a great impact on research utilization in long-term care.

5. *Professional development.* Staff nurses were highly motivated to learn principles and strategies of geriatric nutrition. However, with no formal in-service programs, rewards for continuing education or certification, professional library/on-line facilities, or opportunities to participate in practice standards committees, staff will have little exposure to best practices.

Many of these factors are likely to derail efforts for clinical practice guideline adoption and integration into practice. Experts suggest that identifying barriers and then targeting different strategies to the group, the setting, and the desired practice change will be more effective than using a single strategy to promote the use of best practice protocols (Gross et al., 2001).

SUMMARY

Clinical practice guidelines and protocols are more likely to improve the quality and cost effectiveness of health care, as well as to promote patient satisfaction, when they are up-to-date and are supported by strong evidence from research, clinical expertise, and patient preferences. They should be tailored to the clinical population and setting where they will be used. Protocols need examination prior to use and for continued use. Guidelines with weak underlying evidence will need actual empirical testing to determine if the new practice improves patient outcomes or, at least, has no adverse effects. It is critical that clinical practice guidelines be reexamined when new information on interventions, outcomes, or patient preferences is found during focused literature searches.

Ultimately each professional nurse must review the clinical practice guidelines to assess if these will be applicable to the patient population, the patients' preferences, and the institutional resources and culture. The role of the advanced practice nurse could have a great impact on guideline examination and utilization in long-term care. Nurses have had leadership and involvement in the development of many clinical practice guidelines (i.e., Agency for Healthcare Research and Quality guidelines, University of Iowa research-based practice protocols, and the Hartford Institute's geriatric nursing best practice protocols). The new challenge is to lead the way for examining and testing the geriatric clinical practice guides as part of the process of accepting, integrating, and evaluating continued use as standards of care.

REFERENCES

Amella, E. J., & NICHE faculty. (1999). Eating and feeding difficulties for older persons: Assessment and management. In I. Abraham, M. M. Bottrell, T. Fulmer, & M. D. Mezey (Eds.), *Geriatric nursing protocols for best practice* (pp. 27–39). New York: Springer.

Conn, V. S., Burks, K., Rantz, M., & Knudsen, K. S. (2002). Evidence-based practice for gerontological nursing. *Journal of Gerontological Nursing, 28(2)*, 45–52.

Friedland, D. J., Go, A. S., Davoren, J. B., Shlipak, M. G., Bent, S. W., Subak, L. L. et al. (1998). *Evidence-based medicine: A framework for clinical practice.* Stamford, CT: Appleton & Lange.

Goode, C. J., & Titler, M. G. (1996). Moving research-based practice throughout the health care system. *MEDSURG Nursing, 5(5)*, 380–383.

Gross, P. A., Greenfield, S., Cretin, S., Ferguson, J., Grimshaw, J., Grol, R., et al. (2001). Optimal methods for guideline implementation: Conclusions from Leeds Castle meeting. *Medical Care, 39*(Supp. 2), II-85–II-92.

Haynes, R. B., Hayward, R. S. A., & Lomas, J. (1995). Bridges between health care research evidence and clinical practice. *Journal of the American Medical Informatics Association, 2*, 342–350.

Hayward, R. S. A., Wilson, M. C., Tunis, S. R., Bass, E. B., Guyatt, G., & Evidence-Based Medicine Working Group. (1995). Users' guides to the medical literature: VIII. How to use clinical practice guidelines. A. Are the recommendations valid? *Journal of the American Medical Association, 274(7)*, 570–574.

Kayser-Jones, J., Schell, E., Porter, C., Barbaccia, J. C., Steinbach, C., Bird, W. F., Redford, M., & Pengilly, K. (1998). A prospective study of the use of liquid oral dietary supplements in nursing homes. *Journal of the American Geriatrics Society, 5(3)*, 69–76.

Kayser-Jones, J., & Schell, E. (1997). The effect of staffing on the quality of care at mealtimes. *Nursing Outlook, 45(2)*, 64–72.

Lang, N. M. (1999). Discipline-based approaches to evidence-based practice: A view from nursing. *Joint Commission Journal on Quality Improvement, 25(10)*, 539–544.

Leipzig, R. M. (1998). That was the year that was: An evidence-based clinical geriatrics update. *Journal of the American Geriatrics Society, 46*(8), 1040–1049.

Shaneyfelt, T. M., Mayo-Smith, M. F., & Rothwangl, J. (1999). Are guidelines following guidelines? The methodological quality of clinical practice guidelines in the peer-reviewed medical literature. *Journal of the American Medical Association, 281*(20), 1900–1905.

Shekelle, P. G., Ortiz, E., Rhodes, S., Morton, S. C., Eccles, M. P., Grimshaw, J. M., et al. (2001). Validity of the Agency for Healthcare Research and Quality clinical practice guidelines: How quickly do guidelines become outdated? *Journal of the American Medical Association, 286,* 1461–1467.

Titler, M. G., & Mentes, J. C. (1999). Research utilization in gerontological nursing practice. *Journal of Gerontological Nursing, 25*(6), 6–9.

Titler, M. G., Mentes, J. C., Rakel, B. A., Abbott, L., & Baumler, S. (1999). From book to bedside: Putting evidence to use in the care of the elderly. *Joint Commission Journal on Quality Improvement, 25,* 545–556.

Tonelli, M. R. (2001). The limits of evidence-based medicine. *Respiratory Care, 46,* 1435–1440.

U.S. Department of Health and Human Services. (1995). *Resident Assessment Instrument: MDS Version 2.0* (HCFA State Operations Manual Product No.CP8111). Washington, DC: Author.

Chapter 2

MEASURING PERFORMANCE, IMPROVING QUALITY

Deborah M. Nadzam and Ivo L. Abraham

EDUCATIONAL OBJECTIVES

After completion of this chapter, the reader will be able to:
1. Discuss key components of the definition of quality as outlined by the Institute of Medicine.
2. Describe three challenges of measuring quality of care.
3. Delineate three strategies for addressing the challenges of measuring quality.
4. List three characteristics of a good performance measure.

The main objective of implementing best practice protocols for geriatric nursing is to stimulate nurses to practice with greater knowledge and skill, and thus improve the quality of care to older adults. We can think of this as a process: *Changes in nursing practice → enhanced clinical performance → improved quality.* The other chapters in this book focus on the need to improve geriatric nursing practice, on the tools to do so, and on strategies to put protocols into practice. This chapter focuses on assessing the impact of introducing best practice protocols on quality by measuring performance.

From the very beginning of the NICHE (Nurses Improving Care for Health System Elders) project in the early 1990s (see Fulmer et al., 2002, for an overview), the NICHE team has struggled with the following questions: How can we measure whether the combination of models of care, staff education and development, and organizational change leads to improvements in patient care? How can we provide hospitals and health systems committed to improving their nursing care to older adults with guidance and frameworks, let alone tools for measuring the quality of geriatric care? In turn, these questions generated many other questions: Is it possible to measure quality? Can we identify direct indicators of quality? Or do we have to rely on indirect indicators (e.g., if 30-day readmissions of patients over the age of 65 drop, can we reasonably state that this reflects an improvement in the quality of care?)? What factors may influence our desired quality outcomes, whether these are unrelated factors (e.g., the pressure to reduce length of stay) or related factors (e.g., the severity of illness)? How can we design evaluation programs that enable us to measure quality without adding more burden (of data collection, of taking time away from direct nursing care)? If from research and expert consensus we do know what best practice is, can we ethically justify evaluation designs that provide some patients with best practice and others not? Is it even necessary to go to such "extremes" of scientific rigor when the focus is on changing and monitoring quality of care in specific clinical settings? No doubt, the results from evaluation programs should be useful at the "local" level. Would it be helpful, though, to have results that are comparable across clinical settings (within the same hospital or health system) and across institutions (e.g., as quality benchmarking tools)?

It would be ideal if this chapter provided answers to all of these questions. However, it does not because currently there is no consensus as to how to measure the quality of geriatric nursing care; there may never be. Furthermore, if *the* model of quality measurement were to exist, would it be relevant to all possible clinical sites and implementable without burdensome procedures and resource demands? Would it enable quality improvement at the local level while facilitating comparative analysis across settings? This chapter does provide guidance in the selection, development, and use of performance measures to monitor quality of care as a springboard to quality improvement initiatives. Following a definition of *quality of care,* the chapter identifies several challenges in the measurement of quality. The concept of performance measures as the evaluation link between care delivery and quality improvement is introduced. Next, the chapter offers practical advice on what and how to measure. It concludes with a summary of common measurement problems.

Before we launch into these issues, it is important to reaffirm two key principles. First, at the management level, it is indispensable to measure the quality of geriatric nursing care; however, doing so must help those who actually provide care (nurses) and must impact on those who receive care (elderly patients). Second, measuring quality of care is not the end goal; rather, it is done to enable the continuous use of quality of care information to improve patient care.

DEFINING QUALITY OF CARE

QUALITY OF CARE: A PROCESS, NOT A STATE

The Institute of Medicine (IOM) defines *quality of care* as "the degree to which health services for individuals and populations increase[s] the likelihood of desired health outcomes and are consistent with current professional knowledge" (Kohn, Corrigan, & Donaldson, 2000, p. 222). Note that this definition does not tell us what quality is, but what quality should achieve. This definition also does not say that quality exists if certain conditions are met (e.g., a ratio of x falls to y elderly orthopedic surgery patients, a 30-day readmission rate of z, etc.). Instead, it emphasizes that the likelihood of achieving desired levels of care is what matters. In other words, quality is not a matter of reaching something but, rather, the challenge, over and over, of improving the odds of reaching the desired level of outcomes. Thus, the definition implies the cyclical and longitudinal nature of quality: What we achieve today must guide us as to what to do tomorrow—better and better, over and over.

The IOM definition stresses the framework within which to conceptualize quality: knowledge. The best knowledge to have is research evidence—preferably from randomized clinical trials (experimental studies)—yet without ignoring the relevance of less rigorous studies (nonrandomized studies, epidemiological investigations, descriptive studies, even case studies). Realistically, in nursing we have limited evidence to guide the care of older adults. Therefore, professional consensus among clinical and research experts is a critical factor in determining quality. Furthermore, knowledge is needed at three levels: To achieve quality, we need to know what to do (knowledge about best practice), we need to know how to do it (knowledge about behavioral skills), and we need to know what outcomes to achieve (knowledge about best outcomes).

The IOM definition of quality of care contains several other important elements. "Health services" focuses the definition on the care itself. Granted, the quality of care provided is determined by such factors as knowledgeable professionals, good technology, and efficient organizations, yet these are not the focus of quality measurement. Rather, the definition implies a challenge to health care organizations: The system should be organized in such a way that knowledge-based care is provided and that its effects can be measured. This brings us to the "desired health outcomes" element of the definition. Quality is not an attribute (as in "My hospital is in the top 100 hospitals in the United States as ranked by *U.S. News & World Report*"), but an ability (as in "Only $x\%$ of our elderly surgical patients go into acute confusion; of those who do, $y\%$ return to normal cognitive function within z hours after onset").

In the IOM definition, "degree" implies that quality occurs on a continuum from unacceptable to excellent. The clinical consequences are on a continuum as well. If the care is of unacceptable quality, the likelihood that we will achieve the desired outcomes is nil. In fact, we probably will achieve outcomes that are the opposite of what are desired. As the care moves up the scale toward excellent, the more likely the desired outcomes will be achieved. "Degree" also implies quantification. Although it helps to be able to talk to colleagues about, say, unacceptable, poor, average, good, or excellent care, these terms should be anchored by a measurement system. Such systems enable us to interpret what, for instance, poor care is by providing us with a range of numbers that correspond to "poor." In turn, these numbers can provide us with a reference point for improving care to the level of average: We measure care again, looking at whether the numbers have improved, then checking whether these numbers fall in the range defined as "average." Likewise, if we see a worsening of scores, we will be able to conclude whether we have gone from, say, good to average. "Individuals and populations" underscores that quality of care is reflected in the outcomes of one patient and in the outcomes of a set of patients. It focuses our attention on providing quality care to individuals while aiming to raise the level of care provided to populations of patients.

In summary, the IOM definition of quality of care forces us to think about quality in relative and dynamic rather than in absolute and static terms. Quality of care is not a state of being but a process of becoming. Quality is and should be measurable, using performance measures: "a quantitative tool that provides an indication of an organization's performance in relation to a specified process or outcome" (Schyve & Nadzam, 1998, p. 222).

QUALITY OF CARE IS IN THE EYE OF THE BEHOLDER

If the IOM definition is so helpful, why do different people and different groups think about quality of care in such different ways? Clinicians wonder whether they, as individual practitioners, provide good care and how they can become even better at what they do. They may also question if they work for a good organization, one that consistently provides good care to all its patients and challenges itself to find new and better ways of serving their patients. Health care organizations worry about how they are doing with their patients. Will the patients return? Will they refer family and friends in need of health care? Health care managers worry about reimbursement, accreditation, and contracting, all of which are linked to the institutional level of quality of care. Purchasers and payors of health care try to find ways of balancing quality and cost. Providing the best possible care imaginable may be cost prohibitive, yet too much cost management could have a negative impact on quality. Regulators and accreditors want assurances that safe care is being provided. For them, the issue is not one of top quality but rather of basic and necessary quality. Finally, patients and consumers want assurances. Increasingly, just getting access to health care is a large issue. Once accessed, patients expect their care to be safe. They hope that the care will make them better, or, at least, that suffering will be minimized.

Where do these different views on quality of care come from? This question goes back to the process versus state issue. Quality improvement is a process of attaining ever better levels of care in parallel with advances in knowledge and technology. It strives toward increasing the likelihood that certain outcomes will be achieved. This is the professional responsibility of those who are charged with providing care (clinicians, managers, and their organizations). On the other hand, consumers of health care (patients, but also purchasers, payors, regulators, and accreditors) are much less concerned with the processes in place, as with the results of those processes.

MEASURING QUALITY OF CARE

CHALLENGES

Schyve and Nadzam (1998) identified several challenges to measuring quality. First, the suggestion that quality of care is in the eye of the beholder points to the different interests of multiple users. This issue encompasses both measurement and communication challenges. Measurement and analysis methods must generate information about the quality of care that meets the needs of different stakeholders. In addition, the results must be communicated in ways that meet these different needs. Second, we must have good and generally accepted tools for measuring quality. Thus, user groups must come together in their conceptualization of quality care so that relevant health care measures can be identified and standardized. A common language of measurement must be developed, grounded in a shared perspective on quality that is cohesive across yet meets the needs of various user groups. Third, once the measurement systems are in place, data must be collected. This translates into resource demands and logistic issues as to who is to report, record, collect, and manage data. Fourth, data must be analyzed in statistically appropriate ways. This is not just a matter of using the right statistical methods. More important, user groups must agree on a framework for analyzing quality data to interpret the results. Fifth, health care environments are complex and dynamic in nature. There are differences across health care environments, between types of provider organizations, and within organizations. Furthermore, changes in health care occur frequently, such as the movement of care from one setting to another and the introduction of new technology. Finding common denominators is a major challenge.

Should quality data be made available to the public? A hospital with consistently good quality indicators in geriatric nursing care may not object to publication of its data; it may even see publication as a competitive advantage. On the other hand, a health system with less positive results may want to suppress information until it gets its "geriatric house" in order.

ADDRESSING THE CHALLENGES

These challenges are not insurmountable. However, making a commitment to quality care entails a commitment to putting the processes and systems in place to measure quality through performance measures and to report quality of care results. This commitment applies as much to a quality improvement initiative on a nursing unit as it does to a corporate commitment by a large health care system. In other words, once an organization decides to pursue excellence (i.e., quality), it must accept measurement and reporting and overcome the various challenges. Let us examine how this could be done in a clinical setting.

McGlynn and Asch (1998) offer several strategies for addressing the challenges to measuring quality. First, the various user groups must identify and balance competing perspectives. This is a process of giving and taking: proposing highly clinical measures (e.g., number of pressure ulcers), but also providing more general data (e.g., use of restraints). It is a process of asking and responding: asking management for monthly statistics on medication errors, but also agreeing to provide management with the necessary documentation of why physical restraints have been used for some patients. Second, there must be an accountability framework. Committing to quality care implies that nurses assume several responsibilities and are willing to be held accountable for each of them: (1) providing the best possible care to older patients, (2) examining their own geriatric nursing knowledge and practice, (3) seeking ways to improve it, (4) agreeing to evaluation of their practice, and (5) responding to needs for improvement. Third, there must be objectivity in the evaluation of quality. This requires setting and adopting explicit criteria for judging performance, then building the evaluation process on these criteria. Nurses, their colleagues, and their managers need to reach consensus on how performance will be measured and what will be considered excellent (and good, average, etc.) performance. Fourth, once these indicators have been identified, nurses need to select a subset of indicators for routine reporting. Indicators should give a reliable snapshot of the team's care to older patients. Fifth, it is critical to separate as much as possible the use of indicators for evaluating patient care and the use of these indicators for financial or nonfinancial incentives. Should the team be cost conscious? Yes, but cost should not influence any clinical judgment as to what is best for patients. Finally, nurses in the clinical setting must plan how to collect the data. At the institutional level, this may be facilitated by information systems that allow performance measurement and reporting. Ideally, point-of-care documentation will also provide the data necessary for a systematic and goal-directed quality improvement program, thus eliminating separate data abstraction and collection activities.

The success of a quality improvement program in geriatric nursing care (and the ability to overcome many of the challenges) hinges on the decision as to what to measure. We know that good performance measures must be objective, that data collection must be easy and as burdenless as possible, that statistical analysis must be girded by principles and placed within a framework, and that communication of results must be targeted toward different user groups. Conceivably, we could try to measure every possible aspect of care; realistically, however, the planning for this will never reach the implementation stage. Instead, nurses need to establish priorities by asking these questions: Based on our clinical expertise, what is critical for us to know? What aspects of our care to older patients are high risk or high volume? What parts of our elder care are problem-prone, either because we have experienced difficulties in the past or because we can anticipate problems due to the lack of knowledge or resources? What clinical indicators would be of interest to other user groups: patients, the general public, management, payors, accreditors, and practitioners? Throughout this prioritization process, nurses should keep asking themselves: What questions are we trying to answer, and for whom?

DECIDING HOW TO MEASURE PERFORMANCE

Once they have decided what to measure, nurses in the clinical geriatric practice setting face the task of deciding how to measure performance. There are two possibilities: Either the appropriate measure already exists, or a new performance measure must be developed. Either way, there are a number of requirements of a good performance measure that will need to be applied to the decision process.

WHAT ARE GOOD PERFORMANCE MEASURES?

There are two ways to answer the question Is this a good measure? First, we must decide if the measure is of potential use to the individual nurse and to the organization. Once we have determined the probable utility of the measure, we should review its characteristics to determine if it is a good performance measure in general (e.g., well-defined and tested).

Usefulness

The process of selecting a performance measure begins with two sets of conceptual questions about usefulness:

1. Usefulness of the measure: What do we need to know? What is the measurement purpose of a given performance measure? Do need and purpose match?
2. Usefulness of the measure's output: How do we intend to use the performance measure? Can the measure be used this way?

If we cannot get to a "reasonable yes" on the first set of questions, the performance measure under review may not meet our objectives. By "reasonable yes," we mean that the assessment of the match between our need and the measurement purpose of the measure is not necessarily 100%. Rather, in answering this question, we should evaluate to what extent the measure can be adapted to our needs, or to what extent we and our team can adapt to the measure. The second set of questions, about the usefulness of the output of the measure, pertains to the relevance of the measure to the quality of care program. Does the measure give performance results that can be applied to our efforts to improve care to older adults?

Characteristics of Performance Measures

Now that we have determined that the measure will be of use to the organization, we should evaluate the key characteristics of the measure to ensure that it is adequately defined, tested, and operational. Several characteristics are described below.

Targets improvement. The measure and its output need to focus on improvement, not merely the description of something. It is not helpful to have a very accurate measure that just tells the status of a given dimension of practice. Instead, the measure needs to inform us about current quality levels and relate them to previous and future quality levels. It needs to be able to compute improvements or declines in quality over time so that we can plan for the future. For example, to have a measure that only tells the number of medication errors in the past month would not be helpful. Instead, a measure that tells what types of medication errors were made, perhaps even with a severity rating indicated, compares this to medication errors made during the previous months, and shows in numbers and graphs the changes over time will enable us to do the necessary root cause analysis to prevent more medication errors in the future.

Precisely defined and specified.　The measure needs to be clearly defined, including the terms used, the data elements collected, and the calculation steps employed. Imagine that we want to monitor falls on the unit. The initial questions would be What is considered a fall? Does the patient have to be on the floor? Does a patient slumping against the wall or onto a table while trying to prevent himself or herself from falling to the floor constitute a fall? Is a fall due to physical weakness or orthostatic hypotension treated the same as a fall due to tripping over an obstacle? The next question would be Over what time period are falls measured: a week, a fortnight, a month, a quarter, a year? The time frame is not a matter of convenience, but of accuracy. To be able to monitor falls accurately, we need to identify a time frame that will capture enough events to be meaningful and interpretable from a quality improvement point of view. If the surgical units of the hospital register on average only 1 fall event per week, using 1 week as the unit of time will be insufficient: (1) Most likely, in most weeks there will be a report that 1 fall occurred, and it will be impossible to see trends of improvement or decline over time. (2) In weeks in which no falls occurred, an improvement over the last week that a fall occurred would be reported, and we might mistakenly believe that this is a true improvement, when, in fact, it may be nothing else than random variation over time. Likewise, (3) in weeks in which 2 or 3 falls occurred, we would be confronted with reports showing a 100% or 200% increase in events. Thus, the time period used for calculating the incidence of falls should be defined as a function of the event being measured, not in function of absolute time or convenience.

Consider in this regard seasonal events, as the case of nosocomial infections illustrates. A performance measure related to nosocomial infections should begin with a clear definition of what counts as a case and how the diagnosis should be made. Next, the time period for incidence calculations must be selected. Again, we do not want the time period to be too restrictive, yet we do not want it to be too long (preventable new cases might be occurring while we wait for results). In addition, we must consider the seasonal nature of noso-comial infections: They are more likely in late fall, throughout the winter, and into early spring. Thus, the measure should be able to give seasonal reports, not only from one season to the next, but by comparing a current season with the same season in years past. Purists may even argue that the measure should be sensitive to regional differences in climate, to regional population density (com-munity-acquired infections being transmitted across hospitalized patients), and to patient density in the hospital (the closer the patients, the higher the risk). The latter illustrates the importance of the degree of granularity of any performance measure: how focused should it ultimately be—not for the sake of accuracy itself, but for the sake of supporting the geriatric nursing quality program.

Validity, sensitivity, and specificity. It is important that information be obtained about the validity of a measure. *Validity* refers to whether the measure "actually measures what it purports to measure" (Wilson, 1989, p. 355). For example, if we are concerned that elderly patients who underwent an emergency (as opposed to elective) total hip replacement are discharged too early, perhaps without ade-quate immediate postsurgical rehabilitation, prevention of coagula-tion problems, prevention of postsurgical anemia, and prevention of wound infection. Our colleagues argue that these are the patients that often return with infected wounds, blood clots, and so on. One colleague suggests asking the medical records department for 30-day readmission rates for all patients age 65 and over. Would this be a valid measure; that is, would it truly measure the risks associ-ated with premature discharge of hip patients? A gross measure like 30-day readmissions may not be valid for the quality of care issue at hand. Instead, we may want to think of a selective 30-day readmis-sion rate that focuses specifically on the patients in our unit (and compares them with other patients), the reasons for their readmis-sion, and whether these reasons reflect the type of surgery, the associated risks, and the elderly status of the patients.

Sensitivity and specificity refer to the ability of the measure to cap-ture all true cases of the event being measured, and only true cases. We want to make sure that a performance measure identifies true cases as true and false cases as false and does not identify a true case as false or a false case as true. Sensitivity of a performance measure is the likelihood of a positive test when a condition is present. Lack of sensitivity is expressed as false-positives: The indicator calculates a condition as present when in fact it is not. Specificity refers to the likelihood of a negative test when a condition is not present. False-negatives reflect lack of specificity: The indicators calculate that a condition is not present when in fact it is. Consider the case of depression and the recommendation in chapter 11 to use the Geriatric Depression Scale, in which a score of 11 or greater is indicative of depression. How robust is this cut-off score of 11? What is the likelihood that someone with a score of 9 or 10 (i.e., negative for depression) might actually be depressed (false-negative)? Similarly, what is the likelihood that a patient with a score of 13 would not be depressed (false-positive)?

Reliability.   Reliability means that results are reproducible; the indicator measures the same attribute consistently across the same patients and across time. Reliability begins with a precise definition and specification, as described earlier. A measure is reliable if different people calculate the same rate for the same patient sample. The core issue of reliability is measurement error, or the difference between the actual phenomenon and its measurement: The greater the difference, the less reliable the performance measure. For example, suppose that we want to focus on pain management in elderly patients with end-stage cancer. One way of measuring pain would be to ask patients to rate their pain as *none, a little, some, quite a bit,* or *a lot.* An alternative approach would be to administer a visual analog scale, a 10-point line on which patients indicate their pain levels. Yet another approach would be to ask the pharmacy to produce monthly reports of analgesic use by type and dose. Generally speaking, the more subjective the scoring or measurement, the less reliable it will be. If all these measures were of equal reliability, they would yield the same result.

Interpretable.   Several of the examples given earlier imply the criterion of interpretability. A performance measure must be interpretable; that is, it must convey a result that can be linked to the quality of clinical care. First, the quantitative output of a performance measure must be scaled in such a way that users can interpret it. For example, a scale that starts with 0 as the lowest possible level and ends with 100 is a lot easier to interpret than a scale than starts with 13.325 and has no upper boundary except infinity. Second, we should be able to place the number within a context. Suppose we are working in a hemodialysis center that serves quite a large proportion of end-stage renal disease (ESRD) patients over the age of 60—the group least likely to be fit for a kidney transplant yet with several years of life expectancy remaining. We know that virtually all ESRD patients develop anemia (Hb < 11 g/dL), which in turn impacts on their activities of daily living (ADL) and independent activities of daily living (IADL) performance. In collaboration with the nephrologists, we initiate a systematic program of anemia monitoring and management, relying in part on published best practice guidelines. We want to achieve the best practice guideline of 85% of all patients having hemoglobin levels equal to or greater than 11 g/dL. We should be able to succeed because the central laboratory provides us with Hb levels, which allows us to calculate the percentage of patients at Hb of 11 g/dL or greater.

Risk-adjusted. Some patients are sicker than others; some have more comorbidities; some are older and frailer. No doubt, we could come up with many more risk variables that influence how patients respond to nursing care. Good performance measures take this differential risk into consideration. They create a "level playing field" by adjusting quality indicators on the basis of the (risk for) severity of illness of the patients. It would not be fair to the health care team if the patients on the unit are a lot sicker than those on the unit a floor above. The team is at greater risk for having lower quality outcomes, not because they provide inferior care, but because the patients are a lot sicker and are at greater risk for a compromised response to the care provided. The sicker patients are more demanding in terms of care, and ultimately are less likely to achieve the same outcomes as less ill patients.

Easy to collect. The many examples cited earlier also refer to the importance of using performance measures for which data are readily available, can be retrieved from existing sources, or can be collected with little burden. The goal is to gather good data quickly without running the risk of having "quick and dirty" data.

In control. Performance measures are indicators of quality. It is essential that these indicators reflect nursing practice and can be influenced by nursing care if they in fact do relate to nursing care. Quality scores cannot be improved if the measures are based on variables beyond nurses' control.

It is essential that we consider these characteristics as we review existing performance measures or develop our own new measure.

COMMON PROBLEMS WITH PERFORMANCE MEASUREMENT AND QUALITY IMPROVEMENT PROGRAMS

The consequences of poor planning or poor performance measure selection are ineffective performance measurement and improvement programs. Specific implications from the list of characteristics of good measures, as well as other program planning challenges, are described below. This is not intended to be an exhaustive list of issues that can influence the success of a quality of care improvement program. For example, the persons involved in the program have a tremendous effect on improvement efforts; including the right people in planning and interpreting results is critically important to successful use of the data. The challenges below are primarily focused on the measures themselves.

1. *Lack of focus:* a measure that tries to track too many criteria at the same time or is too complicated to administer, interpret, or use for quality monitoring and improvement
2. *Wrong type of measure:* a measure that calculates indicators the wrong way (e.g., uses rates when ratios are more appropriate, uses a continuous scale rather than a discrete scale, measures a process, when the outcome is measurable and of greater interest)
3. *Unclear definitions:* a measure that is too broad or too vague in its scope and definitions (e.g., population is too heterogeneous, no risk adjustment, unclear data elements, poorly defined values)
4. *Too much work:* a measure that requires too much clinician time to generate the data or too much manual chart abstraction
5. *Reinventing the wheel:* a measure that is a reinvention rather than an improvement of a performance measure
6. *Events not under control:* measure focuses on a process or outcome that is out of the organization (or the unit's) control to improve
7. *Trying to do research rather than quality improvement:* is done data collection and analysis are done for the sake of research

rather than for improvement of nursing care and the health and well-being of the patients

8. *Poor communication of results:* the format of communication does not target and enable change

9. *Uninterpretable and underused:* uninterpretable results are of little relevance to improving geriatric nursing care

USING EXISTING MEASURES

We begin the process of deciding how to measure by reviewing existing measures. There is no need to reinvent the wheel, especially if good measures are out there. Nurses should review the literature, check with national organizations, and consult with colleagues. Yet we should not adopt existing measures blindly. Instead, we need to subject them to a thorough review using the characteristics identified above. Also, health care organizations that have adopted these measures can offer their experience.

DEVELOPING NEW MEASURES

It may be that, after an exhaustive search, we cannot find measures that meet the various requirements outlined above. We decide instead to develop our own in-house measure. Here are some important guidelines:

1. *Zero in on the population to be measured.* If we are measuring an undesirable event, we must determine the group at risk for experiencing that event, then limit the denominator population to that group. If we are measuring a desirable event or process, we must identify the group that should experience the event or receive the process. Where do problems tend to occur? What variables of this problem are within our control? If some are not within our control, how can we zero in even more on the target population? In other words, we exclude patients from the population when good reason exists to do so (e.g., those allergic to the medication being measured).

2. *Define terms.* This is a painstaking but essential effort. It is better to measure 80% of an issue with 100% accuracy than 100% of an issue with 80% accuracy.

3. *Identify and define the data elements and allowable values required to calculate the measure.* This is another painstaking but essential effort. The 80/100 rule applies here as well.

4. *Test the data collection process.* Once we have a prototype of a measure ready, we must examine how easy or difficult it is to get all the required data.

SUMMARY

There is no mystery to the process of performance measurement and improvement. However, it is hard work—from identifying what to measure, to selecting the measures, collecting the data, analyzing and presenting results, and implementing change. This chapter has focused primarily on the first steps: the measurement of a quality of care program. When determining whether the measures taken are good for the staff and the organization, three things matter:

1. It works for the organization.
2. It is well defined, tested, and applied.
3. Quality improvement happens.

REFERENCES

Fulmer, T., Mezey, M., Bottrell, M., Abraham, I., Sazant, J., Grossmann, C., & Grisham, E. (2002). Nurses improving care for health system elders (NICHE): Using outcomes and benchmarks for evidence-based practice. *Geriatric Nursing, 23,* 121–127.

Kohn, L. T., Corrigan, J. M., & Donaldson, M. S. (Eds.). (2000). *To err is human: Building a safer health system.* Washington, DC: National Academy Press.

McGlynn, E. A., & Asch, S. M. (1998). Developing a clinical performance measure. *American Journal of Preventative Medicine, 14*(35), 14–21.

Schyve, P. M., & Nadzam, D. M. (1998). Performance measurement in healthcare. *Journal of Strategic Performance Measurement, 2*(4), 34–42.

Wilson, H. S. (1989). *Research in nursing* (2nd ed.). Reading, MA: Addison-Wesley.

Chapter 3

ASSESSMENT OF FUNCTION

Denise M. Kresevic and Mathy Mezey

EDUCATIONAL OBJECTIVES

On completion of this chapter, the reader should be able to

1. Identify physical functioning as an important clinical indicator of health/illness, response to treatment, and need for services.
2. Describe common components of standardized functional assessment instruments.
3. Identify unique challenges to gathering information from older adults regarding functional assessments.

Physical functioning is a dynamic process of interaction between individuals and their environments and is influenced by motivation, physical capacity, illness, cognitive ability, and the external environment including social supports. Functional assessments serve as the common language of health for patients, family members, and health care providers of older adults. The ability to manage day-to-day activities such as eating, bathing, ambulating, managing money, and keeping track of medications serves as the foundation of safe, independent functioning for all adults. However, changes in functional status are more common in older adults with chronic and acute illnesses. These changes have important implications for nursing care across settings, but especially during hospitalization.

31

BACKGROUND

It is estimated that between 20% and 40% of all elders experience functional decline during hospitalization. These declines appear to be multifactorial and at least in part preventable. Common risk factors for functional decline include injuries, acute illness, medication side effects, depression, malnutrition, and decreased mobility, from the use of physical restraints to associated iatrogenic complications such as incontinence, falls, and pressure sores. In one randomized clinical trial of hospitalized elders, the daily nursing assessment of ability to perform bathing, dressing, grooming, toileting, transferring, and ambulation during routine nursing care yielded information necessary for maintenance of function in self-care activities (Landefeld, Palmer, Kresevic, Fortinsky, & Kowa, 1995).

Assessment of function includes a systematic process of identifying the older person's physical abilities and need for help. This information is especially important for nurses in planning and evaluating care. Nurses are in a pivotal position in all care settings to assess elders' functional status by direct observation during routine care and through information gathered from the individual patient, the patient's family, and any other long-term caregivers. Including critical components of functional assessments into routine assessments in the acute care setting can provide (1) baseline information to benchmark patients' response to treatment as they move along the continuum from acute care to rehabilitation or from acute to subacute care; (2) information regarding care needs and eligibility for services, including safety needs, physical therapy needs, and posthospitalization needs; and (3) information on quality of care. The ongoing use of a standardized functional assessment instrument promotes systematic communication of patients' health status between care settings and allows units to compare their level of care with other units in the facility and to measure outcomes of care (see Table 3.1). This chapter addresses the goals and the need for functional assessment of older adults in acute care, and it provides a clinical practice protocol to guide nurses in the functional assessment of older adults (Box 3.1).

Although gathering information about functional status is a critical indicator of quality care in geriatrics, it is not always a task easily accomplished. Older persons often present to the care setting with multiple medical conditions resulting in fatigue and pain. In addition, sensory aging changes, particularly to vision and hearing,

TABLE 3.1 Functional Assessment of Older Adults

Dimension	Assessment parameter	Standardized instrument	Nursing strategies
ADLs			
Bathing Dressing Eating Toileting Hygiene Transferring	Self-report of patient, family, or home nurse Direct observation while in the hospital	Katz ADL (Katz et al., 1963) ADL Situation test (Skurla et al., 1988) Functional status (Lowenstein et al., 1989) Performance test of ADL (Kurianski & Gurland, 1976)	Encourage active participation in ADLs and assist as needed Orient to unfamiliar environment Encourage to be out of bed Ambulate daily Consult with PT/OT for strengthening exercises and adaptive behavior
Mobility			
Transferring	Self-report of patient, family, or home nurse regarding ability and frequency of performance		Encourage active and passive range of motion Encourage and assist out-of-bed ambulation

(continued)

TABLE 3.1 Functional Assessment of Older Adults *(continued)*

Dimension	Assessment parameter	Standardized instrument	Nursing strategies
Mobility *(continued)*			
Walking	Observe: Balance Gait distance Capacity	"Get Up and Go" test (Mathias, Nayak, & Isaacs, 1986)	Physical therapy; consult for exercises and equipment Refer to community exercise programs Refer for visual testing
IADLs Housework Transportation Medications Food preparation Shopping Managing finances	Self-report of patient, family, or home nurse Direct observation Simulated evaluation (e.g., evaluation by OT for kitchen safety)	Lawton IADL (Lawton & Brody, 1969) Medication Management test (Gurland et al., 1994)	Community referral for housework/shopping, etc. Vision screening Identify community resources for Home meals Transportation Pharmacy delivery Pill counters

ADLs = activities of daily living; IADLs = instrumental activities of daily living; PT/OT = physical therapist/occupational therapist

---

BOX 3.1   Nursing Standard of Practice Protocol: Assessment of Function in Acute Care

---

The following nursing care protocol has been designed to help bedside nurses to monitor function in elders, to prevent decline, and to maintain the function of elders during acute hospitalization.

Objective: The goal of nursing care is to maximize the physical functioning, prevent or minimize decline in ADL function, and plan for future care needs.

I. BACKGROUND
   A. Functional status of individuals describes the capacity and performance of safe ADLs. Functional status is a sensitive indicator of health or illness in elders and therefore a critical nursing assessment.
   B. Some functional decline may be prevented or ameliorated with prompt and aggressive nursing intervention (e.g., ambulation, enhanced communication, adaptive equipment, and attention to medications and dosages).
   C. Some functional decline may occur progressively and is not reversible. This decline often accompanies chronic and terminal disease states such as degenerative joint disease, Parkinson's disease, and dementia.
   D. Functional status is influenced by physiological aging changes, acute and chronic illness, and adaptation to the physical environment. Functional decline is often the initial symptom of acute illness such as infections (e.g., pneumonia and urinary tract infection). These declines are usually reversible and require medical evaluation.
   E. Functional status is contingent on motivation, cognition, and sensory capacity, including vision and hearing.
   F. Risk factors for functional decline include injuries, acute illness, medication side effects, depression, malnutrition, decreased mobility (including the use of physical restraints), and changes in environment or routines.
   G. Additional complications of functional decline include loss of independence, falls, incontinence, malnutrition, decreased socialization, and increased risk for long-term institutionalization and depression.
   H. Recovery of function can also be a measure of return to health, such as for those individuals recovering from exacerbations of cardiovascular or respiratory diseases and acute infections.

(continued)

BOX 3.1   Nursing Standard of Practice Protocol: Assessment of Function in Acute Care *(continued)*

I. Functional status evaluation assists in planning future care needs posthospitalization, such as short-term skilled care and home care.
II. ASSESSMENT PARAMETERS
   A. Comprehensive functional assessment of elders includes independent performance of basic ADLs, social activities, or IADLs, the assistance needed to accomplish these tasks, and the sensory ability, cognition, and capacity to ambulate.
      1. Basic activities of daily living
         a. Bathing
         b. Dressing
         c. Grooming
         d. Eating
         e. Continence
         f. Transferring
      2. Instrumental activities of daily living
         a. Meal preparation
         b. Shopping
         c. Medication administration
         d. Housework
         e. Transportation
         f. Accounting
      3. Mobility
         a. Ambulation
         b. Pivoting
   B. Elderly patients may view their health in terms of how well they can function rather than in terms of disease alone.
   C. The clinician should document baseline functional status and recent or progressive decline in function.
   D. Function should be assessed over time to validate capacity, decline, or progress.
   E. Standard instruments selected to assess function should be efficient to administer and easy to interpret. They should provide useful practical information for clinicians and be incorporated into routine history taking and daily assessments.
   F. Interdisciplinary communication regarding functional status, changes, and expected trajectory.
   G. Multidisciplinary team conferences including patient and family whenever possible.

BOX 3.1 *(continued)*

III. CARE STRATEGIES
  A. Strategies to maximize functional status
    1. Maintain individual's daily routine. Help to maintain physical, cognitive, and social function through physical activity and socialization. Encourage ambulation, allow flexible visitation, including pets, and encourage reading the newspaper.
    2. Educate elders, family, and formal caregivers on the value of independent functioning and the consequences of functional decline.
      a. Physiological and psychological value of independent functioning
      b. Reversible functional decline associated with acute illness
      c. Strategies to prevent functional decline: exercise, nutrition, and socialization
      d. Sources of assistance to manage decline
    3. Encourage activity, including routine exercise, range of motion, and ambulation to maintain activity, flexibility, and function.
    4. Minimize bed rest.
    5. Explore alternatives to physical restraints use.
    6. Judiciously use medications, especially psychoactive medications, in geriatric dosages.
    7. Assess and treat for pain.
    8. Design environments with handrails, wide doorways, raised toilet seats, shower seats, enhanced lighting, low beds, and chairs of various types and height.
    9. Help individuals regain baseline function after acute illnesses by using exercise, physical therapy consultation, nutrition, and coaching.
    10. Obtain assessment for physical and occupational therapies needed to help regain function.
  B. Strategies to help older individuals cope with functional decline
    1. Help older adults and family members determine realistic functional capacity with interdisciplinary consultation.
    2. Provide caregiver education and support for families of individuals when decline cannot be ameliorated in spite of nursing and rehabilitative efforts.
    3. Carefully document all intervention strategies and patient response.
    4. Provide information to caregivers on causes of functional decline related to acute and chronic conditions.

(continued)

BOX 3.1   Nursing Standard of Practice Protocol: Assessment of Function in Acute Care *(continued)*

    5. Provide education to address safety care needs for falls, injuries, and common complications. Short-term skilled care for physical therapy may be needed; long-term care settings may be required to ensure safety.

    6. Provide sufficient protein and caloric intake to ensure adequate intake and prevent further decline. Liberalize diet to include personal preferences.

    7. Provide caregiver support community services, such as home care, nursing, and physical and occupational therapy services, to manage functional decline.

IV. EXPECTED OUTCOMES

  A. Patients can:

    1. Maintain safe level of ADL and ambulation

    2. Make necessary adaptations to maintain safety and independence including assistive devices and environmental adaptations

  B. Providers can demonstrate:

    1. Increased assessment, identification, and management of patients susceptible to or experiencing functional decline

    2. Ongoing documentation and communication of capacity, interventions, goals, and outcomes

    3. Competence in preventive and restorative strategies for function

  C. Institution can demonstrate:

    1. Incidence and prevalence of functional decline will decrease in all care settings

    2. Decrease in morbidity and mortality rates associated with functional decline

    3. Decreased use of physical restraints

    4. Decreased incidence of delirium

    5. Increase in prevalence of patients who leave hospital with baseline or improved functional status

    6. Decreased readmission rate

    7. Increased early utilization of rehabilitative services (occupational and physical therapy)

    8. Support of institutional policies/programs that promote function:

      a. Caregiver educational efforts

      b. Walking programs

    9. Environments that reflect designs sensitive to older adults

   10. Evidence of continued interdisciplinary assessments, care

can threaten the accuracy of responses. Ideally, information regarding functional status should be elicited as part of the routine history. Patients should be made as comfortable as possible, with frequent rest periods allowed. Adaptive aids such as glasses and hearing aids should be applied. Often family members accompany the older person and can assist in answering questions regarding function. It is important for patients and family members to understand that baseline functional levels as well as recent changes in function need to be reported. Many older adults may be reluctant to report declines in function, fearing that such reports will threaten their autonomy and independent living.

Functional assessments are constantly conducted by nurses every time they notice that a patient can no longer pick up a fork or has difficulty walking. A comprehensive functional assessment leads to more than simply noticing a change in activity or ability, however. In a systematic manner, nurses need to assess the ability of a patient to perform activities of daily living (ADLs) in the context of the patient's baseline functional status and hospitalization status. Any decrease in functional status should prompt an immediate search for underlying causes.

A variety of instruments/methods are available for conducting functional assessments. The Katz ADL index (Mezey, Rauckhorst, & Stokes, 1993) has been the most widely used in a variety of settings. It has established reliability and is easy to use, by gathering information on observation of bathing, dressing, eating, transferring, continence, and grooming. The Katz ADL index is easily incorporated into history and physical assessment flowsheets and takes little time to complete. Elders are evaluated according to levels of independence. The Barthel index for physical functioning (Mahoney & Barthel, 1965; Mezey et al., 1993) includes bathing, grooming, continence, stair climbing, and the ability to propel a wheelchair. This instrument has been useful in rehabilitation settings to monitor improvements over time. The Barthel instrument allows differentiation among task performance, including amount of help and amount of time needed to accomplish each task. The Older Americans Resource and Services (OARS) instrument for physical function (Burton, Damon, Dillinger, Erickson, & Peterson, 1978; Kane & Kane, 2000) is similar in scope of measurement to the Katz scale, including bathing, dressing, grooming, and continence. However, unlike the Katz instrument, which uses caregiver observation, the OARS instrument relies on self-report. Self-reports of capacity may be less valid than observations of performance, with some elders overestimating or underestimating actual capacity (Kidd et al., 1995). The Functional Independence Measure (FIM™) was designed to assess "the burden of care" in six areas: self-care, transfers, sphincter control, locomotion, communication, and social cognition. This instrument has been used to assess outcomes of patients with orthopedic and neurologic conditions. Information may be gathered by phone, mail, self-report, or proxy report using the appropriate version. Each item is scored from 1 to 7, with 1 indicating a need for total assistance and 7 completely independent in a timely and safe manner.

The assessment of instrumental activities of daily living (IADLs), including the ability to prepare meals and administer medications safely, may not be observed during an acute hospitalization, although assessment of capacity in these domains has important implications for planning for posthospitalization services. Regardless of the instrument used, basic ADL and IADL function should be assessed for each patient, including capacity for dressing, eating, transferring, toileting, hygiene, and ambulation. Appropriate assessment instruments should be readily available on acute care units. To adequately assess function, sensory capacity and cognitive capacity must be established.

AMBULATION

The ability to walk is a critical parameter for functional assessment. Some instruments used to assess ambulation, balance, and gait are sensitive measures of mobility (Applegate, Blass, & Franklin, 1990); however, they are also complex and time consuming to use. Direct observation of an individual's ability to get out of bed, sit in a chair, assume a standing position, and steadily walk a short distance, with or without assistive devices, is important to ensure safety in ADL capacity (Applegate et al., 1990; Cress et al., 1995). Direct observation of transfer and ambulation should include an assessment of speed of performance, hesitancy, stumbling, swaying, grabbing for support, or unsafe maneuvers such as sitting too close to the edge of a chair or dizziness while pivoting (Tinetti & Ginter, 1988). The "Get Up and Go" test (Table 3.2) can be used by nurses for ambulation assessments during routine daily activities of older individuals (Applegate et al., 1990). Assessment of unsafe transfers or ambulation indicates the need to begin immediate restorative therapies to prevent injuries and falls.

TABLE 3.2   The "Get Up and Go" Test for Gait Assessment in Elderly Patients

Have the patient sit in a straight-backed high-seat chair.

Instructions for patient:
1. Get up (without use of armrests, if possible).
2. Stand still momentarily.
3. Walk forward 10 ft (3 m).
4. Turn around and walk back to chair.
5. Turn and be seated.

Factors to note:
   Sitting balance
   Transfers from sitting to standing
   Pace and stability of walking
   Ability to turn without staggering

Source: Adapted from Applegate et al. (1990), with permission.

SENSORY CAPACITY

Evaluation of the potential impact of sensory changes on the performance of ADLs is often underestimated. A simple test for functional vision is to have elders read a headline from the newspaper. A moderate impairment can be noted if only the headline can be read (Tinetti & Ginter, 1988). Another way to assess vision is to have older persons read prescription bottles. Glasses should be available and cleaned. Inability to read raises issues of literacy. Often overlooked is the number of older people who may not be able to read but are too embarrassed to reveal that information.

Hearing ability is essential to function and cognition. Individuals with decreased hearing may be inaccurately labeled as cognitively impaired. Hearing aids may not have been sent to the hospital with the elder. The family should obtain these. Hearing acuity may be validated by asking patients to identify the sound of a ticking watch. The "whisper test" may also be used. This is performed by whispering 10 words while standing 6 inches away from the individual. Inability to repeat 5 of the 10 words indicates a need for further assessment of hearing acuity. Occlusion of the external ear canal by cerumen may be found on visualization, an easily treatable problem in decreased hearing acuity (Mathias, Nayak, & Isaacs, 1986). Individuals with hearing deficits that are detected as part of bedside assessment should be referred for additional assessment and treatment, including hearing aids. Headphone amplifier devices may be useful and are an inexpensive item to stock on nursing units in hospitals.

COGNITIVE CAPACITY

Cognitive function is a major factor in a person's functional capacity. Baseline cognitive function is important to assess. However, such assessments most often initially rely on information provided by family members because acute illness may be clinically manifested as acute confusional states and does not reflect baseline cognitive function (Kurianski & Gurland, 1976). Nurses can assess components of cognitive function (including attention, language, and memory) during interviews and routine care, although anxiety and illness may be complicating factors. Fluctuating attention may indicate an acute reversible impairment (delirium) or temporary reactions to hospitalization. An acute change in cognition should be evaluated for an underlying acute medical problem. In chapter 7 of this book, Marquis Foreman and colleagues provide guidelines for cognitive assessment in a clinical practice protocol.

CAUSE OF FUNCTIONAL DECLINE

All instances of functional decline should be assessed for an underlying cause. Patients experiencing any acute loss of independence in ADLs should be thoroughly assessed for acute illness. In the presence of acute illness (e.g., urinary tract infection, pneumonia, or recovery after surgery), impaired ADLs are expected to return to baseline with appropriate care and rehabilitation as the illness resolves. Comprehensive musculoskeletal or neurologic examination, laboratory tests, or referral for a therapeutic trial of physical or occupational therapy may be needed.

USE OF ASSESSMENT INFORMATION

Knowledge of ADLs and IADLs, including shopping, housework, finances, food preparation, medication administration, and transportation, is an important part of comprehensive discharge planning (Woolf, 1990). In summary, for older people, the evaluation of function represents the cornerstone of good nursing care and affords a sound baseline by which to provide information essential to plan for continued care across settings.

CASE STUDY 1

Mrs. Brown, a 93-year-old widow, was admitted to a general medical surgical nursing unit after her daughter found her at home, clothing in disarray and mumbling incoherently. A chest x-ray in the emergency room revealed pneumonia, and her blood work revealed severe dehydration with elevated serum sodium and blood urea nitrogen levels. Mrs. Brown's daughter assured the nursing staff that her mother had been living alone independently and caring for her own physical needs before this episode of illness.

As soon as Mrs. Brown arrived on the unit, she began screaming for her daughter. Despite attempts to help Mrs. Brown to walk, she was unable to take more than one or two steps before she froze in place. The nursing staff, fearful of a fall, used a vest restraint to keep Mrs. Brown in the chair. She developed incontinence and refused food and fluids, despite efforts by the nurse's aide to feed her. She continued to scream for her daughter all evening. The night nurse convinced the physician on call to order haloperidol 5 mg stat for agitation. Rather than mitigating or reducing Mrs. Brown's agitation, it escalated throughout the night. Exhausted, she fell asleep in the early morning hours.

The next day, Mrs. Brown's daughter arrived with her mother's glasses, hearing aid, and walker. That afternoon, with her glasses and hearing aid on, Mrs. Brown began to ask what had happened to her. She drank two glasses of juice and ate a bowl of chicken soup. Using her wheeled walker, she was able to ambulate independently to the bathroom and even to the nurse's station to find a newspaper. An early comprehensive assessment and history taking that included contact with her daughter might have prevented the fear, confusion, and agitation Mrs. Brown experienced on her first day of hospitalization.

CASE STUDY 2

Mr. Goode is an 86-year-old retired college history professor who is well known for his accomplishments as a collegiate football player. His wife of 60 years died last year. He lives alone in a one-floor condominium. His daughter and son live in the same city. He has a cleaning lady who comes once a week. He has been receiving Meals-on-Wheels; he admits to being a terrible cook. Mr. Goode has been driving only short distances during the daytime since his cataract surgery 15 years ago. He rides his stationary exercise bike daily to keep up his "boyish" figure.

Mr. Goode has a long history of cardiac disease, including two myocardial infarctions and a coronary bypass graft 20 years ago. He has degenerative joint disease that affects his hips and knees, and 10 years ago he underwent bilateral knee replacements. Twenty years ago he had prostate surgery for enlargement. His current medications include lisinopril 5 mg, furosemide 20 mg, and potassium chloride 8 mEq qod, acetaminophen 650 mg bid, and analgesic balm as needed.

Mr. Goode is admitted to the emergency room extremely short of breath; the cleaning lady had called 911. He has crackles in his lungs and 4+ pitting edema of his legs. He is placed on oxygen and given IV Lasix. A Foley catheter is placed, and an IV of D$_5$½NS at 50 cc per hour is started. On admission to the nursing unit, he requires assistance to move from the cart to the bed. He complains of nausea, weakness, and knee pain. His physician orders bedrest and Benadryl 25 mg hs prn for sleep.

On hospital day 2, Mr. Goode refuses to get out of bed because of knee pain. He requests assistance with his bathing and eating. His weight has decreased 2 pounds, and he has decreased crackles in his lungs. His daughter arrives with his glasses, hearing aids with batteries, and pillboxes. His medication boxes are still filled from the previous 5 days. His laboratory results return. His urine is positive for bacteria, red and white cells, and leukoesterase, confirming a urinary tract infection. An electrocardiogram is negative for an acute myocardial infarction. A chest x-ray confirms acute congestive heart failure and pneumonia. He is placed on antibiotics.

During team rounds, his orders are changed to the following: out of bed and ambulate in hallway bid, discontinue Foley catheter and Benadryl, wean oxygen. His nurses review his baseline ADL function and current function and request a physical therapy consultation to evaluate safe ambulation and a social work consultation to evaluate self-care ability and home care services. The patient requests analgesic balm for his knees. Fall precautions are initiated, including frequent prompted voiding.

On hospital day 4, Mr. Goode ambulates out to the nurse's station and announces that he feels much better and is ready to go home. His progress is reviewed on team rounds. The physical therapy evaluation reveals that he is capable of ambulating and transferring independently and safely, and the therapist recommends a continued home exercise program. The social worker has shared information with Mr. Goode and his son regarding the "life line" and check-in phone calls every evening. Nutrition services recommended a low-salt diet, and a nurse has reviewed medications with Mr. Goode and his daughter. A pillbox is filled in the pharmacy. Mr. Goode's daughter will check the pillbox weekly. Mr. Goode is ready for discharge from the hospital and will return to his condominium because he has returned to his baseline ADLs.

ACKNOWLEDGMENT

Supported by a grant from the John A. Hartford Foundation.

REFERENCES

Abrams, W. B., & Berkow, R. (Eds.). (1990). *The Merck manual of geriatrics.* White House Station, NJ: Merck, Sharp & Dohme.

Applegate, W. B., Blass, J., & Franklin, T. (1990). Instruments for the functional assessment of older patients. *New England Journal of Medicine, 322,* 1207–1214.

Burton, R. M., Damon, W. W., Dillinger, D. C., Erickson, D. J., & Peterson, D. W. (1978). Nursing home rest and care: An investigation of alternatives. In E. Pfeiffer (Ed.), *Multidimensional functional assessment: The DARS methodology.* Durham, NC: Duke Center for Study of Aging Human Development.

Cress, M. E., Schectman, K. B., Mulrow, C. D., Fiatarone, M. A., Gerety, M. B., & Buchner, D. M. (1995). Relationship between physical performance and self perceived physical function. *Journal of the American Geriatric Society, 43,* 93–101.

Gurland, B. J., Cross, I., Chen, C., Wilder, D. E., Pine, Z. M., Lantigua, R. A., & Fulmer, T. (1994). A new performance test of adaptive cognitive functioning: The medication management (MM) test. *International Journal of Geriatric Psychiatry, 9,* 875–885.

Kane, R. A., & Kane, R. L. (2000). *Assessing older persons: Measures, meaning, and practical applications.* New York: Oxford.

Katz, S., Ford, A. B., Moscokowitz, R. W., Jackson, B. A., & Jaffe, M. W. (1963). Studies of illness and the aged: The index of ADL. A standardized measure of biological and psychosocial function. *Journal of the American Medical Association, 185,* 914–919.

Kidd, D., Stewart, G., Baldry, J., Johnson, J., Rossiter, D., Petruckevitch, A., & Thompson, A. (1995). The Functional Independence Measure: A comparative validity and reliability study. *Disability and Rehabilitation, 17*(1), 10–14.

Kurianski, J., & Gurland, B. (1976). The performance test of activities of daily living. *International Journal of Aging and Human Development, 7,* 343–352.

Landefeld, S. C., Palmer, R. M., Kresevic, D. M., Fortinsky, R. I., & Kowa, J. (1995). A randomized trial of care in a hospital medical unit especially designed to improve the functional outcomes of acutely ill older patients. *New England Journal of Medicine, 332,* 1338–1344.

Lawton, M. P., & Brody, E. M. (1969). Assessment of older people: Self-maintaining and instrumental activities of daily living. *Gerontologist, 9,* 179–186.

Lowenstein, D. A., Amigo, E., Duara, R., Guterman, A., Hurwitz, D., Berkowitz, N., et al. (1989). A new scale for the assessment of functional status in Alzheimer's disease and related disorders. *Journal of Gerontology, 44,* 114–121.

Mahoney, F. L., & Barthel, D. W. (1965). Functional evaluation: The Barthel index. *Maryland State Medical Journal, 14,* 61–65.

Mathias, S., Nayak, U. S., & Isaacs, B. (1986). Balance in elderly patients: The "Get Up and Go" test. *Archives of Physical and Medical Rehabilitation, 67,* 387–389.

Mezey, M. D., Rauckhorst, L. H., & Stokes, S. A. (1993). *Health assessment of the older individual.* New York: Springer Publishing Co.

Skurla, E., Rogers, J. C., & Sunderland, T. (1988). Direct assessment of activities of daily living in Alzheimer's disease: A controlled study. *Journal of the American Geriatric Society, 36,* 97–103.

Tinetti, M. E., & Ginter, S. F. (1988). Identify mobility dysfunctions in elderly patients: Standard neuromuscular examination or direct assessment? *Journal of the American Medical Association, 259,* 1190–1193.

Woolf, S. H. (1990). Screening for hearing impairment. In R. B. Goldbloom & R. S. Lawrence (Eds.), *Preventing disease: Beyond the rhetoric* (pp. 331–346). New York: Springer-Verlag.

Chapter 4

EXCESSIVE SLEEPINESS

Mary Grace Umlauf, Eileen R. Chasens, and Terri E. Weaver

EDUCATIONAL OBJECTIVES

On completion of this chapter, the reader should be able to
1. Identify the signs of excessive sleepiness (ES) and rate these symptoms using a standardized numerical scale.
2. Describe the signs and symptoms for the most common causes of ES in older adults: obstructive sleep apnea, restless leg syndrome, insomnia, and narcolepsy.
3. Plan appropriate interventions for the patient with ES.
4. Provide nursing care that incorporates sleep hygiene measures.
5. Educate patients and families about sleep disorders and sleep hygiene measures.

Excessive sleepiness (ES), sometimes called excessive daytime sleepiness, is a common symptom in the elderly. Distinct from fatigue, which is the increased difficulty of sustaining a high level of performance, ES refers to the inability to maintain alertness and is characterized by hypersomnolence. Causes for ES include age-related changes in sleep pattern and architecture, sleep disorders, other

47

medical and psychological disorders, medications, environmental factors, and altered social patterns. It remains unclear how much of the changes in sleep patterns encountered by older adults are due to normal physiological alterations, pathological events, sleep disorders, or poor sleep hygiene. In the acute care setting, the patient with ES will be more complicated when either the underlying causes of ES are not yet diagnosed or the plan of care does not reflect maintenance of ongoing treatments for ES.

The primary purpose of this chapter is to provide a basic foundation in sleep disorders, because this content traditionally has not been included in standard nursing curricula and because many practicing nurses have no background in the content area. Nurses in the acute care setting must be able to identify, screen, and refer patients for sleep disorders because other health care providers are similarly uninformed about these serious conditions. Additionally, sleep hygiene measures and the ongoing treatment of existing sleep disorders must be incorporated into the plan of care for older adults to preserve and conserve sleep in all settings: acute care, primary care, and in the home.

CONSEQUENCES OF EXCESSIVE SLEEPINESS

Estimates from the most recent national poll assert that 47 million American adults do not get the minimum amount of sleep they need to be alert the next day. Many respondents (37%) said that they were so sleepy during the day that it interfered with their daily activities at least a few days a month, and others (16%) had problems with sleepiness at least a few days a week (National Sleep Foundation, 2002).

The primary consequences of sleepiness are decreased alertness, delayed reaction time, and decreased cognitive performance. Complicating the clinical importance of ES is the commonly held belief that daytime sleepiness is an acceptable behavior for older adults. This misperception prevents elders from seeking medical attention for ES and reduces the likelihood that health care providers will evaluate, treat, or refer patients who present with clear symptoms of ES. The causes of ES may also be contributing to the circumstances and/or conditions that bring the patient to the health care provider in the first place. Thus, the problem of ES is not just an issue of making a diagnosis and treatment. There are many effective treatments for sleep disorders, but the first step toward reducing ES is to identify, quantify, and aggressively treat this condition in the older adult by incorporating sleep-enhancing interventions in the plan of nursing care and by referring the patient to a doctor who specializes in sleep medicine.

Recent studies show that daytime sleepiness is significantly associated with declining cognitive function (Cohen-Zion et al., 2001) and cardiovascular disease events (Newman et al., 2000b; Whitney et al., 1998). Obstructive sleep apnea (OSA) has been found to have negative, yet reversible, effects on attention, learning abilities, planning capacities, categorizing activities, and verbal fluency (Naegele et al., 1998). Approximately 56,000 car crashes per year are attributed to falling asleep at the wheel (Garabino, Nobili, Beelke, DeCarli, & Ferrillo, 2001; George & Smiley, 1999; Masa, Rubio, & Findley, 2000; Young, Blustein, Finn, & Palta, 1997). Thus, when ES is seen concomitantly with accidental or workplace injury, cardiovascular morbidity, or cognitive impairment, sleep-related causes should be considered.

PHYSIOLOGICAL CHANGES IN SLEEP THAT ACCOMPANY AGING

Normal changes in sleep that occur as part of human development should be differentiated from pathological conditions that increase in prevalence with aging. Although older adults require as much sleep as younger persons, the distribution of sleep in older adults may not be a single consolidated period at night but rather may consist of nighttime sleep and daytime napping (Bliwise, 2000; Richardson, Carskadon, & Orav, 1982; Roehrs, Carskadon, Dement, & Roth, 2000). Although older adults may spend more time in bed, there is a decrease in the actual time they spend sleeping. Older adults have increased sleep latency, or the time it takes to fall asleep, impaired sleep maintenance because of arousals, and more difficulty in returning to sleep if awakened during the night. There is decreased stage 3 and 4 "deep sleep" and an increase in the percentage of stage 1 "lighter sleep." Older adults are more likely to awaken because of environmental factors such as noise or because of physiological factors of pain or nocturia. Although older women report more complaints of sleep disturbances than older men, an analysis of women's sleep studies indicates that their sleep is less disturbed than men's sleep (Rediehs, Reis, & Creason, 1990).

SLEEP DISORDERS: CAUSES OF EXCESSIVE DAYTIME SLEEPINESS

OBSTRUCTIVE SLEEP APNEA

Sleep apnea is both an age-related and an age-dependent condition, with an overlap in both distributions in the 60 to 70 age range (Bliwise, King, & Harris, 1994). As many as 24% of those over the age of 65 have been identified with sleep apnea, predominantly of the obstructive type (Ancoli-Israel, Kripke, & Mason, 1987). OSA is a condition in which there is intermittent pharyngeal obstruction producing cessation of respiratory airflow (for at least 10 seconds) and often oxygen desaturation. The arousal subsequent to the apneic event restores upper airway patency that permits breathing and airflow to resume. According to the American Academy of Sleep Medicine Task Force (1999), OSA is diagnosed when these events occur at a rate of greater than 5 per hour of sleep accompanied by snoring, gasping, daytime sleepiness, and impaired daytime functioning. However, it is not uncommon for patients with severe symptoms to experience multiple awakenings in one night. These multiple awakenings severely fragment sleep, preventing deep sleep (stages 3 and 4) and rapid eye movement (REM) sleep necessary for healthy mental and physical functioning. Age-related risk factors for OSA in older adults include obesity and being overweight, decreased thyroid function, increased collapsibility of the upper airway, decreased lung capacity, altered ventilatory control, decreased muscular endurance, and altered sleep architecture (Bliwise, 2000). However, evidence is mounting to support the existence of a link between disordered breathing and insulin resistance, a contributing factor to weight gain and diabetes (Ip et al., 2002; Punjabi et al., 2002; Tasali & VanCauter, 2002).

Treatments for sleep apnea include continuous positive airway pressure (CPAP), surgical procedures designed to increase the posterior pharyngeal area, oral appliances, and weight reduction, when obesity is a contributing factor. CPAP is the most effective treatment for OSA, producing improvements in neurobehavioral performance, daytime sleepiness, snoring, and quality of life (Grunstein & Sullivan, 2000).

INSOMNIA

Insomnia includes complaints of delayed sleep onset, premature waking after sleep onset, and very early arousals that result in a shortened total sleep time. Recent studies comparing younger and older adults found that the elderly (> 65 years) have approximately a 1.5 times higher prevalence of sleep difficulty. In addition, women are more likely than men to report insomnia-like symptoms (Zorick & Walsh, 2000). Although it remains unclear whether insomnia is an organic, psychological, pharmacological, chronobiological, or behavioral problem, it has been associated with cardiovascular, respiratory, gastrointestinal, renal, and musculoskeletal disorders. Insomnia may be transient or chronic, and the perception of sleep duration may not correspond to objective assessment. The frequent awakenings suggestive of insomnia may be a conditioned arousal response due to environmental or behavioral cues. Anxiety associated with emotional conflict, stress, recent loss, feeling insecure at night, or change in living arrangement can also produce insomnia. The general anxiety and conditioned arousal response at sleep onset associated with insomnia may prompt more frequent use of hypnotic medication. Although the use of hypnotics may produce temporary symptom relief, they also affect sleep architecture and consequently deterioration in the quality of sleep. Thus, a cycle of dependency can occur when hypnotics are prescribed. The shortest acting drugs are most appropriate, and there remains a need to initiate sleep hygiene measures (Ancoli-Israel, 2000). When insomnia can be traced to pain, such as with arthritis, strategies must be added to pain management to promote sleep onset such as a nonsteroidal anti-inflammatory drugs (NSAIDs) before bedtime.

RESTLESS LEG SYNDROME AND PERIODIC LEG MOVEMENTS

Restless leg syndrome (RLS) is a disorder characterized by an almost irresistible urge to move the limbs. It is usually associated with disagreeable leg sensations, is worse during inactivity, and often interferes with initiating and maintaining sleep. The cause of primary RLS is not well defined, but it appears to have a familiar pattern, increases in incidence with age, and has been linked to metabolic, vascular, and neurologic causes. As a secondary condition, RLS may be caused by iron deficiency anemia, uremia, neurologic lesions, diabetes, Parkinson's disease, and rheumatoid arthritis, and is a side effect of certain drugs (e.g., tricyclic antidepressants, selective serotonin reuptake inhibitors [SSRIs], lithium, dopamine blockers, and xanthines). Although RLS is diagnosed by reviewing the patient history and symptoms, periodic leg movement disorder

(PLMD) is diagnosed by a sleep study. PLMD, also known as nocturnal myoclonus, is an involuntary flexion of the leg and foot that produce microarousals, as well as full arousals, from sleep. Treatment for RLS and PLMD includes the use of dopaminergic medications, opioids, benzodiazepines, and iron supplements.

NARCOLEPSY

Narcolepsy is characterized by uncontrollable daytime "sleep attacks," with sleep-onset REM periods, excessive daytime sleepiness, cataplexy (abrupt loss of muscle tone), sleep paralysis of skeletal muscles on falling asleep or awakening, and sleep-onset hallucinations. Although the symptoms frequently first develop in young and middle-aged adults, the mean time for diagnosis is 15 years, with frequent misdiagnosis of depression. Diagnosis is made by clinical symptoms and either a short sleep latency or the presence of two or more sleep-onset REM periods on the Multiple Sleep Latency Test. Persons with uncontrolled sleepiness need to be cautioned to avoid potentially dangerous activities, such as driving, until their symptoms are under control (Guilleminault & Anagnos, 2000; Littner et al., 2001).

ASSESSMENT OF ES

There are several valid and reliable clinical measures that can be used to assess ES. One of the most commonly used is the Epworth Sleepiness Scale (Johns, 1992), which has been broadly disseminated on the Internet in recent years (see Table 4.1). The likelihood of having OSA can be determined using the Multivariable Apnea Prediction Index (Maislin et al., 1995). The Functional Outcomes of Sleep Questionnaire (Weaver et al., 1997) can be employed to assess the impact of daytime hypersomnolence on functional status, and the Pittsburgh Sleep Quality Index (Buysse, Reynolds, Monk, Berman, & Kupfer, 1989) is beneficial in the assessment of insomnia. Because it is so readily available, many sleep clinicians use the Epworth Sleepiness Scale to rate the severity of somnolence during common soporific activities, such as sitting and reading, watching television, and riding in a car. The Epworth Sleepiness Scale is easy to administer and to score, and it has scoring parameters to indicate when sleepiness clearly warrants a more complete evaluation by a sleep

TABLE 4.1   The Epworth Sleepiness Scale

Instructions to the patient: The following questionnaire will help you measure your general level of daytime sleepiness. It asks you to rate the likelihood that you would doze off or fall asleep during different, routine, daytime situations. Answers to the questions are rated on a scale from 0 to 3, with 0 meaning you would never doze off or fall asleep in a given situation, and 3 meaning that there is a very high likelihood that you would doze off or fall asleep in that situation. How likely are you to doze off or fall asleep in the following situations listed, in contrast to just feeling tired? Even if you haven't done some of these things recently, think about how they would have affected you. Use the following scale to choose the most appropriate number for each situation:

0 = would never doze
1 = slight chance of dozing
2 = moderate chance of dozing
3 = high chance of dozing

Situation	Circle your score 0–3			
Sitting and reading	0	1	2	3
Watching television	0	1	2	3
Sitting inactive in a public place, for example, a theater or meeting	0	1	2	3
As a passenger in a car for an hour without a break	0	1	2	3
Lying down to rest in the afternoon	0	1	2	3
Sitting and talking to someone	0	1	2	3
Sitting quietly after lunch (when you've had no alcohol)	0	1	2	3
In a car, while stopped in traffic	0	1	2	3

Score Results:
  1–6   Getting enough sleep
  4–8   Tends to be sleepy but is average
  9–15   Very sleepy and should seek medical advice
  > 16   Dangerously sleepy

Source: Johns (1992).

specialist. A sleep history may be obtained by using questionnaires in Tables 4.2 and 4.3. In a sleep laboratory setting, ES can be measured by electrophysiologic tests such as the Multiple Sleep Latency Test, which measures how long it takes to fall asleep, and the Maintenance of Wakefulness Test, which tests the ability to stay awake. Table 4.4 presents the criteria for the severity of sleepiness developed by the American Academy of Sleep Medicine Task Force (1999). Most important in the assessment of ES is an evaluation of the patient's knowledge and performance of sleep hygiene measures to complement clinical findings(see Table 4.5).

INTERVENTION/CARE STRATEGIES

The first line of defense against ES is a lifestyle that promotes and ensures adequate sleep and rest. Although there is a natural drive to sleep, environment and habituation play an important part in being able to obtain quality sleep. There are many facets to sleep hygiene, and each element bears review and reinforcement over time. Regardless of health status, the sleep hygiene measures outlined in Table 4.5 are just as important for older adults as they are for children, adolescents, and other adults.

Secondarily, nurses in acute care settings must be able to identify sleep disorders among their patients. Sleep disorders are not just bothersome; they can complicate care and pose important risks if they are not managed or diagnosed. ES is only the general symptoms of a more specific problem for a given individual. Developing individualized plans of care for patients must include both active treatment of known sleep disorders and incorporation of the sleep hygiene measures.

CASE STUDY

Mr. S. has come to the emergency room of a community hospital on a Saturday morning complaining of chest pain during the previous night. He has run out of nitroglycerin and needs a refill. His primary care physician is no longer in the community, and Mr. S. had not made plans to find another physician in the interim. He is in no acute distress, and he denies any chest pain at this time.

TABLE 4.2 Sleep History

Basic sleep history questions	Follow-up questions	Sleep disorders to consider
• Do you have any difficulty falling asleep?	• What time do you usually go to bed? Fall asleep? • What prevents you from falling asleep? • Review intake of alcohol, nicotine, caffeine, medications.	• Shift work/sleep schedule disorders • Psychophysiologic insomnia • Restless leg syndrome • Psychiatric disorders • Substance/medication related disorders
• Are you having any difficulty sleeping until morning?	• Review of depressive symptoms: weight loss, sadness, recent losses, and so on	• Depression
• Are you having difficulty sleeping throughout the night?	• How often do you waken? • How long are you awake? • Do you have any pain, discomfort, or shortness of breath during the night? • What prevents you from falling back to sleep?	• Insomnia • Medical causes of sleep disturbance • Obstructive sleep apnea
• Have you or anyone else ever noticed that you snore loudly or stop breathing in your sleep?	• Are you sleepy or tired during the day? • Review risk factors such as obesity.	• Obstructive sleep apnea
• Do you find yourself falling asleep during the day when you don't want to?	• Review answers to questions above. • If you laugh or get angry, do you feel weak (as if you might fall down or drop what you are holding)? • Do your legs kick or jump around while you sleep?	• Functional impairment resulting from sleep disorder • Narcolepsy • Periodic leg movement disorders

Adapted from Owens (2000).

TABLE 4.3   I SNORED

I	Insomnia—an inability to fall asleep that may be amenable to sleep hygiene measures or may be a sign of clinical depression
S	Snoring and sleep quality—clues to sleep apnea, which causes sleep fragmentation
N	Not breathing—witnessed apneas reported by family or friends are important diagnostic clues.
O	Older or obese—both conditions are risk factors for obstructive sleep apnea.
R	Restorative or refreshing sleep—poor quality sleep is absent in many sleep disorders.
E	Excessive daytime sleepiness—a strong urge to sleep during inappropriate times
D	Drugs and alcohol—over-the-counter (OTC) and prescribed drugs may cause sleepiness or cause sleep disturbances. Also, many older adults self-medicate with OTC drugs to manage their symptoms.

Adapted from Harding (2000).

Mr. S. is a 73-year-old male who is moderately overweight (height—5'9", weight—210 pounds, body mass index [BMI] = 35). He is hypertensive (sitting blood pressure [BP]—154/98) and takes several medications to control his blood pressure (amlodipine, lanoxin, hydrochlorothiazide/lisinopril, pravastatin, and enteric coated aspirin). He is not diabetic and has no symptoms of UTI. Mr. S. was widowed 2 weeks ago and admits that he has not had time to attend to his own health problems for some time.

HISTORY AND SYMPTOMS

Mr. S. reports, "I have no energy. I can sleep anytime and any-where, but I am tired all the time. I fell asleep while driving on the highway last week and nearly ran off the road." He reports the fol-lowing: wakes unrefreshed, morning headaches, sleep disturbed by nocturia 4 times per night, heartburn at night, legs jerk during sleep, has difficulty staying awake, fell asleep while driving during daytime, loss of energy, cannot go to church or movies without falling asleep, takes over-the-counter (OTC) sleeping pill 3 or 4 times

TABLE 4.4   Severity Criteria for Sleepiness

Mild	• Episodes of unwanted sleepiness or involuntary sleep episodes occur only during activities when little attention is required. • Occurs while watching television, reading, or traveling as a passenger in a moving vehicle.
Moderate	• Episodes of unwanted sleepiness or involuntary sleep occur during activities when some attention is required. • Moderate impairment of social and occupational function occurs as a result of sleepiness. • Occurs during activities such as attendance at concerts, presentations, and meetings.
Severe	• Episodes of unwanted sleepiness or involuntary sleep occur when more active attention is required. • Marked impairment of social and occupational function. • Occurs while eating, walking, standing, or driving; may occur during conversations or sex.

American Academy of Sleep Medicine Task Force (1999).

a week, takes frequent naps, consumes > 6 cups coffee per day, uses alcohol on weekends. He has a history of snoring (> 20 years) and was a smoker until 12 years ago.

ASSESSMENT

Mr. S. has severe daytime ES and symptoms of OSA. Sleep hygiene habits are poor: He self medicates with caffeine, as a daytime stimulant; he uses alcohol and OTC hypnotics to reduce spontaneous arousals at night. He is obese, and obesity is a contributing factor to OSA. Nocturia and systemic hypertension are associated with OSA, which also increases the risk of stroke and heart attack. Clearly, this patient is a driving risk even during daylight hours. Although depression can cause sleep disruption, this patient's medical history and symptom report are compelling and warrant a referral to a sleep specialist for evaluation and treatment.

INTERVENTIONS

The immediate interventions is a referral to a sleep specialist. Intermediate interventions include weight loss, instruction on

TABLE 4.5   Sleep Hygiene Measures

- Use the bed only for sleeping (or sex).
- Develop consistent and rest-promoting bedtime routines.
- Maintain the same bedtime and waking time every day.
- Exposure to bright sunlight is desirable upon awakening but should be avoided just prior to bedtime.
- Upon awakening, get up out of bed slowly, no matter what time it is.
- If awakened during the night, avoid looking at the clock; frequent time checks will heighten anxiety and make sleep onset more difficult.
- Avoid naps entirely or limit naps to 10 to 15 minutes' duration.
- Sleep in a cool, quiet environment.
- Patients who cannot sleep after 15 or 20 minutes should get up and go into another room, read, or do a quiet activity, using dim lighting until they are sleepy again. (Do not watch television, which emits a bright light.)
- Sleeping alone is more restful than sleeping with another person or pets. If pets or bed partners add to the problem, move to the couch for a couple of nights, and restrict pets from sharing the bed.
- Prior to bedtime, avoid the following:
  - caffeine and nicotine after noon
  - alcohol intake (> 3 drinks)
  - large meals or exercise 3 to 4 hours before bedtime
  - emotional upset or emotionally charged activities

sleep hygiene measures, and recommendations to avoid sedating OTC drugs (alcohol), which can exacerbate OSA symptoms, and driving long distances, especially if alone or at night, until after the treatment of OSA has begun. If the patient receives treatment by positive airway pressure and is compliant, he may be more successful at weight loss efforts, which can improve hypertension and glucose control. In addition, the effective treatment of OSA often improves nighttime symptoms of gastric reflux and nocturia.

The result of an overnight polysomnography test was the diagnosis of severe OSA. The physician ordered CPAP treatment.

OUTCOME

Six months after starting CPAP, Mr. S. has lost 30 pounds and has already had CPAP pressures and antihypertensive medications titrated downward. His blood pressure has dropped to 132/88, and he seldom has nocturia or naps. He no longer feels tired and has taken several car trips without feeling sleepy. Mr. S. also states that he is "about ready" to start dating. He reports, "I did not know how tired I was until I started on this breathing machine at night. I will admit, a few nights I haven't used it. But the next day, I always know that I made a mistake by skipping the night before."

SUMMARY

Failing to identify, diagnose, and treat ES has important implications for older adults. Findings from the Sleep Heart Health Study show that mild to moderate sleep-disordered breathing (SDB) is associated with cardiovascular disease (Nieto et al., 2000; Newman et al., 2000b) and reduced vitality, and severe SDB is more broadly associated with poorer quality of life (Baldwin et al., 2001). Motor vehicle accidents (George, 2001) and falls (Brassington, King, & Bliwise, 2000) are some of the obvious consequences of untreated sleep problems. Sleep medicine is a relatively new specialty, and most health care providers have never had any education about sleep disorders. Because nurses are in the position of observing patients while they sleep, they have even more reasons to become informed about sleep disorders that affect patient outcomes on a daily basis.

BOX 4.1   Nursing Standard of Practice Protocol

GOAL: Optimal state of alertness while awake, with optimal quality and quantity of sleep during the patient's preferred sleep interval.

I. BACKGROUND/STATEMENT OF PROBLEM—Excessive Sleepiness (ES)
    A. Definition: Excessive sleepiness (somnolence, hypersomnia, and excessive daytime sleepiness): A subjective report of difficulty in maintaining the alert awake state, usually accompanied by a rapid entrance into sleep when the person is sedentary (American Academy of Sleep Medicine, 2001).
    B. Etiology and Epidemiology
       1. ES may be due to difficulty initiating sleep, impaired sleep maintenance, or waking after sleep onset, inability to return to sleep, or sleep fragmentation.
       2. Sleep disorders may be either dyssomnias or parasomnias and are associated with mental, neurologic, or other medical disorders. ES is primarily a function of both quality and quantity of sleep and has been documented in 20% of elders (n = 4578 over age 65) in the Cardiovascular Health Study (Whitney et al., 1998).
       3. Daytime sleepiness is the only sleep symptom associated with mortality, incident of cardiovascular disease morbidity and mortality, myocardial infarction, and congestive heart failure, particularly among women (Newman et al., 2000a).
       4. According to the most recent "Sleep in America" poll drawn from a home telephone survey (National Sleep Foundation, 2002), 27% of Americans categorize their sleep as fair or poor.
       5. Patients in acute care settings are more likely to have problems with ES and sleep disorders. For example, Ancoli-Israel and colleagues (1987, 1991) found undiagnosed OSA in 24% of independent living elders (over age 65), 33% of elders in acute care settings, and 42% of elders in nursing home settings.
II. PARAMETERS OF ASSESSMENT
    A. A careful history should be taken that includes both the patient and family members. People who share living and sleeping spaces can provide important information about sleep behavior that the patient may not be able to convey.
    B. Several sleep history strategies have been developed by the National Heart, Lung, and Blood Institute (NHLBI). (See Tables 4.2 and 4.3).
    C. For patients with a current diagnosis of a sleep disorder, documentation and continuation of ongoing treatments, such as CPAP, should be maintained and reinforced by patient and family education.

BOX 4.1 *(continued)*

III. NURSING CARE STRATEGIES
  A. Manage medical conditions, psychological disorders, and/or symptoms that interfere with sleep, such as depression, pain, hot flashes, anemia, and uremia.
  B. Review and adjust medications that have interactions and/or side effects, including drowsiness and sleep impairment.
  C. Instruct patient on sleep hygiene measures.
  D. Suggest medical referral to a sleep specialist for moderate and severe conditions of ES and/or a clinical profile consistent with major sleep disorders, such as OSA and RLS.
  E. Plan, monitor, and manage patient's sleep disordered breathing with anesthesia or sedative medications, especially home use of positive airway pressure devices.
  F. Assess patient's adherence to prescriptions for sleep hygiene, medications, and devices to support respiration during sleep.
  G. Instruct patient on the use, cleaning, and maintenance of continuous positive airway pressure (CPAP) equipment and masks.
IV. EVALUATION/EXPECTED OUTCOMES
  A. Improved quantity and/or quality of sleep during normal sleep intervals
  B. Reduction in ES and any sequelae
  C. Improved cognitive functioning and functional status, as well as improved social and occupational performance
V. FOLLOW-UP MONITORING
  Depending on the diagnosis, follow-up monitoring may include long-term reinforcement of the original interventions, along with support of the patient by the sleep specialist to adhere to prescriptions.
  A. Rebound sleepiness may be noted during the initial treatment phase. This occurs because of sleep deprivation and should subside over time. Follow-up monitoring should include ongoing assessment of napping and sleepiness.
  B. If obesity has been a complicating health factor, weight reduction may be a desirable patient goal in the long term. With a reduction in daytime sleepiness, activity level should increase. Treatment of sleep disorders should include planning for strategic changes in lifestyle such as regular exercise, which is consistent with cardiovascular rehabilitation and long-term diabetic control.
  C. Sleep hygiene measures should be continually reassessed.

RESOURCES

National Institutes of Health, National Center on Sleep Disorders Research—the most recent information on sleep disorders. Includes brochures that may be downloaded or printed for distribution to patients or health care providers.
Web site for patients and the general public:
http://www.nhlbi.nih.gov/health/public/sleep/index.htm
Web site for health care professionals:
http://www.nhlbi.nih.gov/health/prof/sleep/index.htm

New Abstracts and Papers in Sleep—excellent resource for finding the most recent research on sleep disorders and their treatments. Services include:

Weekly personalized e-mail
Alerts of new citations
Author abstracts
Compilation of the current week's literature in sleep
Archival accumulation of the current year's literature in sleep
Search and retrieval capabilities customized for sleep
Computer-generated reprint request forms
Notification of topical information pertaining to particular areas of interest
http://www.websciences.org/bibliosleep/NAPS/

American Academy of Sleep Medicine—this organization for sleep professionals is also a great source of information for the public.
http://www.aasmnet.org/

Narcolepsy Network, 277 Fairfield Road, Suite 310B, Fairfield, NJ 07004; (973) 276-0115
http://www.websciences.org/narnet/

Restless Leg Syndrome Foundation, 4410 19th Street, NW, Suite 201, Rochester, MN 55901
http://www.rls.org

The Sleep Syllabus—*The Basics of Sleep Behavior* is a comprehensive syllabus that considers sleep and its functions and describes the processes that occur in the brain during sleep. The syllabus is designed for undergraduates, graduate students, medical students, and postdoctoral scholars.
http://www.sleephomepages.org/sleepsyllabus/

Clinical Guidelines for Sleep Disorders—the American Academy of Sleep Medicine has established clinical guidelines for the diagnosis and treatment of the major sleep disorders. These guidelines are customarily published in the journal *Sleep*, but they are made available to the professional public on the Web site:
   http://www.aasmnet.org/practiceparameters.htm

REFERENCES

American Academy of Sleep Medicine Task Force. (1999). Sleep-related breathing disorders in adults: Recommendations for syndrome definition and measurement techniques in clinical research. *Sleep, 22,* 667–689.

Ancoli-Israel, S. (2000). Insomnia in the elderly: A review for the primary care practitioner. *Sleep, 23*(Suppl 1), S23–30.

Ancoli-Israel, S., Kripke, D. F., & Mason, W. (1987). Characteristics of obstructive and central sleep apnea in the elderly: An interim report. *Biological Psychiatry, 22,* 741–750.

Baldwin, C. M., Griffith, K. A., Nieto, F. J., O'Connor, G. T., Walsleben, J. A., & Redline, S. (2001). The association of sleep-disordered breathing and sleep symptoms with quality of life in the Sleep Heart Health Study. *Sleep, 24,* 96–105.

Bliwise, D. L. (2000). Normal aging. In M. H. Kryger, T. Roth, & W. C. Dement (Eds.), *Principles and practice of sleep medicine* (3rd ed., pp. 26–42). Philadelphia: W. B. Saunders.

Bliwise, D. L., King, A. C., & Harris, R. B. (1994). Habitual sleep durations and health in a 50–65 year old population. *Journal of Clinical Epidemiology, 47,* 35–41.

Brassington, G. S., King, A. C., & Bliwise D. L. (2000). Sleep problems as a risk factor for falls in a sample of community dwelling adults aged 65–99 years. *Journal of the American Geriatric Society, 48,* 1234–1240.

Buysse, D. J., Reynolds, C. F., III, Monk, T. H., Berman, S. R., & Kupfer, D. J. (1989). The Pittsburgh Sleep Quality Index: A new instrument for psychiatric practice and research. *Psychiatry Research, 28,* 193–213.

Cohen-Zion, M., Stepinowsky, C., Marler, M., Shochat, T., Kripke, D. F., & Ancoli-Israel, S. (2001). Changes in cognitive function associated with sleep disordered breathing in older people. *Journal of the American Geriatrics Society, 49,* 1622–1627.

Garabino, S., Nobili, L., Beelke, M., DeCarli, F., & Ferrillo F. (2001). The contributing role of sleepiness in highway vehicle accidents. *Sleep, 24,* 203–206.

George, C. F. (2001). Reduction in motor vehicle collisions following treatment of sleep apnea with nasal CPAP. *Thorax, 56,* 508–512.

George, C. F., & Smiley, A. (1999). Sleep apnea and automobile crashes. *Sleep, 22,* 790–795.

Grunstein, R., & Sullivan, C. (2000). Continuous positive airway pressure for sleep breathing disorders. In M. H. Kryger, T. Roth, & W. C. Dement (Eds.), *Principles and practice of sleep medicine* (3rd ed., pp. 894–912). Philadelphia: W. B. Saunders.

Guilleminault, C., & Anagnos, A. (2000). Narcolepsy. In M. H. Kryger, T. Roth, & W. C. Dement (Eds.), *Principles and practice of sleep medicine* (3rd ed., pp. 676–686). Philadelphia: W. B. Saunders.

Harding, S. (2000). I SNORED. Retrieved April 5, 2002, from http://www.aasmnet.org/AASM2003/Products/(Harding)ISNORED.pdf

Ip, S. M., Lam, B., Ng, M., Lam, W. K., Tsang, K. W., & Lam, K. S. (2002). Obstructive sleep apnea is independently associated with insulin resistance. *American Journal of Respiratory and Critical Care Medicine, 165,* 670–676.

Johns, M. W. (1992). Reliability and factor analysis of the Epworth Sleepiness Scale. *Sleep, 15,* 376–381.

Littner, M., Johnson, S. F., McCall, W. V., Anderson, W. M., Davila, D. D., Hartse, K., et al. (2001). Practice parameters for the treatment of narcolepsy: An update for 2000. *Sleep, 24,* 451–466.

Maislin, G., Pack, A. I., Kribbs, N. B., Smith, P. L., Schwartz, A. R., Kline, L. R., Schwab, R. J., & Dinges, D. F. (1995). A survey screen for prediction of apnea. *Sleep, 18,* 158–166.

Masa, J. F., Rubio, M. & Findley, L. J. (2000). Habitually sleepy drivers have a high frequency of automobile crashes associated with respiratory disorders during sleep. *American Journal of Respiratory and Critical Care Medicine, 162,* 1407–1412.

Naegele, B., Pepin, J. L., Levy, P., Bonnet, C., Pellat, J. & Feurstein, C. (1998). Cognitive executive dysfunction in patients with obstructive sleep apnea syndrome (OSAS) after CPAP treatment. *Sleep, 21,* 392–397.

National Sleep Foundation. (2002). Sleep in America Poll. Retrieved April 4, 2002, from http://www.sleepfoundation.org/2002poll.html

Newman, A. B., Nieto, F. J., Guidry, U., Lind, B. K., Redine, S., Pickering, T. G., et al. (2000a). Relation of sleep-disordered breathing to cardiovascular disease risk factors: The Sleep Heart Health Study. *American Journal of Epidemiology, 154,* 50–59.

Newman, A. B., Spiekerman, C. F., Enright, P., Lefkowitz, D., Manolio, T., Reynolds, C. F., et al. (2000b). Daytime sleepiness predicts mortality and cardiovascular disease in older adults. The Cardiovascular Health Study Research Group. *Journal of the American Geriatrics Society, 8,* 115–123.

Nieto, F. J., Young, T. B., Lind, B. K., Shahar, E., Samet, J. M., Redline, S., et al. (2000). Association of sleep-disordered breathing, sleep apnea and hypertension in a large community-based study. *Journal of the American Medical Association, 283,* 1829–1836.

Owens, J. (2000). Why take a sleep history? Retrieved April 5, 2002, from http://www.aasmnet.org/MEDSleep/author.htm

Punjabi, N. M., Sorkin, J. J., Katzel, I., Goldberg, A., Schwartz, A., & Smith, P. L. (2002). Sleep-disordered breathing and insulin resistance in middle aged and overweight men. *American Journal of Respiratory and Critical Care Medicine, 165,* 677–682.

Rediehs, M. H., Reis, J. S., & Creason, N. S. (1990). Sleep in old age: Focus on gender differences. *Sleep, 13,* 410–424.

Richardson, G. S., Carskadon, M. A., & Orav, E. J. (1982). Circadian variation of sleep tendency in elderly and young adult subjects. *Sleep, 5,* S82–S94.

Roehrs, T., Carskadon, M. A., Dement, W. C., & Roth, T. (2000). Daytime sleepiness and alertness. In M. H. Kryger, T. Roth, & W. C. Dement (Eds.), *Principles and practice of sleep medicine* (3rd ed., pp. 43–52). Philadelphia: W. B. Saunders.

Tasali, E., & VanCauter, E. (2002). Sleep-disordered breathing and the current epidemic of obesity: Consequence or contributing factor? *American Journal of Respiratory and Critical Care Medicine, 165,* 562–563.

Weaver, T. E., Laizner, A. M., Evans, L. K., Maislin, G., Chugh, D. K., Lyon, K., et al. (1997). An instrument to measure functional status outcomes for disorders of excessive sleepiness. *Sleep, 20,* 835–843.

Whitney, C. W., Enright, P. L., Newman, A. B., Bonekat, W., Foley, D., & Quan, S. F. (1998). Correlates of daytime sleepiness in 4578 elderly persons: The Cardiovascular Health Study. *Sleep, 21,* 27–36.

Young, T., Blustein, J., Finn, L., & Palta, M. (1997). Sleep-disordered breathing and motor vehicle accidents in a population-based sample of employed adults. *Sleep, 20,* 608–613.

Zorick, F. J., & Walsh, J. K. (2000). Evaluation and management of insomnia: An overview. In M. H. Kryger, T. Roth, & W. C. Dement (Eds.), *Principles and practice of sleep medicine* (3rd ed., pp. 615–623). Philadelphia: W. B. Saunders.

_____ Chapter **5**

MEALTIME DIFFICULTIES

Elaine J. Amella

EDUCATIONAL OBJECTIVES

On completion of this chapter, the reader should be able to
1. Describe older adults who are at high risk for inadequate nutrition and hydration related to problems at mealtime.
2. Identify physiological parameters that are used to assess the nutritional status of older adults.
3. Discuss methods that can facilitate mealtime independence for older adults.
4. Identify ways to maximize contextual cues both in the home and in the institution that could facilitate positive mealtimes for disabled or cognitively impaired older adults.
5. Identify members of the interdisciplinary team who could facilitate mealtimes.

Although maintenance of good nutrition is important throughout the life span, it is critical during older age, especially if chronic illness is present. A focus of *Healthy People 2010* (U.S. Department of Health and Human Services [USDHHS], 2000) concerns reducing chronic illness related to nutrition (e.g., diabetes and osteoporosis), increasing the number of older adults who achieve a healthy weight, and increasing food security, that is, having adequate finances to afford a healthy diet. Of the top 10 causes of death (Mineo & Smith, 2001), a lifetime of good nutrition would positively affect 9 causes, accidents being the outlier. Although the definitions of nutritional deficiency syndromes vary, nearly 1 out of 3 older Americans may be at risk for malnutrition (USDHHS, 2002). Malnutrition is commonly characterized by an inability to ingest, metabolize, or acquire an adequate amount of protein or calories for anabolism. However, there is a growing realization that obesity (resulting from overconsumption) also contributes to both poor morbidity and functional impairment and is a significant nutritional problem in older adults (Jensen, McGee, & Binkley, 2001). Additionally, inadequate fluid intake contributes to functional and cognitive impairment as well as increased morbidity.

Numerous cultural and religious rituals influence the way that food is consumed; thus, the meaning of food and the way it is shared often supplant the nutritional value of the calories consumed by individuals. Therefore, examining mealtime and food as merely an exercise necessary to acquire needed nutrients misses the critical social aspect of mealtime. However, persons entrusted with serving or assisting with meals often frame meals only in the context of nutritional requirements, examining nutritional requirements only when an individual experiences unplanned outcomes such as a weight loss or gain. Additionally, alterations in nutritional health may indicate unrecognized disease states or adverse reactions to medications, unmet assistive needs, or psychological problems. The professional nurse plays a critical role in recognizing and assessing problems with nutrition, eating, feeding, and hydration in implementing a plan of care that involves education and supervision of caregivers, and in making appropriate referral to the interdisciplinary team.

RECOGNITION OF MEALTIME PROBLEMS

Nutritional issues are addressed by two prominent screening tools: the Mini Nutritional Assessment (MNA) (Guigoz, Vellas, & Garry, 1997; Rubenstein, Harker, Salva, Guigoz, & Vellas, 2001) and DETERMINE Your Health (White et al., 1992). Both have been used for screening community-dwelling older adults, but only the MNA has been shown to be valid and reliable in institutions and in several countries (Donini et al., 2002). The MNA also allows formulation of an assessment and treatment plan from initial findings. Instruments that measure the amount of assistance required at meals generally rate disability as mild, moderate, or severe, but make no attempt to define areas of strength that may be amenable to intervention or maintenance (Reuben, Greendale, & Harrison, 1995).

As individuals age, the likelihood of functional impairment increases. With increased frailty and deconditioning, loss of function follows a predictable pattern, with the ability to feed oneself the last activity of daily living (ADL) to be lost (Katz, Ford, Moskowitz, Jackson, & Jaffe, 1963). Based on type of care received, it was estimated that 25.5% of older adults living in the community receive informal and formal caregiving, and 50.9% of those living in institutions receive assistance with three to six ADLs, which would include help with meals (Spector, Fleishman, Pezzin, & Spillman, 2000). Although self-feeding must be promoted for all persons for as long as possible, techniques for promotion of independence at meals are often not used by both formal and informal caregivers, which reinforces dependence at mealtimes.

For persons who have multiple sensory changes or cognitive loss or who have well-established dining rituals, institutional mealtime routine may make food unacceptable and interfere with intake. Different religions may have strict requirements for preparation and blessing of food before it can be consumed (Tesoro, 2002). Individuals who follow dietary restrictions for religious reasons may not eat when religious rules have not been observed. In general, most cultures promote the washing of hands before meals; this may not be offered in institutional settings.

Older adults who are terminally ill should be consulted regarding preferences for food and fluid intake and may make their wishes known regarding treatment with artificial nutrition and hydration via an advance directive. If the elder loses the capacity for decision making, the proxy for health care decisions should be consulted rather than the provider assuming responsibility for the management of nutritional care.

DIAGNOSIS AND MANAGEMENT OF EATING AND FEEDING PROBLEMS

For older persons, weight is considered the "fifth vital sign," as so many health problems present initially with weight loss or gain.

Initially, both height and weight are measured to calculate body mass index (BMI), a much more sensitive indicator of nutritional problems than weight alone. BMI is determined by dividing the weight in kilograms by the height in meters squared. Normal BMI for the elderly ranges from 22 to 27, which is higher than that for young and middle-aged adults (White, Ham, & Lipschitz, 1991). Height changes in the elderly. Therefore, it is imperative that height should be measured either by standing or extrapolated from arm span or knee height (Estimating Stature, 1990).

White female ages 60 to 80 years—weight (kg) = [knee height (cm) x 1.09] + [MAC (cm) x 2.68] – 65.51 (margin of error is +/– 11.42 kg)

White males age 60 to 80 years—weight (kg) = [knee height (cm) x 1.10] + [MAC (cm) x 3.07] – 75.81 (margin of error is +/– 11.46 kg)

MAC = mid-arm circumference

The review of systems and physical examination must focus on key areas that influence eating and hydration status. The nurse should pay particular attention to the need for adaptive equipment, including eyeglasses, hearing aids, and special utensils needed to maintain independence. Because good oral health is the best predictor of good nutritional status in older adults, oral health and hygiene should be assessed initially and consistently, and include regular preventive care and/or treatment by a dentist. If food texture needs to be altered due to a physical condition, such as dysphagia after a stroke, a speech and language pathologist should be consulted periodically regarding the possibility of advancing the diet to a more palatable and recognizable fare. If no reassessment of swallowing is performed, persons may be kept on diets with modified texture, for example, puree, after the original problem necessitating the change has resolved. Pain, both acute and chronic, should be routinely assessed and palliated. Problems with the gastrointestinal (GI) tract, such as constipation, will compromise the desire to eat. Lack of interest in meals may be a precursor to a change of physical condition; heart failure, chronic obstructive pulmonary disease (COPD) exacerbation, and certain treatments may make food less appealing.

Assessment of swallowing problems includes more than the simple gag reflex (test of cranial nerve X). Inattention to subtle signs that suggest choking may lead to patient aspiration (Amella, 1999a). All patients with known or suspected swallowing problems should be referred to the SLP. Patients who exhibit coughing while drinking fluids should be assessed by an SLP, as dysphagia may occur in the progression of many disorders (e.g., Parkinson's and other neuro-muscular disorders and advancing dementia). Video fluoroscopy is helpful in diagnosing swallowing disorders; however, the patient must be able to cooperate with the examination. Patients are assessed for proper sitting posture, upper body strength, fine and gross motor movement, and head and neck strength by the occupa-tional therapist.

Medications may interact with food, altering absorption of key nutrients. Additionally, psychotropic and other neuroleptic drugs may negatively influence the patient's ability to eat, be fed, or safely ingest food. Tardive dyskinesia resulting from long-term use of older psychotropic drugs makes it difficult to chew and swallow food. Consultation with a clinical pharmacologist is important.

INTAKE

The most accurate assessment of intake requires weighing and recording all food consumed. Using a food diary or calorie count confirms problems. The count should be conducted over a 3-day period, with one of those days being on the weekend. Requesting the patient or patient's family to assist in compiling the food diary will help emphasize the critical importance of eating. The registered dietitian should be involved in designing individualized intake records that can accurately assess the patient's intake. Within the institution, a 72-hour calorie count is routine. Because nursing assis-tants often underreport the percentage of food consumed, teaching needs to occur that demonstrates ways to estimate consumption. The professional nurse needs to regularly monitor the assistants' ability to approximate food eaten.

Because of physiological changes such as a decrease in lean mus-cle mass, an inability to concentrate urine, changes in the diurnal pattern of urine production, and a depressed thirst response, as well as the use of medications that directly or indirectly influence body fluids, most older adults teeter on the verge of dehydration. Dehydration quickly becomes a critical problem during periods of ill-ness and is often a secondary diagnosis on admission to a hospital. The assessment of hydration must be performed in all older people and should include the recall or monitoring of fluids ingested. Please see Mentes (2000) for a detailed protocol on hydration management.

The elderly may present differently than their younger counter-parts when dehydrated. The symptoms of dehydration are often subtle and may include irritability, confusion or change in usual cog-nitive function, lethargy, low urine output, constipation or fecal impaction, infection, fatigue, or muscle weakness (e.g., suddenly unable to assist in standing when usually able). Additionally, the physical signs on exam are different in the elderly, particularly the frail. Poor skin turgor on the forehead or sternum is a better indica-tor of dehydration than the forearm because of changes with age. Additionally, observation of the mouth and lips (mucous membranes) for dryness is a good indicator of dehydration in the elderly patient. Mental status testing may reveal a subtle change in baseline, or families may note that "Mom doesn't seem herself today." Checking for orthostatic hypotension for a fall in blood pressure from lying to standing of 10 to 15 mm Hg systolic and/or a rise in pulse by 15 beats per minute (Reese, 2001) is often indicative of dehydration. However, a drop in systolic blood pressure is a more reliable indica-tor than heart rate, as heart rate does not always increase in the presence of dehydration.

Numerous biochemical parameters can be used to determine ade-quacy of nutritional intake. For older persons, laboratory diagnos-tics that best define nutritional status are serum albumin, prealbu-min, transferrin, and serum cholesterol (Jensen et al., 2001), as well as hemoglobin, hematocrit, B_{12} levels, and total lymphocyte count. Low levels may indicate underlying pathology or malnutrition relat-ed to inadequate consumption of nutrients or undiagnosed wasting disorders (Verdery, 1997). Laboratory testing to assess for dehydra-tion includes serum sodium (hypo- or hypernatremia), potassium (hyperkalemia), creatinine (not as reliable in elderly persons), blood urea nitrogen, urine specific gravity, and urine electrolytes.

COGNITION/BEHAVIORAL DEFICITS

Cognitive deficits impair the ability to eat and drink. Persons with severe cognitive impairments may develop refuse-like or aversive behavior that affects their ability to be assisted at meals (Amella, 2002). Watson (1996) developed a psychometrically sound instru-ment, the ED-FedQ, to measure the declining ability to consume food offered related to resistance. Nurses can use the principles of this instrument to determine the stage of eating behavior. In the earlier stages, more active behaviors are displayed (e.g., the individual pushes food away or turns his or her head away from the feeder). In later stages, passive behaviors occur, as the patient does not swallow and allows food to fall from his or her mouth. In late-stage dementia, a primitive and less forceful swallow pattern may develop. The upper airway is not well protected, making the use of bottle or syringe-type feeding not only undignified but ineffective and unsafe.

As one of the most common causes of weight loss in the elderly, depression should be investigated in persons who manifest problems with eating or decline to be assisted with meals. Some medications prescribed for depression, for example, the selective serotonin reuptake inhibitors (SSRIs), may depress the appetite in the elderly, while tricyclic antidepressants may potentiate appetite. Additionally, failure to thrive (FTT), a diagnosis once reserved for children, is now recognized as a major factor in frailty and weight loss in older persons (Verdery, 1997). Loss of skeletal muscle mass (sacropenia) may make the process of eating and digestion difficult (Jensen et al., 2001). Thus, for very frail persons, a circular process of decompensation ensues, with loss of muscle mass leading to further inability to eat and metabolize food.

Obesity among older adults can be difficult to resolve if complicated by immobility related to illness, a sedentary lifestyle, or an eating disorder. Visceral adipose tissue increases with age and is an independent risk factor for insulin resistance (Cases & Barzilai, 2001). Diets that incorporate either very-low-energy calories or are protein sparing are not recommended for older adults (Jensen & Rogers, 1998). An interdisciplinary strategy is optimal in helping older persons design healthy weight loss goals that are consistent with recommendations for macro- and micronutrients. Use of pharmacological agents for weight loss is usually not recommended in older adults.

ENVIRONMENT/AMBIENCE

Because of the strong social and cultural components of eating, where one dines is sometimes as important as what one eats. Simply, staff should ask themselves, Would I want to eat my next meal where the patient is eating? If the answer is no, then steps should be taken to improve the dining area. Small changes in the dining environment may make large improvements in a patient's capacity and motivation to eat or be fed (VanOrt & Phillips, 1995).

Use of flatware and china plates, cups and saucers help to cue the patient. Removing dishes from the tray and placing them directly on either a tablecloth or a placemat of contrasting or darker color provide visual cues and the food as the patient's own. When the caregiver places the tray in front of himself or herself, then reaches across to give the food to the patient, the patient may interpret this as eating from another person's plate.

In addition to avoiding medicalization of the eating space, nurses should be alert for all the possible interruptions and disruptions that occur during the patient's meal. The number of interruptions during meals, even by persons walking in and out of the room, can be linked to lower intake. When less than 50% of the meal is consumed, nurses should attempt to assess events surrounding that meal.

RELATIONSHIP WITH CAREGIVER AT MEALS

Above all, dining is a shared experience. Successful completion of the meal is dependent on who assists or feeds the patient and the interpersonal process that person uses to interact with the patient (Amella, 2002, 1999b). Caregivers who are able to let the patient set the tempo of the meal and allow others to make choices will be more effectual. Unfortunately, time is a costly commodity within institutions. It is critical that the nurse (with the assistance of the SLP if the patient has swallowing problems) teach the patient's family, friends, and nonprofessional caregivers how to safely assist the patient while preserving the patient's dignity and social aspects of the meal. These persons should be periodically supervised while assisting the patient. Touching and smiling have been correlated with improved intake (Eaton, Mitchell-Bonair, & Freidman, 1986). Facing the patient on the same plane preserves the social aspects of dining and therefore may have aesthetic value. Patients may need to be assisted into a functional eating posture or have assistive devices developed by the occupational or physical therapist to facilitate self-feeding.

Cuing is critical for patients with neuromuscular diseases or dementia. Whenever finger foods are given, they should be placed in the patient's hand. The caregiver may even assist by putting the patient's hand and arm through the motions a few times while repeating simple cues. Pantomime of gestures helps to pattern the most effective eating strategies. Sitting more able patients next to less able ones offers another opportunity for modeling appropriate behavior. Family-style dining (foods placed in serving dishes rather than on trays) offers an environmental context that is more akin to remembrances of meals past.

The patient should be allowed and encouraged to feed himself or herself, to whatever degree possible. Adaptive equipment should be clean and readily available. Caregivers should be instructed in techniques that facilitate the social aspects of meals and set the stage for the task of eating. They should also be familiar with an individualized plan of care that fosters independence. The ideal model of practice is one that supports an individual in his or her attempts to eat independently for as long as possible.

CASE STUDY

Mrs. Simpson is an 84-year-old African American female who is admitted to a busy acute care unit with the following diagnoses: heart failure (New York Heart Association stage III), poorly controlled hypertension, and long-standing osteoarthritis. Her medications prior to admission included hydrochlorothiazide 25 mg daily, enalapril 20 mg twice daily, and naproxen 250 mg twice daily. She denies allergies. She was hospitalized for a hysterectomy 35 years ago, heart failure 3 times in the past 4 years, and pneumonia 6 months ago.

Mrs. Simpson has been widowed for 20 years and lives alone in her own home in a rural community. She sees her provider yearly and usually gets her medications refilled over the phone. She is up-to-date on immunizations and screenings. Because of a lack of insurance, it has been over 10 years since she has visited her dentist for an adjustment of her full dentures. She wears bifocals that were last adjusted 4 years ago. Members from her Seventh-Day Adventist church help with household chores and shopping; however, she basically spends her days alone. Her son lives out of state, and 2 years ago Mrs. Simpson's youngest daughter died of cancer, an event that Mrs. Simpson says "changed my life forever."

During the past 6 months, Mrs. Simpson has unintentionally lost 15 pounds, going from her usual weight of 180 to 165 pounds (75 kg). Her height is 63 inches (1.6 m). Over the past 3 days, though, she has gained back approximately 5 pounds (BMI = 75 kg/1.6 m^2 = 29.3). Vital signs today are 162/94 (without orthostasis), 98.0 (temperature), 95 (heart rate), 18 (respiratory rate). In the past 3 days, Mrs. Simpson experiences shortness of breath when walking > 20 feet; she is unable to climb stairs or do light housework, and she notes swelling in both her ankles in the morning. She also has a loss of appetite and is able only to snack. Both knees and her right hip are usually quite painful (rates as 8–9 out of 10 on a pain scale where 0 = no pain and 10 = worst pain imaginable) by midafternoon. She has been more tearful lately, although she tries to distract herself by reading the Bible. Dietary recall shows a diet high in salt and fat. A brief examination shows moist oral mucosa with poorly fitting dentures, adequate swallow, good skin turgor on the sternum, bilateral crackles at the lung bases, presence of an S_3 heart sound, 2+ edema bilaterally to midcalf, and enlarged knees with limited range of motion.

During her hospital stay, Mrs. Simpson is gently diuresed, and a beta-blocker is added. Nurses advocate for better pain control, and the naproxen is changed to Oxycontin, with great improvement in function and diminished frequency and quality of pain. This also decreases the opportunity for development of renal problems and edema, which are associated with NSAIDs. The nursing staff noted that Mrs. Simpson was picking at her tray. In collaboration with the registered dietitian, a 3-day calorie count revealed a diet low in protein, high in carbohydrates and fat, and not meeting her nutritional needs based on level of stress. Upon questioning, Mrs. Simpson revealed her religious preference for a vegetarian diet, and an appropriate order was given. Additionally, after her heart failure was controlled, an improvement in appetite was noted. A depression screen was performed using the Geriatric Depression Scale, which showed moderate depression. An antidepressant that does not have anorectic side effects was started. A dental consultation was initiated and will be covered through a community outreach program. The social worker made a referral to a local senior center that provides transportation and offers a nutrition program for two meals daily and opportunities for socialization. Mrs. Simpson named her son as her health care proxy and completed advance directives that included her wishes for artificial nutrition and hydration. Although Mrs. Simpson needs to continue to lose weight to control her heart failure and increase mobility, a weight loss of 15 pounds is more than 5% of her body weight (15/180 = 8.3%), so if other interventions fail, a more aggressive workup will be initiated to determine a possible cause for the weight loss.

BOX 5.1   Protocol Mealtime Difficulties: Assessment and Management

Guiding principles:
1. The adequate intake of nutrients is necessary to maintain physical and emotional health.
2. Mealtime is a not only an opportunity to ingest nutrients but to maintain critical social aspects of life.
3. The social components of meals will be observed, including mealtime rituals, cultural norms, and food preferences.
4. Persons will be encouraged and assisted to self-feed for as long as possible.
5. Persons dependent in eating will be fed with dignity.
6. End-of-life decisions by the individual or his or her proxy regarding the provision or termination of food and fluid will be respected.
7. The quality of mealtime is an indicator of quality of life and care of an individual.
A. BACKGROUND
   1. Definitions:
      a. *Feeding* is "the process of getting the food from the plate to the mouth. It is a primitive sense without concern for social niceties" (Katz, Downs, Cash, & Grotz, 1970, p. 21).
      b. *Eating* is "the ability to transfer food from plate to stomach through the mouth" (Katz et al., 1970, p. 21). Eating involves the ability to recognize food, the ability to transfer food to the mouth, and the phases of swallowing.
      c. *Anorexia* is characterized by a refusal to maintain a minimally normal body weight (American Psychiatric Association, 1994, p. 539). May have physiological basis in the elderly.
      d. *Dehydration* is "a decrease in total body water" (Reese, 2001, p. 183).
      e. *Dysphagia* is "an abnormality in the transfer of a bolus from the mouth to the stomach" (Groher, 1997, p. 1).
      f. *Apraxia* is an inability to carry out voluntary muscular activities related to neuromuscular damage. As it relates to eating and feeding, it involves loss of the voluntary stages of swallowing or the manipulation of eating utensils.
      g. *Agnosia* is the inability to recognize familiar items when sensory cuing is limited.
   2. Etiology of problems with eating:
      a. *Myopathies:* myasthenia gravis, scleroderma, congenital weakness, spasms of the esophagus

BOX 5.1 *(continued)*

b. *Neurogenic:* movement disorders, especially Parkinson's disease; amyotrophic lateral sclerosis; dementia, especially Alzheimer's disease; stroke with lesions of the upper motor neurons, brainstem, inferior portions of the precentral gyrus, or the posterior portion of the inferior frontal gyrus; cranial neuropathies related to cancer or diabetes
c. *Systemic infections:* anorexia related to infections or sepsis
d. *Mechanical disorders:* severe cervical spondylosis in C4 to C7 with osteophytes; tracheotomy tubes; significant kyphosis; poor dentition
e. *Psychological:* depression, anorexia, failure to thrive
f. *Iatrogenic:* adverse drug reactions, especially tardive dyskinesia; poor or absent oral care; lack of adaptive equipment; untreated pain; use of physical restraints that limit ability to move, position, or self-feed; improper chair or table surface or discrepancy of chair to table height; use of wheelchair in lieu of table chair; use of disposable dinnerware, especially for patients with cognitive or neuromuscular impairments

B. ASSESSMENT
1. Assessment with elder and caregivers:
    a. Rituals used before meals (e.g., hand washing and toilet use); dressing for dinner.
    b. Blessings of food or grace, if appropriate
    c. Religious rites or prohibitions observed in preparation of food or before meal begins (e.g., Muslim, Jewish, and Seventh-Day Adventist; consult with pastoral counselor, if available)
    d. Cultural or special cues—family history, especially rituals surrounding meals
    e. Preferences as to end-of-life decisions regarding withdrawal or administration of food and fluid in the face of incapacity, or request of designated health-proxy; ethicist or social worker may facilitate process (see chapter 15).
2. History and physical assessment (focused) coordinated with nursing and medicine:
    a. Weight and height—on admission to determine body mass index (weight in kg/height in m^2); thereafter, weight taken at least every 7 days if a diagnosis of alteration in nutritional status exists. Weight loss/gain strategy devised by registered dietitian with input from provider, if appropriate.

(continued)

BOX 5.1   Protocol Mealtime Difficulties: Assessment and Management *(continued)*

---

    b. Skin—lesions, turgor, dryness, hair loss
    c. Neurologic—cranial nerves V, VII, IX, X, XI, XII (involved in swallowing)
    d. Sensory limitations—vision, smell, taste, hearing
    e. Oral cavity—cleanliness; dentition, including caries at root and surface; fit of denture or other oral appliances; lesions; condition of gums and tongue. Refer to dentist for evaluation and treatment.
    f. Neck—capacity to swallow. Refer to speech and language pathologist for thorough assessment.
    g. Respiratory—restrictive disease limiting ability to eat or tolerate larger quantities of food, oxygen desaturation during meals, exercise intolerance. Refer to respiratory therapist, if appropriate.
    h. Cardiac—presence of heart failure, stages III or IV, or poorly controlled angina, indicating intolerance of any activity.
    i. Gastrointestinal (GI)—GERD (gastroesophageal reflux disease), hiatal hernia, hypo- or hyperactive bowel (constipation or diarrhea), abdominal pain or tenderness, diverticular disease
    j. Strength and coordination—neuro and musculoskeletal exam (i.e., sitting posture, use of upper extremities including ROM [range of motion], tremors, and fine motor movements). Refer to occupational and physical therapist for assessment, as appropriate.
    k. Psychological—affective disorders, especially depression
    l. Pain—general and localized, especially in jaw, mouth, throat, and GI
    m. Endocrine—fasting blood sugar, microalbuminemia, and thyroid-stimulating hormone in weight loss, for undiagnosed/poorly controlled diabetes and thyroid disease
    n. Medications—sedation, abnormal movements, and dehydration. Pharmacologist to determine polypharmacy.
  3. Intake (precise measurement needed as estimates can be inaccurate):
    a. Calorie count for 3 days (including one weekend day, if in community)
    b. Weighing of food (pre- and postmeals, if precise intake is required)
    c. Measurements of dehydration, especially orthostatic hypotension
    d. Biochemical—monitor laboratory diagnostics for abnormalities

BOX 5.1 *(continued)*

e. Diet history—designed by registered dietitian and completed by nursing staff

4. Cognition after diagnosis established through neuropsychological testing:
   a. Aphasia—cannot verbally express preferences
   b. Apraxia—cannot manipulate utensils and food prior to eating; cannot manipulate food within mouth/swallow
   c. Agnosia—cannot recognize utensils or food
   d. Amnesia—forgets having eaten; does not recognize need to eat
   e. Anorexia—lack of desire to eat, possible physiological basis

5. Environment/ambience:
   a. Dining or patient room—personal trappings versus institutional environment; no treatments or other activities occurring during meals; no distractions
   b. Tableware—use of standard dinnerware (e.g., china, glasses, cup and saucer, flatware, tablecloth, napkin vs. disposable tableware and bibs)
   c. Furniture—elders seated in armed chair; table-appropriate height versus eating in wheelchair or in bed
   d. Noise level—environmental noise from music, caregivers, and television is minimal; personal conversation between patient and caregiver is encouraged
   e. Light—adequate and nonglare-producing versus dark, shadowy, or glaring
   f. Odor—familiar smells of food prepared versus all food prepared away from elder or medicinal smells and waste
   g. Adaptive equipment—available, appropriate, and clean; caregivers and/or elder knowledgeable in use. Occupational therapist assists in evaluation.

6. Relationship with caregiver:
   a. Social atmosphere—meal sharing versus accomplishment of task
   b. Position of caregiver relative to elder—eye contact; seating so caregiver faces elder patient in same plane
   c. Pacing and choice—caregiver allows elder to choose food and determine tempo of meal; relies on elder's preference whenever known, voiced, or expressed through gestures and/or sounds
   d. Cueing—caregiver cues elder whenever possible with words or gestures

(continued)

BOX 5.1   Protocol Mealtime Difficulties: Assessment and Management *(continued)*

---

    e. Self-feeding—encouragement to self-feed with multiple methods versus assisted feeding to minimize time

C. EVALUATION OF EXPECTED OUTCOMES
  1. Individual:
    a. Diet assessment on admission to unit or service documented
    b. Weight and height measured initially, and weight measured at least weekly
    c. Assessment of patient, context, and caregiver interaction after meals in which less than 50% of food offered is consumed
    d. Diagnostic workup, care, and treatment by interdisciplinary team, if deviations from expected nutritional norms exist
    e. Corrective and supportive strategies reflected in plan of care
    f. Quality of life issues emphasized in maintaining social aspects of dining
    g. End-of-life decisions regarding nutrition respected
  2. Health care provider:
    a. System disruptions at mealtimes minimized
    b. Family and paraprofessional staff informed and educated to patient's special needs to promote safe and effective meals
    c. Maintenance of normal meals and adequate intake for the patient reflected in care plan
    d. Competence in diet assessment; knowledge of and sensitivity to cultural norms of mealtimes reflected in care plan
  3. Institution:
    a. Documentation of nutritional status and eating and feeding behavior meets expected standard
    b. Alterations in nutritional status, eating and feeding behaviors assessed and addressed in a timely manner
    c. Referrals to interdisciplinary team (geriatrician, advanced practice nurse [NP/CNS], dietitian, speech therapist, dentist, occupational therapist, social worker, pastoral counselor, ethicist) appropriate
    d. Nutritional, eating, and/or feeding problems modified to respect individual wishes and cultural norms

D. FOLLOW-UP to MONITOR CLOSELY
  1. Providers' competency to monitor nutritional status and eating and feeding behaviors
  2. Documentation of nutritional status, eating and feeding behaviors
  3. Documentation of care strategies, and follow-up of alterations in nutritional status and eating and feeding behaviors

---

See Mentes (2000) for a detailed, evidence-based hydration management protocol; see also the "Try This" Series on Nutrition and Hydration (www.hartfordign.org).

REFERENCES

Amella, E. J. (2002). Resistance at mealtimes for persons with dementia. *Journal of Nutrition, Health and Aging, 6*(2), 117–122.

Amella, E. J. (1999a). Dysphagia—the differential diagnosis in long-term care. *Primary Care Practice, 3*(2), 135–149.

Amella, E. J. (1999b). Factors influencing the amount of food consumed by nursing home residents with dementia. *Journal of the American Geriatrics Society, 47,* 879–885.

American Psychiatric Association. (1994). *Diagnostic and Statistical Manual of Mental Disorders* (4th ed.). Washington, DC: Author.

Cases, J. A., & Barzilai, N. (2001). Biology of fat in aging. In G. L. Maddox (Ed.), *The Encyclopedia of Aging* (3rd ed., pp. 124–125). New York: Springer.

Donini, L. M., de Felice, M. R., Tassi, L., de Bernardini, L. Pinto, A., Giusti, A. M., & Cannella, C. (2002). A proportional and objective score for the Mini Nutritional Assessment in Long-Term Geriatric Care. *Journal of Nutrition Health and Aging, 6,* 141.

Eaton M., Mitchell-Bonair, I. L., & Freidman, E. (1986). The effects of touch on nutritional intake of Chronic Brain Syndrome patients. *Journal of Gerontology, 41,* 611–616.

Estimating stature from knee height. (1990). Columbus, OH: Ross Laboratories.

Groher, M. E. (1997). *Dysphagia: Diagnosis and Management* (3rd ed.). Boston: Butterworth-Heimemann.

Guigoz, Y., Vellas, B., & Garry, P. J. (1997). Mini Nutritional Assessment: A practical assessment tool for grading the nutritional state of elderly patients. In B. J. Vellas, P. J. Garry, & J. L. Albarede (Eds.) *Facts, Research and Interventions in Geriatrics: Nutrition in the Elderly* (3rd ed., pp. 15–60).

Jensen, G. L., McGee, M., & Binkley, J. (2001). Nutrition in the elderly. *Gastroenterology Clinics, 30*(2), 313–334.

Jensen, G. L., & Rogers, J. (1998). Obesity in older persons. *Journal of the American Dietetic Association, 98*(11), 1308–1311.

Katz, S., Downs, T. D., Cash, H. R., & Grotz, R. C. (1970). Progress in the development of the Index of ADL. *The Gerontologist, 10,* 22.

Katz, S., Ford A. B., Moskowitz, R.W., Jackson, B. A., & Jaffe, M. W. (1963). The Index of ADL: A standardized measure of biological and psychological function. *Journal of the American Medical Association, 185,* 915–919.

Mentes, J. (2000). Hydration management protocol. *Journal of Gerontological Nursing, 26,* 6–15.

Mineo, A. M., & Smith, B. L. (2001). Death: Preliminary data for 2000. In *National Vital Statistics Reports, 49*(12). Hyattsville, MD: National Center for Health Statistics.

Reese, J. L. (2001). Fluid volume deficit—dehydration: Isotonic, hypotonic and hypertonic. In M. L. Maas, K. C. Buckwalter, M. D. Hardy, T. Tripp-Reimer, M. G. Titler, & J. P. Specht (Eds.), *Nursing Care of the Older Adult: Diagnoses, Outcomes and Interventions* (pp. 183–200). St. Louis: Mosby.

Reuben, D.B., Greendale, G.A., & Harrison, G. G. (1995). Nutrition screening in older persons. *Journal of the American Geriatrics Society, 43,* 415–425.

Rubenstein, L. Z., Harker, J. O., Salva, A., Guigoz, Y., & Vellas, B. (2001). Screening for undernutrition in geriatric practice: Developing the Short-Form Mini–Nutritional Assessment (SF-MNA). *Journal of Gerontology: Medicine,* 56A, M366–M372.

Spector, W. D., Fleishman, J. A., Pezzin, L. E., & Spillman, B. C. (2000). *The characteristics of long-term care users* (AHRQ Pub. No. 00-0049). Rockville, MD: Agency for Healthcare Quality and Research.

Tesoro, E. (2002). *Religion and Food: An EU Project.* Retrieved from http://www.eat-online.net/english/education/religion_and_food/religious_determinants.htm

U.S. Department of Health and Human Services (USDHHS). (2002). *Focus on your Health: Senior Nutrition* [On-line]. Retrieved from http://www.aoa.dhhs.gov/nutrition/Focus-On-Senior-Nutrition

U.S. Department of Health and Human Services (USDHHS). (2000). *Healthy People 2010* [On-line]. Retrieved from http://www.health.gov/healthypeople

VanOrt, S., & Phillips, L. R. (1995). Nursing interventions to promote functional feeding. *Journal of Gerontological Nursing, 21*(10), 6–14.

Verdery, R. (1997). Clinical evaluation of Failure to Thrive in older people. *Clinics in Geriatric Medicine, 13,* 769–778.

Watson, R. (1996). The Mokken scaling procedure (MSP) applied to the measurement of feeding difficulty in elderly people with dementia. *International Journal of Nursing Studies, 33,* 385–393.

White, J. V., Dwyer, J. T., Posner, B. M., Ham, R. J., Lipschitz, D. A., & Wellman, N. S. (1992). Nutrition Screening Initiative: Development and implementation of the public awareness checklist and screening tools. *Journal of the American Dietetic Association, 92,* 163–167.

White, J., Ham, R., & Lipschitz, D. (1991). Consensus of the Nutrition Screening Initiative: Risk factors and indicators of poor nutritional status in older Americans. *Journal of the American Dietetic Association, 91,* 783–787.

Chapter 6

URINARY INCONTINENCE

Annemarie Dowling-Castronovo and Christine Bradway

EDUCATIONAL OBJECTIVES

On completion of this chapter, the reader should be able to:
1. Discuss the transient and established etiologies of urinary incontinence (UI).
2. Describe the core components of a nursing assessment for UI in hospitalized elders.
3. Identify two major treatment strategies for UI.
4. List limited indications for indwelling catheter use.

Urinary incontinence (UI) affects more than 17 million adults in the United States and is most often defined as the involuntary loss of urine sufficient to be a problem (Fantl et al., 1996; National Association for Continence, 1998). A critical review of the literature by Skelly and Flint (1995) reveals an 11% to 90% prevalence rate of

Adapted from the chapter in the original edition by C. Bradway, S. Hernley, and the NICHE Faculty. (1999). Urinary incontinence in older adults. In Abraham, I., Bottrell, M., Fulmer, T., & Mezey, M., Eds. *Geriatric nursing protocols for best practice.* New York: Springer Publishing Co.

UI in individuals with dementia. Whereas the highest prevalence rate occurs in institutionalized older adults, 15% to 53% of home-bound elderly and at least 11% of older adults admitted to acute care suffer from UI (Fantl et al., 1996; McDowell et. al, 1999).

In addition to being a common geriatric syndrome, UI significantly affects health-related quality of life (HRQOL). For example, adverse consequences of UI include social isolation, depression, and falls (Bogner et al., 2002; Brown, 2000; Norton, 1982; Shumaker, Wyman, Uebersax, McClish, & Fantl, 1994; Wolf, Riolo, & Ouslander, 2000). This emphasizes the need to assess and treat UI when addressing other medical problems such as depression and falls.

Nurses are in a key position to identify and treat UI in hospitalized elders. This chapter reviews the etiologies and consequences of UI, with an emphasis on the most common types of UI encountered in the acute care setting. Assessment parameters and care strategies are highlighted, and a nursing standard of practice protocol is presented.

ASSESSMENT OF THE PROBLEM

Adverse physiologic consequences of UI commonly encountered in acute care facilities include an increased potential for urinary tract infections (UTIs) and indwelling catheter use, dermatitis, skin infections, and pressure ulcers (Jackson, 1997; Sier, Ouslander, & Orzeck, 1987). Moreover, UI that results in functional decline predisposes older individuals to complications associated with bed rest and immobility (Harper & Lyles, 1988).

Continence is a complex, multidimensional phenomenon influenced by anatomical, physiological, psychological, and cultural factors (Gray, 2000). Thus, continence requires intact lower urinary tract function, cognitive and functional ability to recognize voiding signals and use a toilet or commode, the motivation to maintain continence, and an environment that facilitates the process (Jirovec, Brink, & Wells, 1988).

Micturition (urination) involves voluntary as well as reflexive control of the bladder, urethra, detrusor muscle, and urethral sphincter. When the bladder volume reaches approximately 400 milliliters, stretch receptors in the bladder wall send a message to the brain, and an impulse for voiding is sent back to the bladder. The detrusor muscle then contracts, and the urethral sphincter relaxes to allow urination (Gray, Rayome, & Moore, 1995; McDowell et al., 1999).

Normally, the micturition reflex can be inhibited voluntarily (at least for a time) until an individual desires to void or finds an appropriate place for voiding. Urinary incontinence occurs as the result of a disruption at any point during this process. Age-associated changes including a decrease in bladder capacity, benign prostatic hyperplasia (BPH) in men, and menopausal loss of estrogen in women can affect lower urinary tract function and predispose older individuals to UI (Bradway & Yetman, 2002).

The Agency for Healthcare Research and Quality (Fantl et al., 1996) identifies the following types of UI: transient (acute) and established (chronic) UI. Transient UI is characterized by the sudden onset of potentially reversible symptoms. Causes of transient UI include delirium, infections (e.g., untreated UTI), atrophic vaginitis, urethritis, pharmaceuticals, depression or other psychological disorders that affect motivation or function, excessive urine production, restricted mobility, and stool impaction or constipation (which creates additional pressure on the bladder and can cause urinary urgency and frequency). Hospitalized older adults are at risk of developing transient UI, and with shorter hospital stays they are also at risk of being discharged without resolution of the UI. Transient UI is often preventable, or at least reversible, if the underlying cause for the UI is identified and treated. (Fantl et al., 1996).

Established UI has either a sudden or a gradual onset and is often present prior to hospital admission. However, health care providers or family caregivers may discover it initially during the course of an acute illness, hospitalization, or an abrupt change in environment or daily routine (Palmer, 1996). Types of established UI include stress, urge, overflow, and functional UI.

Stress UI is defined as an involuntary loss of urine associated with activities that increase intra-abdominal pressure. Symptomatically, individuals with stress UI usually present with complaints of small amounts of daytime urine loss that occur during physical activity or with increased intra-abdominal pressure (e.g., coughing and sneezing). Stress UI is more common in women, but it can be found in older men with postprostatectomy incontinence. (Fantl et al., 1996).

Urge UI is characterized by an involuntary urine loss associated with a strong desire to void (urgency). In addition to urgency, signs and symptoms of urge UI most often include urinary frequency, nocturia, enuresis, and UI of moderate to large amounts. Bladder changes associated with aging make older adults particularly prone to this type of UI (Fantl et al., 1996).

Overflow UI is an involuntary loss of urine associated with overdistention of the bladder. It may be caused by an underactive detrusor muscle or outlet obstruction leading to overdistention and overflow. Individuals with overflow UI often describe dribbling, urinary retention or hesitancy, urine loss without a recognizable urge, or an uncomfortable sensation of fullness or pressure in the lower abdomen. A common condition associated with this type of UI is BPH (Fantl et al., 1996).

Functional UI is caused by nongenitourinary factors, such as cognitive and physical impairments that result in an inability for the individual to be independent in voiding. For example, acutely ill hospitalized individuals may be challenged by a combination of an acute illness and environmental changes. This, in turn, makes the voiding process too complex, resulting in a functional type of UI (Fantl et al., 1996).

ASSESSMENT PARAMETERS

Nurses play a key role in assessing and managing UI in hospitalized elders. Because UI is an interdisciplinary issue, collaboration with other members of the health care team is essential. Basic history and examination techniques are presented here, along with a nursing standard of practice protocol.

When a patient is admitted, nursing history should include questions to determine if the individual has preexisting UI or risk factors for developing UI while hospitalized. Questions should focus on the characteristics of incontinence: time of onset, frequency, and severity of the problem. Questions also should review the past health history and address possible precipitants of UI, such as coughing, functional decline, and acute illness. Nurses should inquire about lower urinary tract symptoms, such as nocturia, hematuria, and hesitancy, as well as current management strategies for the UI. The presence and rationale for an indwelling urinary catheter should be documented. A bladder diary or voiding record is the gold standard for obtaining objective information about the patient's voiding pattern, incontinent episodes, and severity of the UI. There are numerous voiding records available. Figure 6.1 presents an example of a voiding record. Advanced practice nurses or urologic/continence specialists can assist nursing staff with interpretation and offer suggestions regarding nursing interventions based on information

Sample Bladder Record

Name_____ Date_____

Instructions: Place a check in the appropriate column next to the time you urinated in the toilet or when an incontinence episode occurred. Note the reason for the incontinence and describe your liquid intake (for example: coffee, water) and estimate the amount (for example: one cup).

Time Interval	Urinated in Toilet	Had a Small Incontinence Episode	Had a Large Incontinence Episode	Reason for Incontinence Episode	Type/Amount of Liquid Intake
6:00 - 8:00 am					
8:00 - 10:00 am					
10:00 - 12:00 pm					
12:00 - 2:00 pm					
2:00 - 4:00 pm					
4:00 - 6:00 pm					
6:00 - 8:00 pm					
8:00 - 10:00 pm					
10:00pm - 12:00 am					
Overnight					

Number of pads used today _____ Number of episodes _____

Comments_____

FIGURE 6.1 Sample bladder record.

Source: Fantl et al. (1996).

from the diary. A bladder diary completed for even 1 day can help identify patients with bladder dysfunction or those requiring further referral.

A wide variety of medications can adversely affect continence. Nurses should document all over-the-counter, herbal, and prescription medications on admission. Additionally, nurses must closely scrutinize new medications if UI suddenly develops during the patient's hospital stay. Medications that may contribute to iatrogenic (hospital-caused) UI include diuretics (these drugs increase urine volume and urinary urgency) and sedative-hypnotics (sedation may contribute to delirium and functional UI).

Important components of a comprehensive examination include abdominal, genital, rectal, and skin examinations. In particular, the abdominal exam should assess for suprapubic distention indicative of urine retention. Inspection of male and female genitalia can be completed during bathing or as part of the skin assessment. The nurse should observe the patient for signs of perineal irritation, lesions, or discharge. In women, a Valsalva maneuver (if not medically contraindicated) may identify pelvic prolapse (e.g., cystocele, rectocele, or uterine prolapse) or stress UI as a result of increased intra-abdominal pressure with bearing down. Postmenopausal women are especially prone to atrophic vaginitis. Significant findings for atrophic vaginitis include perineal inflammation, tenderness (on occasion, trauma as a result of touch), and thin, pale tissues. Rectal and skin examinations are essential in identifying transient causes such as constipation, fecal impaction, and fungal rashes.

In some cases, diagnostic testing may provide additional information. For example, urinalysis and urine cultures are used to identify a UTI, which may contribute to new onset UI. Postvoid residual (PVR) urine may reveal incomplete bladder emptying. Two ways to accurately evaluate PVR are bladder sonography and catheter insertion after the patient has voided (see Table 6.1).

TABLE 6.1   Postvoid Residual

Instruct the patient to void. Post-void (ideally within 15 minutes or less) measure the residual urine remaining in the bladder by either:
* Bladder Sonography (Scan): noninvasive ultrasound of the suprapubic area identifies the residual amount of urine
* Sterile catheterization: a PVR of greater than 100 cc is considered abnormal and requires further evaluation by a urology specialist

Source: Shinopulos (2000).

Functional, environmental, and mental status assessments are essential components of the UI evaluation in older adults. The nurse should observe the patient voiding, assess mobility, note any use of assistive devices, and identify any obstacles that interfere with appropriate use of toilets or toilet substitutes.

INTERVENTIONS/CARE STRATEGIES IN ACUTE CARE

Palmer's (1994) conceptual model for continence management stresses the need for public education. Adapting this for the acute care environment includes staff education. For example, a brief unit-based in-service followed by patient rounds can be instrumental in identifying patients at risk for UI and those actually experiencing UI.

Transient causes of UI should be investigated, identified, and treated. Individuals with a history of established UI should have usual voiding routines and continence strategies immediately incorporated into the acute care plan, when possible. Nurses play an essential role in initiation of discharge planning and patient/caregiver teaching regarding all aspects of UI. Teaching and discharge planning should begin at admission, be reviewed continually, and be revised as necessary.

Modification of the hospital environment facilitates continence. Call bells should be identified and within easy reach. If limited mobility is anticipated, nursing staff should consider using an elevated toilet or commode seat, male or female urinal, or bedpan. Restraints should be avoided, including side rails (see case studies). Patients should be encouraged and helped to void before leaving the unit for tests. In some instances, patients and staff can use Credé's maneuvers (deep suprapubic palpation) or double voiding techniques (after initial void instruct patients to stand or reposition for a second void) to facilitate bladder emptying. Nurses should obtain referrals to physical and occupational therapy for ambulation aids, gait training, further assessment of activities of daily living associated with continence, and improved muscle strength. Pelvic muscle exercises (PME) can improve stress and urge UI (Bo, Talseth, & Holme, 1999; Sampselle, 1999). Table 6.2 provides helpful tips for instructing patients in PME.

Indwelling urinary catheters should be avoided. Dowd and Campbell (1995) found a UTI incidence of 10% associated with their

TABLE 6.2   Tips for Instructing Patients in Pelvic Muscle Exercises

1. Explain the purpose: Pelvic muscle exercises (PMEs), or Kegel exercises, were developed to help strengthen the pelvic muscles, and can help improve stress and urge UI.
2. Help patients find the correct muscle by either:
   a. verbally explaining that they should gently squeeze the rectal or vaginal muscle, or
   b. manually assisting them to identify the muscle by instructing them to squeeze around your gloved finger during vaginal or rectal examination.
3. Instruct the patient not to squeeze the stomach, buttocks, or thigh muscles (because this only increases intra-abdominal pressure), but to concentrate on isolating the pelvic muscle.
4. Ideally, each exercise should consist of squeezing for 10 seconds and relaxing for 10 seconds. Some patients may need to start with 3 or 5 seconds, and then increase as their muscle gets stronger.
5. Patients should do 50 PMEs per day, and not more than 25 PMEs at once.
6. Patients may notice improvement in 2 to 4 weeks, but not immediately. Reinforce compliance, and initiate a referral for discharge follow-up with a continence specialist.

use. They suggest that unintended infections may have increased length of hospital stay and decreased opportunities for nursing staff to identify continence as a problem. The Wound Ostomy Continence Nurses Society (1996) recommends specific indications for indwelling catheter use, including severe acute illness, urinary retention uncontrollable by other interventions (including medication management and sterile intermittent catheterization), and UI management for patients with stage III–IV pressure ulcers of the trunk. Sterile intermittent catheterization may result in a lower incidence of infection (Terpenning, Allada, & Kauffaman, 1989; Warren, 1997) and may be a viable alternative to placement of an indwelling catheter. Decisions regarding catheterization require careful consideration of the benefits and burdens associated with their use.

CASE STUDY 1

Nurse D. M. received a report on Mr. G., an 86-year-old man with a history of Alzheimer's dementia who was hospitalized for acute mental status changes. The nurse was told that the patient was "pleasantly confused," required full assistance with personal care, and spent most of the day in a Geri-chair. The nurse performed an assessment that revealed the following:

- Patient sleeping in bed with all side rails up, call bell within reach, no urinal in site
- Past medical history (PMH): coronary artery disease, mild hypertension, mild osteoarthritis
- Past social history (PSH): none
- Medications: diphenhydramine (Benadryl) 25 mg qHS prn, enalapril (Vasotec) 5 mg PO QD, multivitamin—1 tablet PO QD, donepezil (Aricept) 10 mg PO QD, Vitamin E 400 IU PO bid
- Vital statistics: blood pressure—114/60, heart rate—72, respiratory rate—14, temperature—98.0° F
- Alert and oriented to self; sleepy; no focal deficits
- Heart rate regular
- Breath sounds clear, slightly decreased at the bases
- Abdomen: +BS (bowel sounds) in all quadrants, soft, nontender, no suprapubic tenderness; left quadrant slightly dull to percussion; last bowel movement unknown
- Dry adult diaper in place

Nurse D. M. learns from the patient's wife (the primary care provider at home) that the patient has experienced occasional urinary leaking in the past but "not to the extent of needing diapers." The nurse helped the patient to a dangling position at the side of the bed. After assessing and evaluating that the patient's muscular strength was strong, ambulation was attempted. The patient ambulated to the bathroom, the adult diaper was removed, and he successfully voided and had a bowel movement. He proceeded to wash his hands and returned to the bedside chair (not the Geri-chair) and enjoyed breakfast. The adult diaper was left off during the time the nurse was there to assist him.

The importance of ongoing nursing assessment was stressed as being vital to quality of care. Had the nurse just transferred the patient to the Geri-chair, he may not have effectively emptied his bowels or bladder. Constipation management in acute care may be effectively managed by providing appropriate fluid/fiber intake and activity as tolerated. The avoidance of diphenhydramine for the elderly was also discussed, as it is known to cause anticholinergic effects, including urinary retention. Diphenhydramine may also cause sedation and a risk for falls.

CASE STUDY 2

Ms. W. is a 92-year-old patient hospitalized for an exacerbation of heart failure. Her past health history is also significant for diabetes mellitus, hypertension, coronary artery disease, and osteoarthritis. Initially, Ms. W. required an indwelling catheter for accurate fluid management. During that time the staff utilized wrist restraints to prevent her from removing intravenous lines and the catheter.

Today the nurse receives a shift report that Ms. W. is ready for discharge. On assessment, the nurse finds Ms. W. lying in bed with all side rails up, and the indwelling catheter has not been discontinued.

Individuals with acute exacerbations of heart failure are at high risk for transient UI and exacerbation of established UI. In addition, these individuals are prone to postural hypotension and polypharmacy as a result of multiple comorbid conditions. During an acute hospital stay, nursing interventions should focus on diuretic management, such as attention to increased voiding needs and appropriate use of urinals, a bedside commode, and other assistive devices. These individuals often require careful fluid and electrolyte management, necessitating the temporary use of an indwelling catheter; however, nursing care should focus on expedient catheter removal. These interventions decrease the risk of catheter-associated urinary tract infections or trauma that may exacerbate UI symptoms (McGann, 2000).

SUMMARY

Although acute care stays are generally short, UI is a significant health problem that should not be overlooked. Behavioral and supportive therapies and patient education should be initiated by nurses if the patient is cognitively, physically, and emotionally able to participate. Moreover, at discharge, hospital nurses have the responsibility to design a plan that includes referral to a continence nurse specialist or physician expert for follow-up.

Continuous quality improvement (CQI) criteria should encompass critical elements in an effective and successful urinary continence program. For example, quality indicators for UI may include appropriate documentation of UI, if the UI is transient or established, if a catheter was used during hospitalization or on discharge, and evidence of documentation of referrals. In addition, the AHRQ

(Agency for Healthcare Research and Quality; formerly AHCPR) Guidelines for UI can be used clinically and facility wide for program development and CQI (Fantl et al., 1996).

Nurses can have a significant impact in improving the assessment and treatment of UI in hospitalized elders. Moreover, nurses can help to promote changes in attitudes toward UI and provide education on individual, facility-wide, community, and national levels.

BOX 6.1   Nursing Standard of Practice Protocol: Urinary Incontinence (UI) in Older Adults Admitted to Acute Care

I. GOAL
  A. Nursing staff will utilize comprehensive assessment and management for patients identified with UI.
  B. Patients with UI will not have UI-associated complications.
II. BACKGROUND
  A. UI is the involuntary loss of urine sufficient to be a problem.
  B. UI affects approximately 17 million Americans and is prevalent in hospitalized elders.
  C. Risk factors associated with UI include immobility, impaired cognition, medications, constipation/fecal impaction, low fluid intake, environmental barriers, diabetes mellitus, and stroke.
  D. Complications of UI are falls, skin irritation leading to pressure ulcers, social isolation, and depression.
  E. Nurses play a key role in assessment and management of UI.
III. ASSESSMENT PARAMETERS
  A. Document the presence/absence of UI for all patients on admission.
  B. Document the presence/absence of an indwelling urinary catheter. Determine appropriate indwelling catheter use: severely ill patients, patient with stage III–IV pressure ulcers of the trunk, urinary retention unresolved by other interventions.
  C. For patients who are incontinent:
    1. Determine whether the problem is transient, established, or both.
    2. Identify and document the possible etiologies of the UI.
    3. Elicit assistance with assessment and management from interdisciplinary team members.

(continued)

BOX 6.1   Nursing Standard of Practice Protocol: Urinary Incontinence (UI) in Older Adults Admitted to Acute Care *(continued)*

IV. NURSING CARE STRATEGIES
   A. General principals that apply to prevention and management of all forms of UI:
      1. Identify and treat causes of transient UI.
      2. Identify and continue successful prehospital management strategies for established UI.
      3. Develop an individualized plan of care using data obtained from the history and physical examination and in collaboration with other team members.
      4. Avoid medications that may contribute to UI.
      5. Avoid indwelling urinary catheters whenever possible.
      6. Monitor fluid intake and maintain an appropriate hydration schedule.
      7. Modify the environment to facilitate continence.
      8. Provide patients with usual undergarments in expectation of continence, if possible.
      9. Prevent skin breakdown by providing immediate cleansing after an incontinent episode and utilizing barrier ointments.
      10. Use absorbent products judiciously.
   B. Strategies for Specific Problems:
      Stress UI:
      1. Teach pelvic muscle exercises (PME) (see Figure 6.1).
      2. Provide toileting assistance and bladder training.
      3. Consider referral to other team members if pharmacologic or surgical therapies are warranted.
      Urge UI:
      1. Implement bladder training or habit training.
      2. Teach PME to be used in conjunction with #1.
      3. Consider referral to other team members if pharmacologic therapy is warranted.
      4. Initiate referrals for those patients who do not respond to the above.
      Overflow UI:
      1. Allow sufficient time for voiding.
      2. Instruct patients in double voiding and Credé's maneuver.
      3. Consider use of external collection devices for men
      4. Provide sterile intermittent or indwelling catheterization.
      5. Initiate referrals to other team members for those patients requiring pharmacologic or surgical intervention.

BOX 6.1   *(continued)*

Functional UI:
1. Provide scheduled voiding or habit training.
2. Provide adequate fluid intake.
3. Collaborate with other team members to eliminate any medications adversely affecting continence.
4. Refer for physical and occupational therapy.
5. Modify environment to be conducive for maintaining independence with continence.

V. EVALUATION OF EXPECTED OUTCOMES
   A. Patients:
      1. Will have fewer or no episodes of UI or complications associated with UI.
   B. Health care providers:
      1. Will document continence status at admission and throughout hospital stay.
      2. Will use interdisciplinary expertise and interventions to assess and manage UI during hospitalization.
      3. Will include UI in discharge planning needs and refer as needed.
   C. Institution:
      1. Incidence and prevalence of acute UI will decrease.
      2. Hospital policies will require assessment and documentation of continence status.
      3. Will provide access to AHCPR (AHRQ) Guidelines for managing acute and chronic UI.
      4. Staff will receive administrative support and ongoing education regarding assessment and management of UI.

IV. FOLLOW-UP TO MONITOR THE CONDITION
   A. Provide patient/caregiver discharge teaching regarding outpatient referral and management.
   B. Incorporate continuous quality improvement criteria into existing program.
   C. Identify areas for improvement, and enlist multidisciplinary assistance in devising strategies for improvement.

RESOURCES

Wound Ostomy Continence Nurses Society
150 South Coast Highway, Suite 201
Laguna Beach, CA 92651
(888) 224-WOCN
http://www.wocn.org
An international society providing a source of networking and research for nurses specializing in enterostomal and continence care

National Association for Continence (NAFC)
(800) BLADDER
http://www.nafc.org/
A not-for-profit organization dedicated to improving the lives of individuals with incontinence

The John A. Hartford Institute for Geriatric Nursing
http://www.hartfordign.org/
This Web site features the "Try This" series, which includes a two-page UI information sheet.

Society of Urologic Nurse and Associates (SUNA)
National Headquarters
East Holly Avenue, Box 56
Pitman, NY 08071-0056
(888) TAP-SUNA
http://www.suna.org/
An international organization dedicated to nursing care of individuals with urologic disorders

REFERENCES

Bo, K., Talseth, T., & Holme, I. (1999). Single blind, randomized controlled trial of pelvic floor exercises, electrical stimulation, vaginal cones, and no treatment in management of genuine stress incontinence. *British Medical Journal, 318,* 487–493.

Bogner, H. R., Gallo, J. J., Sammel, M. D., Ford, D. E., Armenian, H. K., & Eaton, W. W. (2002). Urinary incontinence and psychological distress in community-dwelling older adults. *Journal of the American Geriatrics Society, 50,* 489–495.

Bradway, C., & Yetman, G. (2002). Genitourinary problems. In V. T. Cotter & N. E. Strumpf (Eds.), *Advanced practice nursing with older adults: Clinical guidelines* (pp. 83–102). New York: McGraw-Hill.

Brown, J. S. (2000). Urinary incontinence: Does it increase risk for falls and fractures? Study of Osteoporotic Fractures Research Group. *Journal of the American Geriatrics Society, 48*, 721–725.

Dowd, T. T., & Campbell, J. M. (1995). Urinary incontinence in an acute care setting. *Urologic Nursing, 15*, 82–85.

Fantl, A., Newman, D. K., Colling, J., Delancey, J. O. L., Keeys, C., & Loughery, R. (1996). *Urinary incontinence in adults: Acute and chronic management* (Pub. No. 92-0047). Rockville, MD: Agency for Health Care Policy and Research.

Gray, M. I. (2000). Physiology of voiding. In D. B. Dougherty (Ed.), *Urinary and fecal incontinence: Nursing management* (2nd ed.). St. Louis: Mosby.

Gray, M., Rayome, R., & Moore, K. (1995). The urethral sphincter: An update. *Urologic Nursing, 15*, 40–53.

Harper, C. M., & Lyles, R. M. (1988). Physiology and complications of bed rest. *Journal of the American Geriatrics Society, 36*, 1047–1054.

Jackson, S. (1997). The patient with an overactive bladder—symptoms and quality of life issues. *Urology, 50* (Suppl. 6A), 18–22.

Jirovec, M. M., Brink, C. A., & Wells, T. J. (1988). Nursing assessments in the inpatient geriatric population. *Nursing Clinics of North America, 23*, 219–230.

McDowell, B. J., Engberg, S., Sereika, S., Donovan, N., Jubeck, M. E., Weber, E., & Engberg, R. (1999). Effectiveness of behavioral therapy to treat incontinence in homebound older adults. *Journal of the American Geriatrics Society, 47*, 309–318.

McGann, P. (2000). Comorbidity in heart failure in the elderly. *Clinical Geriatric Medicine, 16*, 631–648.

National Association for Continence (1998, December 4). *Release of findings from consumer survey on urinary incontinence: Dissatisfaction with treatment continues to rise.* Spartansburg, SC: Author.

Norton, C. (1982). The effects of urinary incontinence in women. *International Rehabilitation Medicine, 4*(1), 9–14.

Palmer, M. H. (1994). A health promotion perspective of urinary continence. *Nursing Outlook, 42*, 163–169.

Palmer, M. H. (1996). *Urinary continence: Assessment and promotion.* Gaithersburg, MD: Aspen.

Sampselle, C. M. (1999). Pelvic floor muscle training was the most effective conservative treatment for genuine stress urinary incontinence. *Evidence-based Obstetrics and Gynecology, 1*, 113.

Shinopulos, N. (2000). *Bedside urodynamic testing simple testing for urinary incontinence.* Retrieved May 2, 2002, from http://www.nursing2000.com

Shumaker, S. A., Wyman, J. F., Uebersax, J. S., McClish, D., & Fantl, J. A. (1994). Health-related quality of life measures for women with urinary incontinence: The Incontinence Impact Questionnaire and the Urogenital Distress Inventory, Continence Program in Women (CPW). *Quality of Life Research, 3*, 291–306.

Sier, H., Ouslander J., & Orzeck, S. (1987). Urinary incontinence among geriatric patients in the acute care hospital. *Journal of the American Medical Association, 257,* 1767–1771.

Skelly, J., & Flint, A. (1995). Urinary incontinence associated with dementia. *Journal of the American Geriatrics Society, 43,* 286–294.

Terpenning, M. S., Allada, R., & Kauffaman, C. A. (1989). Intermittent urethral catheterization in the elderly. *Journal of the American Geriatrics Society, 37,* 411–416.

Warren, J. W. (1997). Catheter associated urinary tract infections. *Infectious Disease Clinics of North America, 11*(3), 609–622.

Wolf, S. L., Riolo, L., & Ouslander, J. G. (2000). Urge incontinence and the risk of falling in older women. *Journal of the American Geriatrics Society, 48,* 847–848.

The Wound Ostomy Continence Nurses Society. (1996). *Indwelling catheter fact sheet.* Retrieved March 30, 2002, from http://www.wocn.org/PDF/C_IND-CAT.pdf

Chapter 7

ASSESSING COGNITIVE FUNCTION

Marquis D. Foreman, Kathleen Fletcher, Lorraine C. Mion, and Lark Trygstad

EDUCATIONAL OBJECTIVES

On completion of this chapter, the reader should be able to:
1. List five purposes of a cognitive assessment.
2. Compare and contrast three categories of cognitive decline.
3. Describe the parameters and assessment methods for a comprehensive assessment of cognitive function.
4. Compare and contrast formal and informal methods of assessing cognitive function.

Cognitive functioning encompasses the processes by which an individual perceives, registers, stores, retrieves, and uses information. These processes are vital for the individual to successfully maneuver through an episode of illness. Yet, especially in the elderly, cognitive functioning is particularly vulnerable to insult during an episode of illness. Given the importance and vulnerability of cognitive functioning, nurses' assessments of these processes are critical. The nurse's assessment of an individual's cognitive status can be instrumental in identifying the presence and monitoring the course of specific pathophysiologic states (e.g., dementia, depression, and delirium), determining the individual's readiness to learn, establishing clinical goals, and evaluating the effectiveness of a treatment regimen. However, it is well documented that nurses frequently fail to identify cognitive dysfunction in their patients (Inouye, Foreman, Mion, Katz, & Cooney, 2001). In response to this situation, a standardized practice protocol for assessing cognitive functioning is presented. This is a general approach to the assessment of cognitive functioning that must be adapted to the specifics of the health care setting (e.g., acute care, home care, or long-term care).

ASSESSMENT

To evaluate an individual's cognitive functioning, numerous instruments have been developed. These instruments range from full-scale batteries that require an exquisitely skilled examiner and place intensive demands on the examinee, to instruments that can be done at the bedside and that place little demand on the examiner and examinee. Additionally, some of these instruments are constructed to assess a single process (e.g., attention) in great detail, whereas others assess the spectrum of cognitive processes.

Each approach to assessment has its advantages and disadvantages. An advantage of assessing only a single cognitive process is that it minimizes the demands on the examiner and examinee; however, focusing the assessment on only a single process such as orientation may overlook an important deficit in another area (Dellasega, 1998). Conversely, an assessment of all cognitive processes provides a global indication of the individual's cognitive abilities, but it is time consuming, places intensive demands on the examinee, and may be less sensitive to some aspects of cognition. An extensive review of these instruments is reported elsewhere (Foreman, 1996; Langley, 2000).

SPECIAL CONSIDERATIONS

There are several caveats to consider when selecting an instrument to assess cognitive function. First, consider this question: *What is the purpose of the measurement?* Is the assessment for the purpose of screening, monitoring, or diagnosing? Each of these purposes requires different qualities of an instrument. Screening is conducted to determine whether or not impairment is present; as a result, relatively imprecise methods are acceptable. Also, for the purposes of screening, the exact nature and cause of the impairment are considered irrelevant. Therefore, screening methods will not determine if the impairment is dementia, delirium, or depression, for example. Table 7.1 presents the different clinical features of dementia, delirium, and depression. Conversely, methods useful for diagnostic purposes must provide more precise, detailed, and comprehensive information about an individual's cognitive functioning. Diagnostic methods are used to identify the exact nature and cause of the impairment as well as to indicate the remaining cognitive abilities of the individual. Monitoring activities are to determine cognitive status over time. Such measures generally are useful in documenting an individual's response to treatment.

Closely linked to the purpose of assessment is this question: *How often are the ratings to be made?* Depending on the purpose of the assessment, it may be important to assess the examinee twice. The first assessment should occur in a well-controlled environment to provide information about the individual's maximal abilities, and the second should occur in a more real-world setting to provide an indication of the individual's ability to function relative to performing everyday activities. Monitoring activities typically have multiple assessments. When hospitalized for acute physical illness(es), patients should be assessed at least 3 times a day with standard nursing assessments.

Some instruments are susceptible to learning effects; that is, the examinee can "learn" the correct responses. Some instruments have alternate forms; most do not. Instruments vary greatly relative to these purposes. An instrument that might be best for screening may be useless for diagnosis. Thus, it should not be assumed that these instruments are robust for all purposes. Identify the purpose of the assessment, then select the appropriate instrument according to its strengths and limitations.

The following are additional questions to consider when selecting an instrument: *What level of impairment is to be assessed?* Because there are variable levels of symptomatology and impairment, it is important to select an instrument that is adequate for that level of impairment. An instrument may be highly sensitive only to a part of the spectrum of impairment, that is, sensitive only for mild to moderate impairment and minimally sensitive to differences at the severe range. For example, many instruments will rate an individual

TABLE 7.1 A Comparison of the Clinical Features of Delirium, Dementia, and Depression

Clinical feature	Delirium	Dementia	Depression
Onset	Sudden/abrupt; depends on cause; often at twilight or in darkness	Insidious/slow and often unrecognized; depends on cause	Coincides with major life changes; often abrupt, but can be gradual
Course	Short, diurnal fluctuations in symptoms; worse at night, in darkness, and on awakening	Long, no diurnal effects; symptoms progressive yet relatively stable over time; may see deficits with increased stress	Diurnal effects, typically worse in the morning; situational fluctuations, but less than with delirium
Progression	Abrupt	Slow but uneven	Variable; rapid or slow but even
Duration	Hours to less than 1 month; seldom longer	Months to years	At least 6 weeks; can be several months to years
Consciousness	Reduced	Clear	Clear
Alertness	Fluctuates; lethargic or hypervigilant	Generally normal	Normal
Attention	Impaired; fluctuates	Generally normal	Minimal impairment, but is distractible
Orientation	Generally impaired; severity varies	Generally normal	Selective disorientation
Memory	Recent and immediate impaired	Recent and remote impaired	Selective or "patchy" impairment; "islands" of intact memory; evaluation often difficult due to low motivation

Thinking	Disorganized, distorted, fragmented; incoherent speech, either slow or accelerated	Difficulty with abstraction; thoughts impoverished; judgment impaired; words difficult to find	Intact but with themes of hopelessness, helplessness, or self-deprecation
Perception	Distorted; illusions, delusions, and hallucinations; difficulty distinguishing between reality and misperceptions	Misperceptions usually absent	Intact; delusions and hallucinations absent except in severe cases
Psychomotor behavior	Variable; hypokinetic, hyperkinetic, and mixed	Normal; may have apraxia	Variable; psychomotor retardation or agitation
Sleep/wake cycle	Disturbed; cycle reversed	Fragmented	Disturbed; usually early morning awakening
Associated features	Variable affective changes; symptoms of autonomic hyperarousal; exaggeration of personality type; associated with acute physical illness	Affect tends to be superficial, inappropriate, and labile; attempts to conceal deficits in intellect; personality changes, aphasia, agnosia may be present; lacks insight	Affect depressed; dysphoric mood; exaggerated and detailed complaints; preoccupied with personal thoughts; insight present; verbal elaboration; somatic complaints, poor hygiene, and neglect of self
Assessment	Distracted from task; numerous errors	Failings highlighted by family, frequent "near miss" answers; struggles with test; great effort to find an appropriate reply; frequent requests for feedback on performance	Failings highlighted by individual, frequent "don't knows," little effort; frequently gives up; indifferent toward test; does not care or attempt to find answer

with dementia as having severe cognitive impairment, but they will be unable to differentiate an individual who is totally dependent for care from an individual who can still walk and feed himself or herself.

For what specific subpopulation is the instrument designed? Examples of subpopulations are individuals who are educationally disadvantaged, who speak English as a second language, or who have various physical handicaps. The answer to this question will help to determine the general content and level of functioning that is assessed by the instrument. An instrument for cognitive assessment must also be selected on the abilities or handicaps of the examinee. Lezak (1983) provided an excellent discussion of features to be considered when selecting an instrument for use with individuals with sensorimotor handicaps or those with severe brain damage. Additional characteristics of the examinee to consider are age (some instruments are adversely influenced by age, e.g., measures of depression with a strong focus on somatic symptomatology), health status (acutely ill and hospitalized vs. healthy and living at home), educational level, race, and socioeconomic level.

Who is the examiner? Is the examiner to be a clinician or a lay individual, trained in cognitive assessment or not? Some instruments require the examiner to have extensive knowledge and experience with neuropsychological testing to ensure valid (i.e., truly measuring cognitive function) and reliable (consistently measuring cognitive function the same way) results, whereas others have no requirements of the examiner.

Should subjective (individual self-reports) and objective (observations or testing by the nurse or some other) ratings be distinguished? Again, the answer to this question will be influenced by many of the aforementioned suggestions. For example, if the purpose of the assessment is to determine if the examinee is depressed, having both subjective and objective evidence is critical to making an accurate diagnosis.

How valid and reliable is the scale? This is certainly an important question, but one that does not stand alone. The validity and reliability of any measure are influenced by the purpose of the assessment; the characteristics of the examinee, examiner, and testing environment; and the amount of information that is needed. Trade-offs need to be considered depending on the answers to the above questions.

Once an instrument has been selected, the following aspects should be considered: (1) the characteristics of the environment, (2) the characteristics of the examinee and examiner, and (3) the timing of the assessment. Various characteristics of the assessment environment should be considered to ensure that the results of the assessment accurately reflect the examinee's abilities and not extraneous factors. Overall, the ideal assessment environment should maximize the comfort and privacy of both the examiner and the examinee. With respect to the examinee, the environment should enhance performance by maximizing the examinee's ability to participate in the assessment process (Dellasega, 1998). To accomplish this, the room should be well lit and of comfortable ambient temperature, so that neither party is distracted from the cognitive task. Lighting must be balanced to be sufficient for the examinee to see adequately the examination materials, while not being so bright as to create glare. Care to prevent glare is especially important in the use of laminated materials with elderly examinees. Also, the assessment environment should be free from distractions that can result from extraneous noise, scattered assessment materials, or brightly colored and/or patterned clothing and flashy jewelry on the examiner (Lezak, 1983).

Performing the assessment in the presence of others should be avoided when possible, as the other individual can be distracting. If the other is a significant intimate relative, additional problems arise. For example, when the examinee fails to respond or responds in error, the significant other has been known to provide the answer, or to say such things as "Now, you know the answer to that" or "Now, you know that's wrong." In most instances, the presence of another only heightens anxiety. Rarely does the presence of another facilitate the performance of an examinee on cognitive assessment. However, Dellasega (1998) suggests that for some patients, allowing someone familiar to remain in the room may facilitate the assessment.

In addition, the assessment environment should be emotionally nonthreatening. For example, older adults are especially sensitive to any insinuation that they may have some "memory problem." Therefore, the dilemma for the examiner is to stress the importance of the assessment while taking care not to increase the examinee's anxiety. It is important to create an environment in which the examinee is motivated to perform and to perform well while not being overly anxious and therefore perform poorly. Similarly, it can be counterproductive to describe the assessment as consisting of "simple," "silly," or "stupid" questions. Such explanations tend to diminish the examinee's motivation to perform and only heighten anxiety when errors are committed. Anxiety also is heightened following a series of failures on assessment. Lezak (1983) suggests altering the order of the presentation of items so that the examinee can have some experience with success.

Various characteristics of the examiner and examinee also should be considered. Many of the instruments to assess cognitive functioning can be perceived by the examinee as intrusive, intimidating, fatiguing, and offensive—characteristics that can seriously and negatively affect performance. Consequently, Lezak (1983) recommends a 15- to 20-minute period to establish rapport with the examinee. This period also allows a determination of the examinee's capacity for assessment. For example, this period can be used to establish if the examinee has any special problems that could influence testing or its interpretation (e.g., sensory decrements). With elderly individuals who may have some decrements in sensory abilities, the examiner can improve the examinee's ability to perform through simple methods. For example, if the examinee has any degree of hearing impairment, taking a position across from the examiner or a little to the side may enhance hearing. In this position, the examinee can readily use the examiner's nonverbal communication as well as read the examiner's lips. Both strategies improve communication and thus assessment. Sitting a little to the side of the ear with the better auditory function of the examinee also improves better hearing. Positioning also is important relative to lighting and glare, which were previously discussed.

Cognitive assessment can be fatiguing to both the examiner and the examinee. Thus, examiners are cautioned to be alert for fatigue, as not all examinees will inform the examiner they are becoming fatigued. Lezak (1983) recommends observing for physical evidence of being tired, slurring of speech, motor slowing, and restlessness. When the examinee is fatigued, temporarily terminating the assessment should be considered. Many of the assessment instruments can be administered in sections; however, if the assessment must be terminated in the middle of a section, it would be wise to repeat the entire section.

Clearly, certain times of the day are inappropriate for obtaining a reliable and valid assessment of cognitive functioning. Times of the day that generally should be avoided are immediately upon awakening from sleep, immediately before and after meals, immediately before and after medical diagnostic and therapeutic procedures, and in the presence of discomfort or pain. The timing of the assessment should be selected to best reflect the true abilities of the individual and not extraneous factors.

Interpretation of the results of cognitive assessment is not simple and should consist of more than just the score obtained on testing. The nature and pattern of the examinee's responses to testing; the examinee's behavior during testing; the context of the assessment; the examinee's health history, physical examination, and results of various laboratory and other tests; the educational level, occupation, family history, current living situation, and level of social functioning; and the presence of sensory and/or motor deficits—all must be considered when interpreting the results of the cognitive assessment.

The nature and pattern of the responses to testing can provide valuable information about an individual's cognitive status. Noting the examinee's verbatim responses on testing is often valuable in differential diagnosis. For example, was the examinee not motivated to respond? Did the examinee appear to be capable of performing at a higher level than was attempted? Was "I don't know" a frequent response? If such responses were typical for a given examinee, a likely explanation would be that the individual is depressed.

Also helping to differentiate depression from dementia is the fact that depressed people complain of memory problems more often than do demented people, but they do better on memory tests, show little change in verbal fluency and naming ability, and score within the normal range on tests of intelligence (Langley, 2000). However, depression often occurs in the early stages of dementia, making diagnosis and treatment more complex (Langley, 2000).

Anecdotal notes of the context of testing, the testing environment, and the appearance and demeanor of the examinee during testing also are important for better understanding the performance on testing. Supplementary information from the examinee's health history, physical examination, and laboratory and other tests can provide valuable insight into the individual's performance on testing.

CASE STUDY

RO is a 79-year-old retired nurse who lives with her husband. She was diagnosed with probable Alzheimer's disease several years ago, and with help from their children, neighbors, and friends her husband is able to keep her at home. She is quite mobile and occasionally wanders. Her husband reports that she seems more confused and has had two falls since yesterday. Neither fall resulted in any apparent injury. She has an appointment early next week, but her husband wonders if he should bring her in to see the doctor today. The schedule is very full. As the triage nurse, what do you tell her husband and why?

DISCUSSION

Although at baseline RO has cognitive deficits, there has been a noticeable change in her mental status in the past 24 hours; also, the falls are new and reflect a change in her functional status. Both of these are signs of delirium; therefore, RO should be seen today either at the clinic or in the emergency department.

Delirium is very serious and, in some cases, is a medical emergency. The acute changes in function and mental status signal the need for careful evaluation to identify and treat the cause. Delirium occurs in all age groups but is particularly common in the elderly. About 16% of elderly patients admitted to the hospital are delirious on admission. Patients seen in the emergency room with delirium should be admitted to the hospital unless their cognitive status clears promptly with treatment in that setting.

Delirium is usually a multifactorial syndrome. In some cases, a single drug or illness is the cause. In the majority of cases, however, delirium is the result of the interrelationship between patient vulnerability or predisposing factors such as sensory losses, dementia, limited function, and new or noxious insults such as a new infection, new medication, or becoming dehydrated.

The criteria used to distinguish delirium or acute confusion from other changes in mental status include the following:

- Disturbance of consciousness (reduced clarity and awareness of the environment) with reduced ability to focus, sustain, and shift attention. Patients have trouble following instructions or making sense of their environment, even with cues. They may also get "stuck" on a particular concern or thought.
- A change in cognition: memory deficit, disorientation, language disturbance, or perceptual disturbance. Often associated with disturbances in the sleep/wake cycle and rapidly shifting emotional disturbances, with escalation of the disturbed behavior at night (sundowning). Hallucinations and delusions are common. Patients can be hyperactive and agitated or lethargic and less active. The latter presentation is particularly concerning because it is often not recognized by

health care providers as delirium. The presentation may also be mixed, with the patient fluctuating from one to the other.
* The cardinal sign of delirium is that the above changes occur rapidly over several hours or a few days.

It is important to remember that delirium may occur concurrently with dementia or depression. In fact, demented and depressed patients are at increased risk to develop delirium. Family and caregivers can be invaluable in helping to distinguish cognitive changes in those circumstances when the patient is not well known to you.

When someone becomes delirious, identifying and treating the cause is critical. Supportive and symptomatic interventions to keep the patient safe, to address the underlying cause, and to provide information to help orient and provide meaning to the environment are essential. Delirium is discussed in more detail in the next chapter.

SUMMARY

The determination of an individual's cognitive status is important in the process and outcomes of illness and its treatment. Being competent in the assessment of cognitive functioning requires (1) knowledge and skill as they relate to the performance of a cognitive assessment, (2) sensitivity to the issues that can negatively bias the results of this assessment, (3) accurate and comprehensive documentation of the assessment, and (4) the incorporation of the results of the assessment in the development of the individual's plan of care.

BOX 7.1   Assessing Cognitive Function

A. BACKGROUND
   1. Definition of cognitive function: the processes by which an individual perceives, registers, stores, retrieves, and uses information.
   2. Categories of cognitive change/decline:
      a. The dementias (e.g., Alzheimer's or vascular) are chronic, progressive, insidious, and permanent states of cognitive impairment, generally considered to be irreversible, and unpreventable, although in some instances the progression of theimpairment can be slowed.
      b. Delirium/acute confusion: an acute and sudden impairment of cognition that is considered temporary and reversible; some instances may be preventable, whereas others may only be minimized in severity or duration. There is generally an identifiable, biophysical etiology.
      c. Impairment in thought processes associated with psychiatric disorders (e.g., depression and schizophrenia)
B. ASSESSMENT
   1. Methods of assessment:
      a. Formal—cognitive testing using standardized instruments (e.g., Folstein's Mini-Mental State Examination [MMSE])
         i.   Advantages: standardized; widely used with various individual populations with known reliability and validity in these populations; quick and easy to use; enables comparison across individuals, and nurses.
         ii. Disadvantages: individual performance influenced by pain, education, fatigue, cultural background, and perceptual and physical abilities; as a result, the meaning of the score is not always clear; meaning of change in score is uncertain.
      b. Informal—through structured observations of nurse-individual interactions
         i.   Advantages: minimizes burden of individual and nurse; may have greater meaning about individual's actual cognitive ability/performance.
         ii. Disadvantages: not standardized, therefore, unknown reliability and validity of observations; difficult to make judgments regarding change in an individual's condition; variability in interpretation.
         iii. Can be imputed for formal evaluation

BOX 7.1   *(continued)*

c. Sources of information—obtain data from a variety of sources whenever possible (e.g., family and/or friends, formal caregivers, any individual who has previous intimate knowledge of person).

2. Other considerations for assessment:
   a. Characteristics of the environment for assessment
      i. Physical environment
          • Comfortable ambient temperature
          • Adequate lighting (not glaring)
          • Free of distractions (e.g., should be conducted in the absence of others and other activities)
          • Position self to maximize individual's sensory abilities
      ii. Interpersonal environment
          • Prepare the examinee for the assessment (e.g., what will take place and how long it will take)
          • Initiate the evaluation with nonthreatening conversation to establish patient-professional relationship
          • Use self-paced rate for assessment (i.e., rate set by individual)
          • Emotionally nonthreatening
   b. Timing considerations
      i.   The timing of the assessment should be selected to reflect the actual cognitive abilities of the individual and not extraneous factors
      ii. Assessment may need to be divided to avoid fatigue and the subsequent overexaggeration of deficits
      iii. Times of the day to avoid:
           • Immediately upon awakening from sleep; wait at last 30 minutes
           • Immediately before or after meals
           • Immediately before or after medical diagnostic or therapeutic procedures
           • Presence of pain or discomfort

3. Parameters for assessment:
   a. Alertness/level of consciousness: the most rudimentary cognitive function must be determined first, that is, the basic level of arousal or responsiveness to stimuli. As the level of consciousness declines, the patient is less able to respond. Level of consciousness is determined by interaction with the individual and by determination of the level made on the basis of the individual's best eye, verbal, and motor response to stimuli.

(continued)

BOX 7.1　Assessing Cognitive Function *(continued)*

- Alert—awake and aware of normal external and internal stimuli; able to interact in a meaningful way with the examiner.
- Lethargy or somnolence—not fully alert; individual tends to drift to sleep when not stimulated; diminished spontaneous physical movement; loses train of thought; ideas wander.
- Obtundation—transitional stage between lethargy and stupor; difficult to arouse; meaningful testing futile; requires constant stimulation to elicit response.
- Stupor or semicoma—individual mumbles/groans in response to persistent and vigorous physical stimulation.
- Coma—completely unarousable, no behavioral response to stimuli.

b. Attention: ability to attend/concentrate on stimuli; determined through naturally occurring conversation and daily interaction with individual. Does the individual pay attention to conversation? Can the individual follow through with directions, especially a three-step command? Does the individual have difficulty switching to a new topic? Is the individual easily distracted?

c. Memory: ability to register, retain, and recall information, both new and old. In many instances, the examiner must be able to validate individual response. Orientation is one component of memory function; disorientation may be a consequence of the absence of calendars and clocks rather than of cognitive dysfunction (Dellasega, 1998). Memory can be evaluated through naturally occurring interactions: Does the individual remember your name? Is the individual able to learn and remember new information?

d. Thinking: ability to organize and communicate ideas. Thoughts should be organized, coherent, and appropriate. A person's ability to think can best be determined through naturally occurring interactions and conversations. Conversation should not be disorganized, rambling, incoherent, or fragmented.

e. Perception: presence of misperceptions of environment. Ask questions to determine presence/absence of illusions, delusions, or visual or auditory hallucinations.

f. Psychomotor behavior: two elements are important—the person's general behavior and his or her ability to comprehend and perform simple motor skills. Relative to general

---

BOX 7.1   *(continued)*

---

behavior, direct observation of the individual's ability to sit upright is needed: Does the person sit quietly, or is the person agitated and restless? Are the person's physical movements extraordinarily retarded? Relative to execution ability, ask the individual to perform certain activities of daily living or instrumental activities of daily living, or, using Folstein's MMSE, ask the patient to perform a three-step command or to copy a figure.

  g. Higher cognitive functions: complex neuropsychological functions that are predicated upon the integrity and interaction of the more basic functions previously presented. Can the individual complete a task such as balancing a checkbook?

- Insight: ability to understand oneself and the situation one finds oneself in. Evaluated through naturally occurring conversations or use of standardized tests with the individual. The person should be aware of physical condition warranting hospitalization and the fact that he or she has been hospitalized; the patient should be able to evaluate similarities and dissimilarities.

- Judgment: ability to evaluate a situation (real or hypothetical) and determine an appropriate action; also be observant for nonrational or inappropriate decisions. Evaluated through naturally occurring interactions with the individual or through direct examination using previously constructed hypothetical simulations of events.

4. Interpretation of results:

  a. Performance on formal testing easily influenced by education, motivation, sensory functioning, language (especially when English is a second language), and a distracting environment

  b. Attend to both the nature and pattern of responses as well as to the quantity of errors committed.

C. EVALUATION OF EXPECTED OUTCOMES

1. Individual:

  a. Evidence of assessment upon admission to the unit/service (to include interunit and interinstitutional transfers).

  b. Detection of deviations will be prompt and early, with appropriate care and treatment instituted in a timely manner.

  c. Plans of care will appropriately address corrective and supportive issues in the presence of deviation in cognitive function.

(continued)

BOX 7.1   Assessing Cognitive Function *(continued)*

---

2. Health care provider:
   a. Assessment and documentation of cognitive function upon admission of an older individual to his or her care, as well as daily monitoring for any change in level of alertness or behavior.
   b. Treatment and care that incorporate appropriate strategies to address any deviation in cognitive function and that consider the use of physical and pharmacologic restraint as a last resort.
   c. Competence in cognitive assessment.
   d. Evidence of ability to differentiate among the different types of cognitive change/decline.
3. Institution:
   a. Documentation of cognitive function will increase.
   b. Identification of deviations in cognitive function will increase and occur in a timely manner.
   c. Referral to appropriate advanced practitioners (e.g., geriatric resource nurse, geriatrician, geriatric/gerontological or psychiatric clinical nurse specialist or nurse practitioner, or consultation-liaison service) will increase.
   d. Care of individual with deviations in cognitive function will be modified on the basis of the deviation.
D. FOLLOW-UP TO MONITOR CONDITION
   1. Staff competence in the assessment of cognitive function.
   2. Consistent and appropriate documentation of cognitive assessments.
   3. Consistent and appropriate care and follow-up in presence of deviations in cognitive function.
   4. Nature and origins of deviations will be sought in a timely manner.

REFERENCES

Dellasega, C. (1998). Assessment of cognition in the elderly: Pieces of a complex puzzle. *Nursing Clinics of North America, 33,* 395–405.

Foreman, M. D. (1996). Measuring cognitive status. In M. Frank-Stromborg & S. Olsen (Eds.), *Instruments for clinical research in health care* (2nd ed., pp. 86–113). Wilsonville, OR: Jones and Bartlett.

Foreman, M. D., & Grabowski, R. (1992). Diagnostic dilemma: Cognitive impairment in the elderly. *Journal of Gerontological Nursing, 18*(9), 5–12.

Inouye, S. K., Foreman, M. D., Mion, L., Katz, K. H., & Cooney, L. M., Jr. (2001). Nurses' recognition of delirium and its symptoms. Comparison of nurse and researcher ratings. *Archives of Internal Medicine, 161,* 2467–2473.

Langley, L. K. (2000). Cognitive assessment of older adults. In R. L. Kane & R. A. Kane (Eds.), *Assessing older persons: Measures, meaning, and practical applications* (2nd ed., pp. 65–128). New York: Oxford University Press.

Lezak, M. D. (1983). *Neuropsychological assessment* (2nd ed.). New York: Oxford University Press.

Chapter 8

DELIRIUM: STRATEGIES FOR ASSESSING AND TREATING

Marquis D. Foreman, Lorraine C. Mion, Lark Trygstad, and Kathleen Fletcher

EDUCATIONAL OBJECTIVES

On completion of this chapter, the reader should be able to
1. List the four most common causes of delirium.
2. Describe two characteristics of the etiologic basis of delirium.
3. Identify patients at risk for an episode of delirium.
4. Develop a plan of care for a delirious patient.

Delirium is a prevalent syndrome and one of the major contributors to poor outcomes of health care and institutionalization for older individuals. Delirium is characterized by a disturbance of consciousness with reduced ability to focus, sustain, or shift attention; a change in cognition; or the development of a perceptual disturbance that progresses over a short period of time and tends to fluctuate during the course of the day (American Psychiatric Association, 2000). These disturbances may be manifested by hypervigilance or inattentiveness; disorientation; memory impairment; and illusions, hallucinations, or misperceptions of stimuli. These symptoms are reflected in behavior that appears unusual for the individual or inappropriate to the situation. The severity of these symptoms varies during the day, typically being worse in the evening or when the patient is fatigued (Foreman, Wakefield, Culp, & Milisen, 2001).

With hospitalization, the onset of delirium generally occurs shortly after admission, usually between the second and third days. Few cases of delirium develop after the sixth day of hospitalization (Foreman, 1993), and those that do are typically iatrogenic in nature (Foreman & Bourguignon, 2002). The duration of delirium is highly variable and depends in part on how quickly the delirium and its causes are identified and how promptly and accurately treatment is initiated (Rudberg, Pompei, Foreman, Ross, & Cassel, 1997). Typically, delirium lasts less than 5 days; cases lasting longer than 7 days are rare. However, it is not uncommon for some of the symptoms of delirium to persist for as long as 3 to 6 months (Foreman, 1993; Levkoff et al., 1992, 1994; Rudberg et al., 1997).

Delirious patients more frequently (1) experience adverse reactions to therapeutic doses of medications, (2) fall, (3) develop pressure ulcers, and (4) develop infections. Because of their inability to think clearly, acutely confused patients are unable to care for themselves and frequently exhibit unsafe behaviors; they thus require greater nursing surveillance (Williams, Ward, & Campbell, 1988) and are more frequently physically restrained due to confusion (Sullivan-Marx, 2001). Also, the length of hospitalization is protracted for these patients, frequently beyond that for which hospitals are compensated (Francis, Hilko, & Kapoor, 1993; Pompei et al., 1994; Rizzo, Bogardus, Leo-Summers, Williams, Acampora, & Inouye, 2001).

Despite variability in the etiologic basis of delirium, there is agreement (Inouye et al., 1999; Foreman, 1993; Rapp et al., 2001) about the most common causes of delirium: (1) medication, especially those drugs with anticholinergic properties, or those that have potent central nervous system effects, for example, diphenhydramine (Benadryl); (2) infection, particularly urinary tract and respiratory infections; (3) dehydration and electrolyte imbalance, especially hypo- or hypernatremia and hypo- or hyperkalemia; (4) metabolic disturbances such as azotemia, pH alterations, and nutritional deficiencies; and (5) nontherapeutic environments.

To summarize, the etiologic basis of delirium is (1) multifactorial, comprising physiologic, psychologic, sociologic, and environmental elements, and, (2) dynamic, meaning the causes of delirium vary across time and specific patient populations. Together these characteristics of the etiologic basis of delirium make the diagnosis of specific causes complex and elusive, a diagnostic dilemma that challenges even the most skillful clinicians.

NURSING STRATEGIES FOR DELIRIUM

Once it has been determined that the patient is either at risk for becoming delirious or is already delirious, the question remains, What can be done to either prevent or treat the delirium? The following principles have been set forth to guide the effective prevention and treatment of delirium. The first principle is to minimize risk for delirium by preventing or eliminating the etiologic agent(s). These strategies include administering medications judiciously, preventing infection, maintaining fluid volume, promoting electrolyte balance, encouraging early mobilization, and engaging in cognitively stimulating activities. The second principle is to provide a therapeutic environment and general supportive nursing care (see Table 8.1 for details).

CASE STUDY

Mr. Z. is a 72-year-old patient admitted to your unit for prostate surgery. He is a retired accountant, lives with his wife, and is very active. He drives, plays golf, and regularly participates in activities at the senior center. His type 2 diabetes is well controlled on oral agents. He also has a history of hypertension, moderate hearing loss (hearing aids bilaterally), and previous surgery for hernia repair. He wears glasses. He is alert, oriented, and articulates a good understanding of his upcoming surgery. You care for him again 2 days after surgery. He is confused and picking at the air and oriented to self only. An indwelling urinary catheter and peripheral intravenous line (IV) are in place. In her report, the day shift nurse mentioned she was considering a physical restraint because he was increasingly restless and had tried to get out of bed. As you do your shift assessment, you recognize that he is delirious. What are the signs of delirium? What are some factors that may be contributing to his delirium?

DISCUSSION

The criteria used to distinguish delirium or acute confusion from other changes in mental status include the following:

- Disturbance of consciousness (reduced clarity and awareness of the environment), with reduced ability to focus, sustain, and shift attention. Patients have trouble following instructions or making sense of their environment, even with cues. They may also get "stuck" on a particular concern or thought.
- A change in cognition: memory deficit, disorientation, language disturbance, and/or perceptual disturbance. Symptoms are often associated with disturbances in the sleep/wake cycle and rapidly shifting emotional disturbances, with escalation of the disturbed behavior at night (sundowning). Hallucinations and delusions are common. Patients can be hyperactive and agitated or lethargic and less active. The latter presentation is particularly concerning because it is often not recognized by health care providers as delirium. The presentation may also be mixed, with the patient fluctuating from one to the other.
- The cardinal sign of delirium is that the above changes occur rapidly over several hours or days.

It is important to remember that delirium may occur concurrently with dementia or depression. In fact, those patients are at increased risk to develop delirium. Family and caregivers can be invaluable in helping to distinguish cognitive changes in those circumstances when the patient is not well known to you.

FACTORS THAT MAY CONTRIBUTE TO DELIRIUM

- Age. Older people are at greater risk for delirium, particularly if they have underlying dementia or depression. Physiologic changes occur with aging that can affect the ability of older people to respond to physical and physiologic stress and to maintain homeostasis.
- Anesthesia and other medications. It takes a number of hours for body systems to clear the anesthesia. Older persons have a larger percentage of body fat than younger persons, and many drugs are fat-soluble. This means the drug effects last longer. Also, older people tend to have less water in their cells, and water-soluble drugs will be more concentrated and

have a more pronounced effect. Have any new drugs beside pain medication been added? What is the dose and frequency of the pain medications? Is the dose appropriate for an older person?

- Blood glucose. Mr. Z. is a diabetic, and the stress of surgery can dramatically affect blood sugar control. What have his blood sugars been since surgery?
- Hydration status. Dehydration and electrolyte imbalance are a frequent contributing factor in delirium of hospitalized elders.
- Pain. What is Mr. Z.'s pain control? Poor pain control contributes to restlessness and delirium. Adequate pain control is always the goal. Is the current drug the best for good pain relief in this patient? Are there nonpharmacologic interventions that may help?
- Hypoxia. Mr. Z. is at risk because of limited mobility and possible atelectasis after surgery.
- Sensory deficits. Those with vision and hearing loss are at increased risk for delirium. Are Mr. Z.'s hearing aid and glasses in place?
- Infection or other medical illness. Postoperative infections, intraoperative myocardial infarctions (MIs), or strokes are possible causes of delirium in this case. Could Mr. Z. have a urinary tract infection (UTI) since he is post-prostate surgery and particularly since he has a Foley catheter?
- Unfamiliar surroundings. Particularly for those with sensory deficits, unfamiliar environments can lead to misinterpretations of information.

It is often not one particular factor but the interplay of patient vulnerability (predisposing factors) and precipitating factors that commonly occur during hospitalization.

Mr. Z.'s oxygen saturation, blood glucose values, and vital signs are within normal range. Given your assessment what actions would you take?

- Address safety concerns (e.g., increase surveillance).
- Call the physician immediately and make sure that he or she is aware of your findings; request that he or she come and evaluate the patient.
- Carefully review medications and laboratory work for additional information.

What additional nursing interventions might you consider?

- Frequent reality orientation. This patient had no significant cognitive deficits prior to his surgery. Frequent orientation, reassurance, and help interpreting his environment and what is happening to him should be helpful. (Monitor the patient's reaction. If the patient becomes upset or angry, you will need to modify your approach to one of more reassurance and one of validating the patient's experience rather than reorienting.)
- Are Mr. Z.'s hearing aids and glasses in place? Impaired sensory input contributes significantly to delirium. Also, he may seem more confused than he really is if he is not able to hear what you are saying.
- Invite family/significant others to stay as much as they are able to assist with his orientation and sense of well-being.
- Monitor the effect of family visitation. If the patient has increased agitation or anxiety, then limit the visitation of that individual.
- Mobilize the patient. Mobility assists with orientation and helps prevent problems associated with immobility, such as atelectasis and deep venous thrombosis.
- Judicious use of medications for pain, sleep, or anxiety. If Mr. Z. is having pain, are the drug and dose appropriate for him? A regular schedule of a smaller dose or nonnarcotic pain medication almost always is better than prn dosing. Drugs used to address these issues can exacerbate the delirium. Try nonpharmacologic approaches for sleep and anxiety first.
- Try to provide for adequate sleep: noise reduction at night, soft, relaxing music, warm milk, herbal tea, massage, and rescheduling care so as not to awaken or interrupt sleep.
- Make sure the patient is well hydrated.
- Talk to the doctor about removing the indwelling urinary catheter. Because of his surgery, Mr. Z. may need it now, but it should be removed as soon as possible. Additionally recommend a urinalysis to the doctor to rule out UTI.

Is there any way his delirium could have been prevented?

There is no way to know for sure, but research has shown that recognition of risk factors and the early interventions outlined above to address those risks can significantly reduce the incidence of delirium. This is key to reducing the high morbidity and mortality associated with delirium in the older population.

TABLE 8.1   Nursing Strategies for Delirium

Etiologic agent	Physical findings	Nursing actions

Medications
Anticholinergic preparations:
  Thioridazine
  Amitriptyline
  Neuroleptics
  Tricyclic antidepressants
  Atropine
  Theophylline
  Diphenhydramine
Histamine-2 blocking agents
  Cimetidine
  Ranitidine
Analgesics:
  Meperidine
  Nonsteroidal anti-inflammatory
    agents
  Opiates
Sedative-hypnotics:
  Zolpidem
  Benzodiazepines
Cardiovascular drugs:
  Nifedipine
  Quinidine
  Disopyramide
  Amiodarone
  Beta blockers
	Variable, depending on the specific medication, drug–drug interactions, and the person's underlying health problems and health status	1. Monitor the effects (intended and adverse) of medications. Be especially vigilant for drug interactions. With the onset of any new symptom, first consider it an adverse reaction to a medication (refer to medication protocol in this text).
		2. Regularly evaluate each medication; use only those medications indicated by the patient's status, thereby keeping medication to a minimum.
		3. Monitor for adverse effects, drug–drug, drug–disease, and drug–nutrient interactions, as well as additive effects of drugs (e.g., more than one with anticholinergic effects).
		4. Relieve pain through adequate and appropriate administration of analgesia and alternative nonpharmacologic therapies (see pain management protocol in this text)
		5. Avoid the use of meperidine.

Corticosteroids:
Anti-Parkinsonian agents

Infection
Most common
Urinary tract
Respiratory
Cellulitis
Most overlooked
Mouth
Feet

Symptoms may be vague and nonspecific (e.g., mental status change or functional decline) with significant illness of onset. Change in patient's functional level often seen as first sign of infection in elderly.

Urinary signs and symptoms
Dysuria is frequently absent
Urinary frequency
Urgency
Nocturia
New onset incontinence
Anorexia
U/A +WBC, nitrites
Protein and/or blood dipstick

6. Use nonpharmacologic sleep-enhancing protocols (see sleep protocol in this text).
7. Refer to/notify appropriate advanced practice nurse of house officer and/or pharmacologist for medication review and work-up for underlying cause.
8. Document actions and patient response in hospital record.

1. Determine source and site of infection.
2. Provide adequate fluids (2000 ml per day), unless otherwise contraindicated.
3. Apply cooling techniques as needed and indicated (e.g., remove covers or use cooling mattress/blanket).
4. Monitor for flushed hot skin, tachypnea, tachycardia, seizures, changes in body temperature, and breath sounds q 2 h or as indicated by status of the patient.
5. Monitor intake and output.

(continued)

TABLE 8.1   Nursing Strategies for Delirium (*continued*)

Etiologic agent	Physical findings	Nursing actions
	Respiratory infection: Cough may be dry, productive, or absent Tachypnea Slight cyanosis Anorexia Nausea Vomiting Tachycardia Chills, fever, and elevated WBC may not be present Cultures may be negative Breath sounds: wheezes, crackles, or rhonchi possible	1. For respiratory infections, provide humidified air, cough and deep breathe prn; provide frequent oral hygiene; beta agonistvia nebulizer; chest physiotherapy to mobilize secretions. 2. Monitor oxygen saturation. 3. Administer oxygen prn. 4. Refer to/notify appropriate advanced practice nurse or house officer for further evaluation for underlying medical problem. 5. Document actions and patient response in hospital record.
Dehydration	Hypotension with orthstatic changes Weakness Nausea Oliguria Dry mucous membranes (lips) and skin Poor skin turgor over sternum Lethargy Lightheadedness	1. Determine source of dehydration (e.g., decreased fluid intake or increased fluid output). 2. Check medications as a cause for increased loss of fluids (e.g., diuretics). 3. Check person's ability to swallow or for mechanical problems preventing fluid intake.

Elevations in BUN, HCT, sodium

4. Determine individual's daily fluid needs (Gaspar, 1998), and develop a fluid schedule (Weinberg et al., 1995).
5. Make sure water is in easy reach of the individual.
6. Determine if individual can independently meet fluid needs; if not, place on a fluid schedule.
7. Refer to/notify appropriate advanced practice nurse or house officer.
8. Prepare for fluid replacement and additional diagnostic and therapeutic actions.
9. Continue surveillance of patient q 2–6 h as indicated by patient status.
10. Document actions and patient response in hospital record.

Hypernatremia (> 146 mEq/L)

Weakness
Focal neurologic deficits
Obtundation/stupor
Elevated HCT, BUN, serum osmolarity, urine sodium
Vomiting, diarrhea NG Tube drainage

1. Determine source of hypernatremia:
   Increased water loss (fever, infection, vomiting, diarrhea, diaphoresis), decreased water intake (physical or cognitive limitations), or increased sodium intake

(continued)

TABLE 8.1 Nursing Strategies for Delirium (*continued*)

Etiologic agent	Physical findings	Nursing actions
Hypernatremia (> 146 mEq/L) (*continued*)		2. Evaluate medication causes, e.g., osmotic cathartic (lactulose) 3. Prepare for possible fluid replacement. 4. Restrict activity to maintain energy balance. 5. Continue to monitor parameters q 2 h or as indicated by status of patient. 6. Refer to/notify appropriate advanced practice nurse or house officer. 7. Document actions and patient response in hospital record.
Hyponatremia (< 136 mEq/L)	Orthostatic hypotension Hypothermia Nausea and vomiting Malaise Lethargy Somnolence Decreased serum sodium and osmolality Hyperglycemia Sunken eyes Tachycardia Anorexia Oliguria	1. Determine source of hyponatremia (e.g., inadequate intake of sodium, renal disease, extrarenal fluid loss, e.g., vomiting, diarrhea, fluid restriction, overdiuresis, low-sodium tube feedings). 2. Prepare for electrolyte and possibly fluid replacement. 3. Restrict activity to maintain energy balance. 4. Continue to monitor parameters q 2 h or as indicated by status of patient.

CHF

5. Drug–disease (↑ Na+) interaction oral hypoglycemics, diuretics, antipsychotics, SSRIs (selective serotonin reuptake inhibitor) may potentiate ↓ Na+ further.
6. Refer to/notify appropriate advanced practice nurse or house officer.
7. Document actions and patient response in hospital record.

Hypokalemia (< 3.5 mEq/L)

Muscle weakness
Muscle cramps
Fatigue
Tachyarrhythmias
Atrial-ventricular conduction disturbances

1. Determine source of hypokalemia (e.g., poor nutritional intake of potassium-rich foods, or excessive depletion; nausea, vomiting, and diarrhea; or excessive loss due to the effects of medications such as non-potassium-sparing diuretics).
2. Refer to/notify appropriate advanced practice nurse or house officer.
3. Prepare for electrolyte and possibly fluid replacement.
4. Document actions and patient response in hospital record.
5. Note drug–disease interaction: if also on digoxin, monitor for digoxin toxicity.

(continued)

TABLE 8.1 Nursing Strategies for Delirium (*continued*)

Etiologic agent	Physical findings	Nursing actions
Hypoxia	Tachypnea Cyanosis (peripheral and central) Agitation Increased depth of respirations Decreased oxygen saturation Accessory muscle use Paradoxical breathing pattern	1. Determine source of hypoxia (e.g., infection, COPD, PE, bronchospasm, anemia). 2. Position patient to facilitate air exchange (e.g., high Fowler's position, as tolerated by patient). 3. Restrict/pace activity to reduce additional oxygen requirements. 4. Monitor blood gas results or pulse oximetry. 5. Refer to/notify appropriate advanced practice nurse or house officer. 6. Continue to monitor parameters q 2 h or as indicated by status of patient. 7. Prepare for oxygen administration; use long tubing to maintain mobilization. 8. Document actions and patient response in hospital record.
Environmental change	Variable, depending on whether the environmental change presents as sensory overload or sensory deprivation	1. Provide explanations of nursing care and all diagnostic and therapeutic activities. 2. Position patient in a semi-Fowler's position as tolerated.

3. Minimize abrupt relocations; otherwise, prepare patient by providing explanations of the event; send a health care provider or family member to accompany patient.

4. Offer orienting information as a normal part of daily care and activities.

5. Provide orienting stimuli: clock, watch, calendar, radio, television, and newspapers.

6. Include personal items from home.

7. Encourage social interaction with friends and family.

8. Maintain continuity of care and care environment; limit relocations.

9. Limit the number of staff involved in the care of the patient.

10. Remove meaningless and unnecessary stimuli as soon as possible (e.g., unneeded equipment and supplies, television off when not desired, etc.).

11. Communicate clearly and simply (see Rapp et al., 2001).

12. Refer to/notify appropriate advanced practice nurse or house officer.

(continued)

TABLE 8.1   Nursing Strategies for Delirium *(continued)*

Etiologic agent	Physical findings	Nursing actions
Environmental change *(continued)*		13. Document actions and patient's response in hospital record.
Sensory impairment	Misperceptions of visual and auditory stimuli (e.g., hallucinations, illusions, mistaking objects and persons for others) Diminished hearing acuity Diminished visual acuity	1. Assist patient in accurately interpreting environmental stimuli by having patient use appropriate sensory aids (e.g., eyeglasses or hearing aids); also, ensure that aids are in proper working condition. 2. Eliminate sources of distraction (auditory and visual). 3. Determine source of impairment (e.g., malfunctioning aids or aids not in use, earwax impaction). 4. Speak clearly and slowly; do not shout; repeat key phrases as necessary. 5. Speak directly into the patient's "best" ear. 6. Face the patient when speaking so that lip reading can be used to facilitate understanding as necessary.

7. With written materials, use large print with lighter colored objects on darker backgrounds; place them directly in front of the patient, and use indirect lighting to reduce/eliminate glare.
8. Refer to/notify appropriate advanced practice nurse or house officer.
9. Document actions and patient's response in hospital record.

Inactivity/immobility

Physical weakness
Inactivity/immobility
Functional decline

1. Begin early mobilization, ambulation, or active range-of-motion exercises 3 times a day as tolerated.
2. Make minimal use of immobilizing equipment (e.g., indwelling urinary catheter).
3. Avoid use of physical restraints.
4. Refer to/notify appropriate advanced practice nurse or house officer.
5. Document actions and patient's response in hospital record.

Cognitive impairment

Impaired cognitive function(s)

1. Offer orienting information as a normal part of daily care and activities.

(continued)

TABLE 8.1 Nursing Strategies for Delirium *(continued)*

Etiologic agent	Physical findings	Nursing actions
Cognitive impairment *(continued)*		2. Work with patient to correctly interpret the environment.
		3. Incorporate cognitively stimulating activities as normal part of daily care (e.g., discussion of current events, structured reminiscence, reality orientation, etc.).
		4. Refer to/notify appropriate advanced practice nurse or house officer.
		5. Document actions and patient's response in hospital record.

BUN = blood urea nitrogen; COPD = chronic obstructive pulmonary disease; HCT = hematocrit; PE = pulmonary embolus; O_2 sat = oxygen saturation; SIADH = syndrome of inappropriate antidiuretic hormone; WBC = white blood (cell) count

SUMMARY

Delirium is a common occurrence in many hospitalized elders. With shorter lengths of hospital stays, patients with delirium are frequently discharged before their symptoms are fully resolved (Foreman & Bourguignon, 2002); therefore, discharge planning and family education must reflect safety and monitoring issues. Thus, it is important to promptly identify those patients at risk for delirium or those presently delirious. To do so, nursing assessments must become routine and systematic. In addition, the assessment of cognition should be comprehensive. A standard of practice protocol provides concise information to guide nursing care of individuals at risk of or experiencing delirium.

BOX 8.1   Delirium: Strategies for Assessing and Treating

A. BACKGROUND
 1. Definition: Delirium is a disturbance in consciousness with
    reduced ability to focus, sustain, or shift attention; a change in
    cognition or the development of a perceptual disturbance that
    develop over a short period of time and tend to fluctuate during
    the course of the day (American Psychiatric Association, 2000).
 2. Epidemiology:
    a. Prevalence (upon admission to the hospital): 16%.
    b. Overall incidence during hospitalization: 6% to 55%, typically
       about 20%
       i. Postoperative incidence: 15% to 72%
       ii. Incidence at time of discharge from hospital: 30% to 60%
    c. Onset approximately the third day of hospitalization
    d. Duration typically less than 5 days; however, symptoms of
       delirium can persist 3 to 6 months
 3. Consequences of delirium:
    a. Loss of independence, diminished ability to participate in own
       care, and loss of ability for self-determination
    b. Morbidity: Delirious patients are more likely to develop
       pressure ulcers, fall, have adverse reactions to medications,
       develop infections, become institutionalized, and have
       continued cognitive impairment.
    c. Mortality given equivalent severity of illness: Delirious
       patients are 6 times more likely to die than nondelirious
       patients.
    d. For health care professionals and institutions, acutely
       confused patients are hospitalized for longer periods of time
       and pose an increased demand for and intensity of nursing
       care for which institutions tend not to be adequately
       reimbursed. Hospitals lose on average $30,000 per confused
       patient.
B. RISK FACTORS
 1. Increasing age
 2. Increasing severity of illness
 3. Multiple chronic illnesses with multiple medications
 4. History of cognitive impairment (dementia and depression) or
    previous, experience with delirium
 5. Substance and alcohol use
 6. Sleep deprivation
 7. Immobility
 8. Sensory impairment

BOX 8.1   *(continued)*

C. ASSESSMENT
1. Obtain baseline or premorbid cognitive functioning from family, significant other(s), or another intimate source.
2. Ask patients the following questions when assessing cognitive functioning:
   - Have you noticed any changes in your thinking or memory recently?
   - Recently, have you experienced any strange thoughts?
   Affirmative responses should arouse suspicion of the risk for delirium.
3. Assess parameters specified in Assessing Cognitive Function (see chapter 7); to detect and diagnose delirium, refer to Table 8.2, Assessing for Delirium. To assist in differentiating delirium, dementia, and depression, refer to Table 7.1 in chapter 7.
4. Review current laboratory values, medications, and monitor vital signs and fluid intake and output, to identify the following potential etiologic factors, acute illness, infection (e.g., URI, UTI), medication (e.g., anticholinergic, sedatives, psychotropics, narcotics, H_2 blockers), altered homeostasis (e.g., dehydration and electrolyte imbalance), hemodynamic status (e.g., hypovolemia, hypoxia), and environmental challenge (sensory overload or deprivation).
D. CARE STRATEGIES by etiology, refer to Table 8.1, Nursing Strategies for Delirium, for specifics; a general approach follows.
1. Treat the underlying pathology and contributing factors:
   a. Administer medications judiciously.
   b. Prevent/promptly and appropriately treat infections.
   c. Maintain fluid balance.
   d. Promote electrolyte balance.
2. Provide a therapeutic environment:
   a. Provide appropriate sensory stimulation.
   b. Reassure and reorient patient.
   c. Maintain consistency of caregivers.
   d. Encourage family members or familiar people to be at patient's bedside.
   e. Use sensory aids as appropriate.
   f. Minimize abrupt relocations.
3. Provide general supportive nursing care:
   a. Provide comfort measures.
   b. Protect from hazards of immobility and mobilization.
   c. Provide supportive nursing care for the meeting of basic needs (e.g., toileting, feeding, hydration, pain, etc.)

(continued)

BOX 8.1   Delirium: Strategies for Assessing and Treating *(continued)*

---

    d. Communicate clearly; provide explanations.
    e. Reassure and educate family.
    f. Minimize invasive interventions.
  4. Refer to appropriate advanced practitioners (e.g., geriatric resource nurse, geriatric/gerontological or psychiatric clinical nurse specialist or nurse practitioner, or consultation-liaison service).
E. EVALUATION OF EXPECTED OUTCOMES
  1. Patient:
    a. Improved outcomes of care (e.g., a lowered incidence, duration, severity, and recurrence of delirium; increased functional independence; and decreased mortality)
    b. Cognitive status returns to baseline (predelirious state).
    c. Patient is discharged to same destination as prehospitalization.
  2. Health care provider:
    a. Increased detection of delirium
    b. Prompt implementation of appropriate interventions for delirium
    c. Improved satisfaction in care of hospitalized elderly
  3. Institution:
    a. Decreased overall cost
    b. Decreased length of stays
    c. Decreased morbidity and mortality
    d. Increased referrals and consultation to above specified specialists
    e. Increased provision of quality care
F. FOLLOW-UP TO MONITOR CONDITION
  1. Use of physical and pharmacologic restraints, and sitters; usage to decrease
  2. The incidence, duration, and severity of delirium to decrease
  3. Patient's days with delirium to decrease
  4. Staff competence in recognition and treatment of delirium/delirium
  5. Documentation of the prompt recognition of delirium
  6. Documentation of a variety of interventions for delirium/delirium

TABLE 8.2 Assessing for Delirium

Feature	Assessment parameters	Findings
Alertness	Level of consciousness: observation of behavior and naturally occurring conversation • Alert (normal) • Vigilant (hyperalert) • Lethargic (drowsy but easily aroused) • Stupor (difficult to arouse) • Coma (unarousable)	Fluctuates from stuporous to hypervigilant
Attention	Ability to attend/concentrate: through naturally occurring conversation, observation of behavior, or formal testing using • Digit span, forward and backward • Serial subtraction • Spelling backwards • Clock Drawing Test (Ben-Yehuda, Benter, & Friedman, 1995; Juby, 1999; Kirby, Denihan, Bruce, Coakley, & Lawlor, 2001)	Inattentive, easily distractible; may have difficulty shifting attention from one focus to another; has difficulty keeping track of what is being said
Orientation	Questioning about orientation to person, place, and time: through naturally occurring observation or formal testing	Disoriented to time and place; should not be disoriented to person
Memory	Questioning about recent and remote events; day-to-day observation; Clock Drawing Test	Inability to recall events of hospitalization and current illness; unable to remember instructions; forgetful of names, events, activities, current news, etc.

(continued)

TABLE 8.2 Assessing for Delirium (*continued*)

Feature	Assessment parameters	Findings
Thinking	Naturally occurring conversation	Disorganized thinking; rambling, irrelevant, incoherent conversation; unclear or illogical flow of ideas; unpredictable switching from topic to topic; difficulty in expressing needs and concerns; speech may be garbled
Perception	Recognition of objects and persons; Clock Drawing Test	Perceptual disturbances such as illusions and hallucinations; misperceptions such as calling a stranger by a relative's name
Psychomotor behavior	Observation of behavior: • Hypo- or hyperkinetic • Unusual or inappropriate • Day-to-day interaction	Variable, from sluggish and moving very slowly to restlessness and agitation; behavior that is considered unusual for that individual or inappropriate for the situation

Source: Adapted from Foreman and Zane (1996).

REFERENCES

American Psychiatric Association. (2000). *Diagnostic and Statistical Manual of Mental Disorders* (4th ed., text rev.). Washington, DC: Author.

Ben-Yehuda, A., Bentur, N., & Friedman, G. (1995). The clock drawing test as a cognitive screening tool for elderly patients in an acute-care hospital. *Aging Clinical Experimental Research, 7,* 188–190.

Foreman, M. D. (1993). Delirium in the elderly. *Annual Review of Nursing Research, 11,* 3–30.

Foreman, M. D., & Bourguignon, C. M. (2002). *Delirium in older hospitalized patients: Predisposing, precipitating, perpetuating, and protective factors.* Unpublished manuscript.

Foreman, M. D., Wakefield, B., Culp, K., & Milisen, K. (2001). Delirium in elderly patients: An overview of the state of the science. *Journal of Gerontological Nursing, 27*(4), 12–20.

Foreman, M. D., & Zane, D. (1996). Nursing strategies for delirium in hospitalized elderly patients. *American Journal of Nursing, 96*(4), 44–51.

Francis, J., Hilko, E., & Kapoor, N. (1993). Delirium and prospective payment: The economic impact of confusion [abstract]. *Journal of the American Geriatric Society, 41*(Suppl), SA9.

Gaspar, P. M. (1998, March). *Comparison of four standards used to determine adequacy of water intake among nursing home residents.* Paper presented at the 1998 Midwest Nursing Research Society Conference, Columbus, OH.

Inouye, S. K., Bogardus, S. T., Jr., Charpentier, P. A., Leo-Summers, L., Acampora, D., Holford, T. R., & Cooney, L. M., Jr. (1999). A multicomponent intervention to prevent delirium in hospitalized older patients. *New England Journal of Medicine, 340,* 669–676.

Juby, A. (1999). Correlation between the Folstein Mini-Mental State Examination and three methods of clock drawing scoring. *Journal of Geriatrics Psychiatry and Neurology, 12,* 87–91.

Kirby, M., Denihan, A., Bruce, I., Coakley, D., & Lawlor, B. A. (2001). The clock drawing test in primary care: Sensitivity in dementia detection and specificity against normal and depressed elderly. *International Journal of Geriatrics Psychiatry, 16,* 935–940.

Levkoff, S. E., Evans, D. A., Liptzin, B., Cleary, P. D., Lipsitz, L. A., Wetle, T. T., Reilly, C. H., Pilgrim, D. M., Schor, J., & Rowe, J. (1992). Delirium: The occurrence and persistence of symptoms among elderly hospitalized patients. *Archives of Internal Medicine, 152,* 334–340.

Levkoff, S. E., Liptzin, B., Evans, D. A., Cleary, P. D., Lipsitz, L. A., Wetle, T., & Rowe, J. A. (1994). Progression and resolution of delirium in elderly patients hospitalized for acute care. *American Journal of Geriatric Psychiatry, 2,* 230–238.

Pompei, P., Foreman, M. D., Rudberg, M. A., Inouye, S. K., Braund, V., & Cassel, C. K. (1994). Delirium in hospitalized older persons: Outcomes and predictors. *Journal of the American Geriatrics Society, 42,* 809–815.

Rapp, C. G., & Iowa Veterans Affairs Research Consortium. (2001). Delirium/delirium protocol. *Journal of Gerontological Nursing, 27*(4), 21–33.

Rizzo, J. A., Bogardus, S. T., Jr., Leo-Summers, L., Williams, C. S., Acampora, D., & Inouye, S. K. (2001). Multicomponent targeted intervention to prevent delirium in hospitalized older patients: What is the economic value? *Medical Care, 39,* 740–752.

Rudberg, M. A., Pompei, P., Foreman, M. D., Ross, R. E., & Cassel, C. K. (1997). The natural history of delirium in older hospitalized patients: A syndrome of heterogeneity. *Age and Ageing, 26,* 169–174.

Sullivan-Marx, E. (2001). Achieving restraint-free care of acutely confused older adults. *Journal of Gerontological Nursing, 27*(4), 56–61.

Weinberg, A. D., Minaker, K .L., and the Council on Scientific Affairs, American Medical Association. (1995). Dehydration: Evaluation and management in older adults. *Journal of the American Medical Association, 274,* 1552–1556.

Williams, M. A., Ward, S. E., & Campbell, E. B. (1988). Confusion: Testing versus observation. *Journal of Gerontological Nursing, 14*(1), 25–30.

Chapter 9

PREVENTING FALLS IN ACUTE CARE

Barbara Resnick

EDUCATIONAL OBJECTIVES

On completion of this chapter, the reader should be able to
1. Develop a risk assessment for a falls prevention program in the acute care setting.
2. Perform a comprehensive risk assessment for fall risk in older adults in the acute care setting.
3. Develop an appropriate plan of care for older adults in acute care settings to prevent falls.
4. Complete a comprehensive evaluation of an older patient postfall to include pertinent physical findings postfall and to identify the cause of the fall.
5. Complete an evaluation of a falls prevention program that includes the evaluation of fall rates and injuries.

The majority of all falls that occur in the acute care setting involve individuals over the age of 65 (Halfon, Eggli, Melle, & Vagnair, 2001). For people 65 years of age and over, falls are responsible for one third of deaths due to injury. Hip fractures are a serious consequence of falls in the older adult, with significant morbidity and mortality (Magaziner et al., 2000). The incidence rate of first falls in acute care is 2.2 per 1,000 patient days, and older age was a statistically significant risk for falling. The increased risk of falling in older adults may be due to a number of age-related changes, such as altered visual acuity, decreased reaction time, decreased balance and muscle strength, demineralization of bone, and increased incidence of orthostatic hypotension.

Falls are the single largest category of incidents in acute care settings (Kannus et al., 1999), and approximately 20% of falls result in actual injury to the individual. The fall can result in a subsequent fracture or trauma, soft tissue changes, pneumonia, discomfort, or fear of falling, all of which can cause further decline in functional ability. Falls also are the most common reason that nurses are sued for negligence (Hendrick, Nyhuis, Kppenbrock, & Soja, 1995).

Nurses in the acute care setting have the most contact with patients and are in key positions to evaluate these individuals and implement interventions to decrease falls. Falls may be reduced by following a simple four-step approach: (1) evaluating and identifying risk factors for falls in the older patient, (2) developing an appropriate plan of care for prevention, (3) performing a comprehensive evaluation of falls that occur in the hospital, and (4) performing a postfall revision of plan of care as appropriate.

By definition, a fall is an unintentional change in position resulting in coming to rest on the ground or other lower level (Thapa, Borckman, Gideon, Fought, & Ray, 1996). Incidences in which a patient sits down on the floor deliberately or is settled to the floor with the help of a family member or health care provider should not be considered a fall. In addition, a "near fall" (an episode in which it is believed the individual would have fallen had there not been a staff person nearby for assistance) should likewise not be considered a fall.

The majority of falls occur during routine activities such as bathing and dressing, getting in and out of bed, and going to the bathroom (Resnick, 1999). Hazards within the environment add to the risk of falling in the older adult. Hazards include obstacles in the path, slippery floors, poor lighting, poorly fitting footwear, and the carrying of heavy or bulky objects. The environment, however, is not the sole cause of falls in older adults. Research findings by Norton, Campbell, Lee-Joe, Robinson, and Butler (1997) indicate that only 25% of injurious falls (i.e., those that caused hip fracture) were related to environmental hazards, and for the most part these hazards were not modifiable.

ASSESSMENT

Step 1: Identifying the Risk Factors for Falling

There are many known risk factors associated with falls in the older adult (Table 9.1). These risks can range from a prior history of a fall to a current acute medical problem, medications given, or use of restraints. Each of these risk factors must be carefully considered and entered into the risk assessment tool (Table 9.2) to help determine the degree of risk the individual has related to falling.

A prior history of falls is frequently cited in the literature as a risk factor contributing to falls (Lord & Fitzpatrick, 2001; Tinetti, 1997). Once an older adult has fallen, there is a significant increased risk that he or she will fall again under similar circumstances. A history of recent falls can be assessed by asking the patient and his or her caregivers (Table 9.3). It is helpful to use specific time frames to stimulate memory and facilitate recall.

A major concern with a fall is the subsequent fear of falling that can occur. Fear of falling has been cited as one of the most serious and debilitating psychological consequences of a fall. It is not, however, only those who fall who experience a fear of falling (Arfken, Lach, Birge, & Miller, 1994; Gray-Micelli, 1997). The fear of falling has, in part, been created by increased public awareness of falls in the older adult (Lachman et al., 1998). Moreover, health care providers, out of care and concern for older adults, continually remind them not to get up or ambulate because they might fall (Resnick, 1998). This instills a fear of falling in older adults and may cause them to limit their activity, thereby placing them at greater risk of falling due to deconditioning.

TABLE 9.1   Assessment of Risk Factors Associated with Falls

History of falls
Fear of falling
Bowel and bladder incontinence
Cognitive impairment
Mood
Dizziness
Functional impairment
Medications
Medical problems
Environmental risks

TABLE 9.2   Fall Risk Assessment

Risk	Yes	No
1. Previous falls		
2. Cardiac arrhythmias		
3. Transient ischemic attacks		
4. Stroke		
5. Parkinson's disease		
6. Delirium		
7. Dementia		
8. Depression		
9. Musculoskeletal disorders (e.g., osteoporosis, myopathy)		
10. Altered mobility and/or gait		
11. History of prior fractures		
12. Orthostatic hypotension		
13. Bowel or bladder incontinence		
14. Sensory impairments (vision, hearing, tactile)		
15. Dizziness		
16. Dehydration		
17. Acute illness (e.g., infection)		
18. Use of restraints		
19. Diabetes, particularly with history or risk of hypoglycemia		
20. Polypharmacy		

Score: 0–5 in the Yes column is low risk; 6–10 in the Yes column is moderate risk; 11+ in the Yes column is high risk.

Falls are commonly noted to occur during attempts to get to the bathroom to eliminate or to transfer to a bedside commode (Hendrick et al., 1995). It is useful when evaluating risk of falls in older patients to incorporate within their history taking information about the bowel and bladder function (refer to chapter 6 in this book). The information obtained, such as how often the individual voids at night and whether or not he or she has urgency or urinary incontinence, can be used to develop an appropriate plan of care.

The risk of falling increases in individuals with confusion related to an underlying dementia or an acute delirium. A known diagnosis of dementia accounts for over 50% of falls (Krueger, Brazil, & Lohfeld, 2001; Norwalk, Prendergast, Bayles, D'Amico, & Colvin, 2001). This risk is due to a lack of safety awareness and poor judgment noted in

TABLE 9.3   History of Fall

Name:_____   Date/Time of fall: _____

Description of fall: _____

_____

Fall location:

Room	☐	Bathroom	☐
Facility dining room	☐	Activity room	☐
Facility hallway	☐	Outside	☐
Other	☐		

Please describe: _____

Additional comments:_____

_____

Activity related to fall:

Walking	☐	Transferring	☐
Dressing	☐	Bathing	☐
Toileting	☐	Cooking	☐
Other	☐		

Please describe: _____

Additional comments:_____

_____

Details of fall:

Loss of consciousness	☐	Medication use:	
Dizziness	☐	Hypnotic	☐
		Sedative	☐
		Alcohol	☐

Additional comments:_____

_____

Outcome of fall:

No injury	☐	Musculoskeletal pain	☐
Laceration	☐	Hematoma	☐
Skin tear	☐	Fracture	☐
Other	☐		

Please describe: _____

Additional comments:_____

_____

these individuals. It is essential to evaluate cognitive status at baseline in all older patients using standardized tools such as the Mini Mental State Exam (Folstein, Folstein, & McHugh, 1975; refer to chapter 7). Moreover, it is useful to differentiate between delirium and dementia in these individuals so that appropriate interventions can be made. Delirium is prevalent in acute care settings, and older adults in acute care need to be monitored closely for onset of delirium so that the underlying cause can be identified and resolved as soon as possible.

Dizziness is a prevalent problem in older adults and may be due to diabetes, Parkinson's disease, cerebral vascular accidents or carotid stenosis, orthostatic hypotension, medications, or inner ear problems. Certainly exploring the underlying cause of dizziness is essential so that interventions can be implemented to alleviate or decrease the occurrence of the dizziness. Simple history taking includes asking patients and caregivers if dizziness occurs with position change, such as moving from lying to standing (indicative of orthostatic hypotension) or changes in position of head (indicative of vertigo). These specific questions can help identify the cause of the dizziness. A physical examination should be incorporated into the risk assessment for dizziness and include a lying and standing blood pressure. A drop of 20 mm Hg or more with this position change is indicative of orthostatic hypotension and may be due to a cardiac event, hydration status, or blood loss.

Functional impairment is commonly associated with a fall (Lord & Fitzpatrick, 2001). Patients and caregivers should be asked about or actually evaluated for baseline function using a general assessment tool such as the Katz Index of Activities of Daily Living. Ask patients and caregivers about the use of any assistive devices that facilitate performance of functional activities (e.g., walkers and reachers). Encourage families and caregivers to bring in assistive devices to the hospital for use during recovery. For patients who are able to transfer and ambulate independently, it may also be useful to complete the Tinetti Gait and Balance Measure (1989) to determine the degree of impairment in either gait or balance (Table 9.4).

There are a number of medications that influence gait and balance (Resnick, Cocoran, & Spellbring, 2001). The major drug groups include sedating psychotropic medications such as benzodiazepines, tricyclic antidepressants, phenothiazines, anticonvulsants, salicylates, and antivertigo agents. Moreover, any medication that causes orthostatic hypotension can impair balance and thereby alter gait.

TABLE 9.4   Balance and Gait Evaluation

Tinetti Assessment Tool: Description	
Population:	Adult population, elderly patients
Description:	The Tinetti Assessment Tool is a simple, easily administered test that measures a patient's gait and balance. The test is scored on the patient's ability to perform specific tasks.
Mode of Administration:	The Tinetti Assessment Tool is a task performance exam.
Time to Complete:	10 to 15 minutes
Time to Score:	Time to score is included in time to complete.
Scoring:	Scoring of the Tinetti Assessment Tool is done on a three point ordinal scale with a range of 0 to 2. A score of 0 represents the most impairment, while a 2 would represent independence of the patient. The individual scores are then combined to form three measures: an overall gait assessment score, an overall balance assessment score, and a gait and balance score.
Interpretation:	The maximum score for the gait component is 12 points. The maximum score for the balance component is 16 points. The maximum total score is 28 points. In general, patients who score below 19 are at a high risk for falls. Patients who score in the range of 19–24 indicate that the patient has a risk for falls.
Reliability:	Interrater reliability was measured in a study of 15 patients by having a physician and a nurse test the patients at the same time. Agreement was found on over 85% of the items and the items that differed never did so by more than 10%. These results indicate that the Tinetti Assessment Tool has good interrater reliabilty.
Validity:	Not reported

(continued)

TABLE 9.4   Balance and Gait Evaluation *(continued)*

BALANCE

Patient's Name: _____   Date: _____

Location: _____   Rater: _____

Initial Instructions: Subject is seated in hard armless chair. The following maneuvers are tested.

Task	Description of balance	Possible	Score
1. Sitting balance	Leans or slides in chair	= 0	
	Steady, safe	= 1	
2. Arises	Unable without help	= 0	
	Able, uses arms to help	= 1	
	Able without using arms	= 2	
3. Attempts to rise	Unable without help	= 0	
	Able, requires > 1 attempt	= 1	
	Able to rise, 1 attempt	= 2	
4. Immediate standing balance (first 5 seconds)	Unsteady (staggers, moves feet, trunk sway)	= 0	
	Steady but uses walker or other support	= 1	
	Steady without walker or other support	= 2	

5. Standing balance	Unsteady	= 0
	Steady but wide stance (medial heels > 4 inches apart) and uses cane or other support	= 1
	Narrow stance without support	= 2
6. Nudged (subject at max position with feet as close together as possible, examiner pushes lightly on subject's sternum with palm of hand 3 times)	Begins to fall	= 0
	Staggers, grabs, catches self	= 1
	Steady	= 2
7. Eyes closed (at maximum position #6)	Unsteady	= 0
	Steady	= 1
8. Turning 360 degrees	Discontinuous steps	= 0
	Continuous steps	= 1
	Unsteady (grabs, swaggers)	= 0
	Steady	= 1
9. Sitting down	Unsafe (misjudged distance, falls into chair)	= 0
	Uses arms or not a smooth motion	= 1
	Safe, smooth motion	= 2

(continued)

TABLE 9.4　Balance and Gait Evaluation *(continued)*

GAIT

Patient's Name: _____　**Date:** _____

Location: _____　**Rater:** _____

Initial Instructions: Subject stands with examiner, walks down hallway or across the room, first at "usual" pace, then back at "rapid, but safe" pace (using usual walking aids).

Task	Description of gait	Possible	Score
10. Initiation of gait (immediately after told to "go")	Any hesitancy or multiple attempts to start	= 0	
	No hesitancy	= 1	
11. Step length and height	a. Right swing foot does not pass left stance foot with step	= 0	
	b. Right foot passes left stance foot	= 1	
	c. Right foot does not clear floor completely with step	= 0	
	d. Right foot completely clears floor	= 1	
	e. Left swing foot does not pass right stance foot with step	= 0	
	f. Left foot passes right stance foot	= 1	
	g. Left foot does not clear floor completely with step	= 0	
	h. Left foot completely clears floor	= 1	

12. Step symmetry
- Right and left step length not equal (estimate) = 0
- Right and left step appear equal = 1

13. Step continuity
- Stopping or discontinuity between steps = 0
- Steps appear continuous = 1

14. Path (estimated in relation to floor tiles, 12-inch diameter; observe excursion of 1 foot over about 10 feet of the course).
- Marked deviation = 0
- Mild/moderate deviation or uses walking aid = 1
- Straight without walking aid = 2

15. Trunk
- Marked sway or uses walking aid = 0
- No sway but flexion of knees or back, or spreads arms out while walking = 1
- No sway, no flexion, no use of arms, and no use of walking aid = 2

16. Walking stance
- Heels apart = 0
- Heels almost touching while walking = 1

Gait Score:

Balance + Gait Score:

Medications are frequently listed as a major risk factor for falls in the elderly. The use of any benzodiazepine or other sedative-hypnotic agent and the use of more than four prescription medications have been targeted as risk factors for falls in older adults. Diuretic agents, antihypertensives, and other cardiovascular agents may cause unpredictable fluctuations in blood pressure, with concurrent postural hypotension. Tricyclic antidepressants, phenothiazines, anxiolytics, and narcotics all exhibit central nervous system effects that can lead to impaired cognition, altered reaction time, and decreased coordination. Tardive dyskinesia, which influences gait and balance, has been associated with the phenothiazines and other neuroleptic medications and may persist after these medications are discontinued.

Neurologic problems such as stroke, peripheral neuropathy, and Parkinson's disease, as well as cardiac disease (particularly atrial fibrillation), can put older adults at increased risk of falls because of the impact of these physical problems on function (Resnick, 1999). Musculoskeletal problems such as degenerative joint disease and osteoporosis can alter body position and balance (i.e., increased anteroposterior diameter noted with osteoporosis); this may impair function and put the individual at risk for falls.

Careful assessment of the environment in the acute care setting is very useful for establishing extrinsic risks for falls. All furniture, including beds, should be the proper height for the older adult to transfer. Ideally, the individual's feet should reach the floor comfortably when sitting, and all chairs should have arms to facilitate transfers. Bathrooms should be evaluated for the presence of grab bars, raised toilet seats if necessary, a shower chair, and nonskid mats for the tub/shower.

Risk factors for significant injury from falls should be considered during the risk assessment. These risk factors include current use of antiocoagulants such as Coumadin, Plavix, and aspirin. Use of these agents puts the older adult at increased risk of bleeding following a fall. Patients who have a history of osteoporosis, in particular, are at increased risk of fracture following a fall, with the most common sites being the hip, wrist, and spine. Older adults who have muscle and fat malnutrition are likewise at increased risk of trauma postfall due to the lack of tissue to help absorb the impact of the falls. Hip protectors, such as Safehip™, should be recommended to individuals who are significantly at risk not only for a fall but also for a possible injury postfall.

INTERVENTION/CARE STRATEGIES

STEP 2: DEVELOPMENT OF AN INDIVIDUALIZED FALLS PREVENTION INTERVENTION

Prevention of falls should be considered as part of routine care for all older adults in the acute care setting. Table 9.5 describes ideal routine fall prevention care. The interventions should focus on areas of risk for the individual (Table 9.6), such as environmental challenges, functional limitations, and drug-related problems such as orthostatic hypotension related to a medication or delirium caused by the addition of a sleeping pill. Several approaches to decrease the risk of falls and prevent falls, related to specific problems identified in the initial risk evaluation, will be briefly described.

Identifying those older individuals with a known history of a fall is a quick way to inform all care providers that this individual requires special fall prevention interventions. Identification can be done by using a sticker by the patient's door or on the chart or by using a special color for his or her hospital identification band. Any information obtained about what occurred or what the patient was doing at the time of a fall is also useful.

Acknowledging that there may be a fear of falling and encouraging the patient to discuss feelings related to the fall is a useful way to explore the patient's fear and how it may impact function. In addition, strengthening the individual's belief in his or her ability to safely transfer and ambulate, rather than reinforcing his or her risk of falling, can help to decrease fear and increase participation in functional activities.

Setting up a bladder training program in which the patient is encouraged or helped to ambulate to the bathroom at regular intervals, both day and night, can decrease the risk of falling. Likewise, maintaining regular bowel function will decrease the need for laxatives, which can put the individual at risk for urgently wanting to get to the bathroom and sustaining a fall.

If findings suggest that there is a delirium, reversible causes should be eliminated. Management of cognitive impairment should focus on maintaining a safe environment. This is best done by providing the individual with appropriate cues to help him or her remember how to manage in the environment and by structuring the environment.

TABLE 9.5   Standard Fall Prevention for All Older Adults

1. Familiarize patient with environment (e.g., identify call light and bathroom; may need to label).
2. Maintain call bell in reach, and have patient demonstrate ability to call for the nurse.
3. Place bed in low position with brakes locked.
4. Ensure that footwear is fitted, nonslip, and used properly.
5. Determine appropriate use of side rails based on cognitive and functional status.
6. Use night light.
7. Keep floor surfaces clean and dry.
8. Keep room uncluttered, and make sure that furniture is in optimal condition.
9. Make sure patient knows where personal possessions are and that he or she can safely access them.
10. Ensure adequate handrails in bathroom, room, and hallway.
11. Establish a plan of care to maintain bowel and bladder function.
12. Evaluate effects of medications that increase the individual's risk of falling.
13. Encourage participation in functional activities and exercise at patient's highest possible level; refer to physical therapy as appropriate.
14. Monitor patient regularly.
15. Education patient and family regarding fall prevention strategies.

Ideally, the cause of the dizziness should be identified and eliminated. If the dizziness is related to inner ear/vertigo, the patient can be taught to avoid positions that exacerbate the dizziness, exercises may be instituted, or medications such as meclizine tried (however, the risk of anticholinergic side effects must be considered). In all cases, individuals with dizziness should be encouraged to maintain adequate hydration to prevent exacerbation of the problem. A physical therapy/occupational therapy referral is helpful to facilitate functional activities safely.

Individuals who have had a decline in function after an acute event should be evaluated by physical or occupational therapist as soon as possible. Moreover, nursing care should focus on what the individual is capable of performing and encourage him or her to participate in activities at the highest level possible.

All medications should be reviewed based on their potential for causing a fall. Attempts should be made to decrease the dosages

TABLE 9.6   Interventions to Decrease Risk for Falls

Risk factors	Nursing interventions to decrease risk for the individual
History of falls	Identify the patient as being at risk for falls (may use sticker on chart or door).
Fear of falling	Encourage patient to verbalize feelings. Strengthen self-efficacy related to transfers and ambulation by providing verbal encouragement about capabilities and demonstrating to patient his or her ability to perform safely.
Bowel and bladder incontinence	Set up regular voiding schedule (q 2 h or as appropriate based on patient need). Monitor bowel function, and encourage sufficient fluids and fiber (8 8-ounce glasses daily and 24 grams of fiber). Use laxatives as appropriate.
Cognitive impairment	Evaluate patient for reversible causes of cognitive impairment/delirium, and eliminate causes as relevant. Monitor resident with cognitive impairment at least hourly with relocation of the patient so that nursing staff can observe/monitor regularly. Encourage family member(s) to hire staff or stay with patient continuously. Use monitoring devices if accessible (e.g., bed/chair or exit alarms).
Mood	Encourage verbalization of feelings. Evaluate patient's ability to concentrate and learn new information. Encourage engagement in daily activities. Refer to geriatric psychiatry as appropriate.
Dizziness	Monitor lying, sitting, and standing blood pressure, and continually evaluate for factors contributing to dizziness. Encourage adequate fluid intake (8 8-ounce glasses daily). Set up environment to avoid movements that result in dizziness/vertigo. If diabetic, monitor blood sugars, and facilitate interventions to maintain appropriate blood sugars.

(continued)

TABLE 9.6   Interventions to Decrease Risk for Falls *(continued)*

Risk factors	Nursing interventions to decrease risk for the individual
Functional impairment	Encourage participation in personal care activities at the highest level (i.e., if possible, encourage ambulation to bathroom rather than use of bedpan). Refer to physical and occupational therapy as appropriate. Facilitate adherence to exercise program when indicated.
Medications	Review medications with primary health care provider in the acute care setting, and determine need of each medication. Ascertain that medications are being used at lowest possible dosages to obtain desired results.
Medical problems	Work with primary health care provider in acute care settings to augment management of primary medical problems, such as Parkinson's disease, congestive heart failure, and anemia. Assure patient that medical problems are not a reason to remain in bed and prevent participation in functional activities.
Environment	Remove furniture if patient cannot sit on it and have his or her feet reach the floor. Remove clutter. Make sure furniture and any assistive devices used are in good condition. Make sure lighting is adequate. Make sure safety bars are available in bathroom.

and/or eliminate these drugs when possible. All attempts should be made to manage the older adult's symptoms nonpharmacologically rather than initiating a new medication. For example, in a patient with "sundowning," there are many nonpharmacologic treatment options that may be tried before initiating medications, such as asking the patient's family or a hired caregiver to sit with the individual;

moving the patient closer to the nursing station; and providing the patient with a known, simple activity (eating a sweet granola bar) rather than starting the patient on an anxiolytic medication as the first choice.

Management of underlying medical problems should be optimized. Recognition of sensory problems in the older adult is particularly important, and special consideration should be given to those individuals who report a history of macular degeneration or cataracts, which can significantly impair vision. The environment can then be adjusted to augment what vision the individual has.

In the acute care setting, it is particularly important to familiarize the patient with the new environment. This may need to be done repeatedly, and it may be beneficial to add cues such as large-print signs labeling the bathroom or closet and writing out how to call for a nurse.

EVALUATION

STEP 3: COMPREHENSIVE EVALUATION OF FALLS

Once a patient in the acute care setting has fallen, a comprehensive evaluation should be done to establish harm and the cause of the fall. Table 9.3 provides guidelines for what to evaluate at the time of the fall, and Table 9.7 offers guidelines for a more comprehensive assessment of the patient at the time of the fall to help identify the cause. Table 9.8 provides a guide for evaluating the patient and determining the contributing factors to the fall. This guide helps to identify not only the consequences of the fall but also the potential contributing factors. Although management of the acute problem postfall is essential, it is important to make sure that the initial evaluation of the fall risk and implementation of the plan of care to prevent falls are revised based on the findings from the fall.

STEP 4: REVISION OF THE INITIAL PLAN OF CARE FOR FALLS PREVENTION

Based on the information gleaned from the fall, revisions in the care plan should be made. Older patients are at increased risk for a subsequent fall just based on the fact that they have sustained a fall (Carson & Cook, 2000). Aggressive interventions should be implemented to decrease future falls (Table 9.6).

TABLE 9.7   Comprehensive Evaluation of the Patient at the Time of the Fall

I. Vital signs
   a. Heart rate _____
   b. Heart rhythm: regular _____   irregular _____
   c. Blood pressure: lying _____   standing _____

II. Physical exam
   a. Active, or independent range of motion:
      1. Neck _____ yes _____ no
      2. Shoulders Right: _____ yes _____ no   Left: _____ yes _____ no
      3. Wrists Right: _____ yes _____ no   Left: _____ yes _____ no
      4. Hands Right: _____ yes_____ no   Left: _____ yes _____ no
      5. Hips Right: _____ yes _____ no   Left: _____ yes _____ no
      6. Knees Right: _____ yes _____ no   Left: _____ yes _____ no
      7. Ankles Right: _____ yes _____ no   Left: _____ yes _____ no
      8. Feet Right: _____ yes _____ no   Left: _____ yes _____ no
   b. Observations of resident:
      1. Shortening and external rotation of lower extremities:
         Right: _____ Left: _____
      2. Swelling: Location _____
      3. Redness/bruising: Location _____
      4. Abrasions: Location _____
      5. Pain on movement: Location _____
      6. Shortness of breath: yes _____ no _____
      7. Impaired balance: yes _____ no _____
      8. Loss of consciousness: yes _____ no _____
      9. Change in cognition: yes _____ no _____
   c. Assessment of the environment:
      1. Dim lighting: yes _____ no _____
      2. Glare: yes _____ no _____
      3. Uneven flooring: yes _____ no _____
      4. Wet or slippery floor: yes _____ no _____
      5. Poor fit of seating device: yes _____ no _____
      6. Inappropriate footwear: yes _____ no _____
      7. Inappropriate eyewear: yes _____ no _____
      8. Loose carpet or throw rugs: yes _____ no _____
      9. Use of full-length side rails in bed: yes _____ no _____
     10. Lack of hallway rails in area of fall: yes _____ no _____
     11. Inappropriate assistive devices (fit or condition):
         yes _____ no _____
     12. Lack of grab bars in bathroom: yes _____ no _____
     13. Cluttered areas: yes _____ no _____
     14. Other environmental causes: _____

TABLE 9.8   Fall Prevention Information for Patient and Family

Working Together to Prevent Falls

- Falls can occur, especially when in a new environment and after an acute illness. But here at _____ hospital, we work together to prevent falls and to help you recover quickly and easily.

Fall Prevention Techniques

- Familiarize yourself with your surroundings.
- Get up and move as soon and as much as you can tolerate. This will help you regain and maintain your strength and prevent a fall.
- Feel free to use the rails and supports in the bathroom and hallways that we have provided to help maintain your safety.
- Bring any assistive devices that you use at home into your hospital room, and use these.
- Get up slowly from lying or sitting positions, and count to 10 before you stand or move.
- Wear shoes with good support and that are nonskid; avoid walking in stocking feet or wearing loose-fitting shoes.
- Report spills on your floor, and do not walk in the room until these are removed/cleaned.
- Keep items within your reach or call for assistance rather than leaning toward objects in an unsafe position.
- Call for assistance to go to the bathroom.

If You Fall, Don't Panic

- Stay calm and wait right where you are for help to arrive.
- If you can reach your call light, push that button. If not, call for the nurse to assist you.

The prevention of falls on an acute care unit should include all members of the health care team as well as the patient and his or her family. Patients and their families and/or caregivers are the core of the team; therefore, they should be provided with information on fall-prevention strategies on the unit and what is being done to prevent falls. A simple handout, for example, can explain why a wrist band is a certain color or why the bedrails go halfway down the bed. The philosophy of care on the unit should also be given to patients, families, and caregivers. Ideally, this philosophy should focus on encouraging patients to participate in functional activities at their highest possible level (Table 9.8). This might mean that the individual is encouraged to walk to the bathroom as soon as possible after stabilized from the acute event.

Electronic warning devices such as bed and chair alarms are suggested as an intervention to prevent falls (Pullen, Heikausn & Fusgen, 1999). Alarm systems are designed to alert nursing staff that a patient is getting up from the bed or a chair and for this reason is potentially at risk for falls. Indications for alarm systems include those patients with a history of falls, unsafe bed mobility, cognitive deficits, or confusion; those who are alone in the room; and those who are unable to use the call bell. The efficacy of an alarm system depends on effective technology and the response time of nursing staff. Examples of particular devices and how to obtain them are provided in Table 9.9.

It is important to monitor the outcomes of the fall prevention program and to determine how effective the program actually is in terms of fall and injury reduction. An established policy should assign accountability and responsibility for the ongoing monitoring and reevaluation of fall prevention assessments and interventions, keeping in mind that the fall prevention program should include a multidisciplinary approach. The policy should include (1) assessment criteria and frequency, (2) documentation requirements for assessment and interventions, and (3) methods to communicate changes in the intervention and plan of care. See Table 9.10 for evaluation of the patient postfall. Key elements that are useful to track include fall rate and injury index. Reporting fall rates rather than the number of falls is a more accurate measure of improvement. Fall rates are calculated by dividing the number of falls by patient days, then multiplying by 1,000 (Tinnetti, Williams, & Mayewski, 1986). These rates can vary by type of institution, patient acuity, and clinical service.

Classifications of severity of injury are also important quality indicators. The injury index is calculated by the number of injuries divided by the number of falls multiplied by 100. Hendrick and colleagues (1995) suggest that injuries be categorized into five classes: (1) no injury, (2) minor injury, (3) moderate injury, (4) major injury, and (5) death. Injury rates (classes 2–5) in acute care have been reported to range from 20% to 30% (Rhode, Myers, & Vlahou, 1990). Serious injuries (classes 4 and 5) have been reported to range from 2% to 6% (Morse, 1997). It is useful to report, by unit and overall hospital, the fall rate and injury index. In many cases, the fall rate will increase with the implementation of a fall prevention program because of heightened awareness of falls and increased reporting of fall events. With this phenomenon, however, there may be a decrease

TABLE 9.9 Devices for Fall Prevention

Device	Purpose
Tab alarms	Simplest and least expensive device that is triggered by tugging on a magnetic connection
Motion detectors	Used to detect motion in one part of a room, unit, or facility and alert caregivers
Visitor chimes	Used to sound a chime when there is inappropriate motion or activity in a room or on a unit
Pressure release alarms	Pads, mats, or other devices that go under a mattress or chair and that sound an alarm when there is a change of positioning
Distance devices	Most sophisticated of devices, as they can detect if an individual exceeds a certain distance from a bed or chair

in the injury index because of the increased reporting of minor falls that did not result in injury.

The location, time, and circumstances of a fall, as well as patient risk factors, should also be tracked. This information can help in identifying high-volume or peak time periods or areas where falls occur. These peaks can be reviewed to suggest adjustments in scheduling or routines to help staff further decrease the incidence of falls. Trends across units can then be addressed to augment the individualized approach taken for each patient. Documentation of the use of restraints and bed or chair alarms is also important in order to evaluate the effectiveness of the equipment and the appropriateness of the initial application.

SUMMARY

Implementing a fall prevention program in the acute care setting is both challenging and rewarding. To ensure that such a program will be fully implemented and carried out, all staff must engage in appropriate fall prevention activities. In addition, it may be necessary to provide ongoing education about fall prevention to staff, patients,

TABLE 9.10   Comprehensive Evaluation of the Patient Postfall to Determine the Cause of the Fall

I. Underlying medical problems
    a. Orthostatic hypotension: _____ yes _____ no
       Management: _____
    b. Balance problems: _____ yes _____ no   Management: _____
    c. Dizziness/vertigo: _____ yes _____ no   Management: _____
    d. Other: _____ yes _____ no   Management: _____

II. Medications
    a. Drugs that may contribute to fall:
       Diuretics: _____ yes _____ no   Management: _____
       Cardiovascular medications: _____ yes _____ no
          Management: _____
       Antipsychotics: yes _____ yes _____ no   Management: _____
       Antianxiety agents: _____ yes _____ no   Management: _____
       Sleeping agents: _____ yes _____ no   Management: _____
       Antidepressants: _____ yes _____ no   Management: _____

III. Functional status
    a. Impaired sitting balance: _____ yes _____ no
       Management: _____
    b. Impaired standing balance: _____ yes _____ no
       Management: _____
    c. Independent ambulation: _____ yes _____ no
       Management: _____
    d. Independent toileting: _____ yes _____ no
       Management: _____

IV. Sensory problems
    a. Evidence of impaired vision: _____ yes _____ no
       Management: _____
    b. Evidence of impaired sensation: _____ yes _____ no
       Management: _____
    c. Evidence of impaired hearing: _____ yes _____ no
       Management: _____

V. Psychological status
    a. Evidence of depression: _____ yes _____ no
       Management: _____
    b. Evidence of change in cognition: _____ yes _____ no
       Management: _____
    c. Evidence of impaired judgment: _____ yes _____ no
       Management: _____

and patients' families. Although the challenges of implementation may be great, the rewards are many. The intention of a fall prevention program in acute care is not only to prevent falls, but also to provide patients with nursing care that focuses on improving and maintaining the functional ability of older patients. The step approach presented here provides nurses in the acute care setting with an easy and effective way to implement a fall prevention program and to raise the level of care provided to older patients in the acute care setting.

REFERENCES

Arfken, C., Lach, H., Birge, S., & Miller, J. (1994). The prevalence and correlates of fear of falling in elderly persons living in the community. *American Journal of Public Health, 84,* 565–569.

Carson, M., & Cook, J. (2000). A strategic approach to falls prevention. *Clinical Performance and Quality Health Care, 8,* 136–141.

Folstein, M., Folstein, S., & McHugh, P. (1975). Mini-mental state: A practical method for grading the cognitive state of patients for the clinician. *Journal of Psychiatric Research, 12,* 189–198.

Gray-Miceli, D. (1997). Falling among the aged. *Advance for Nurse Practitioners, 13,* 41–44.

Halfon, P., Eggli, Y., Van Melle, G., & Vagnair, A. (2001). Risk of falls for hospitalized patients: A predictive model based on routinely available data. *Journal of Clinical Epidemiology, 54,* 1258–1266.

Hendrick, A., Nyhuis, A., Kppenbrock, T., & Soja, M. (1995). Hospital falls: Development of a predictive model for clinical practice. *Applied Nursing Research, 8*(3), 129–139.

Kannus, P., Parkkari, J., Koskinen, S., Niemi, S., Palvanen, M., Jarvinen, M. & Vuori, I. (1999). Fall induced injuries and deaths among older adults. *Journal of the American Medical Association, 189,* 1895–1899.

Krueger, P., Brazil, K., & Lohfeld, L. (2001). Risk factors for falls and injuries in a long term care facility in Ontario. *Canadian Journal of Public Health, 92,* 117–120.

Lachman, M. E., Howland, J., Tennstedt, S., Jette, A., Assmann, S., & Peterson, E. W. (1998). Fear of falling and activity restriction: The survey of activities and fear of falling in the elderly (SAFE). *Journal of Gerontology: A Psychological Sciences and Social Sciences, 53,*(1), 43–50.

Lord, S., & Fitzpatrick, R. (2001). Choice stepping reaction time: A composite measure of falls risk in older people. *Journal of Gerontology Biological Sciences Medicine and Science, 56*(10), 627–632.

Magaziner, J., Hawkes, W., Hebel, R., Zimmerman, S., Fox, K, Dolan, M., Felsenthal, G., & Kenzora, J. (2000). Recovery from hip fracture in eight areas of function. *Journal of Gerontology Medical Sciences, 55A*(9), 498–507.

Morse, J. (1997). *Preventing Patient Falls.* Thousand Oaks, CA: Sage.

Norwalk, M., Prendergast, J., Bayles, C., D'Amico, F., & Colvin, G. (2001). A randomized trial of exercise programs among older individuals living in two long term care facilities: The FallsFREE program. *Journal of the American Geriatrics Society, 49,* 859–865.

Norton, R., Campbell, A., Lee-Joe, T., Robinson, E., & Butler, M. (1997). Circumstances of falls resulting in hip fractures among older people. *Journal of the American Geriatrics Society, 45,* 1108–1112.

Pullen, R., Heikaus, C., & Fusgen, I. (1999). Falls of geriatric patients at the hospital. *Journal of the American Geriatrics Society, 47,* 1480–1481.

Ray, W., & Griffin, M. (1990). Prescribed medications, and the risk of falling. *Topics in Geriatric Rehabilitation, 5,* 12–20.

Resnick, B. (1998). Health care practices of the old-old. *American Academy Journal of Nurse Practitioners, 10,* 147–155.

Resnick, B. (1999). Falls in a community of older adults: Putting research into practice. *Clinical Nursing Research, 8,* 251–267.

Resnick, B., Cocoran, M., & Spellbring, A. M. (2001). Gait and balance disorders in the older adult. In A. Adelman & M. Daly (Eds.), *20 common problems in geriatric medicine* (pp. 277–309). New Jersey: McGraw-Hill.

Rhode, J., Myers, A., & Vlahov, D. (1990). Variation in risk for falls by clinical department: Implications for prevention. *Infectious Control Hospital Epidemiology, 11,* 21–22.

Thapa, P., Borckman, K., Gideon, P., Fought, R., & Ray, W. (1996). Injurious falls in risk nonambulatory nursing home residents: A comparative study of circumstances, incidence, and factors. *Journal of the American Geriatrics Society, 44,* 273–278.

Tinetti, M. (1989). Instability and falling in elderly patients. *Seminars in Neurology, 9,* 39–45.

Tinetti, M. (1997). Falls. In C. Cassel et al. (Eds.), *Geriatric Medicine* (3rd ed., pp. 787–799). New York: Springer-Verlag.

Tinetti, M., Williams, T., & Mayewski, R. (1986). Fall risk index for elderly patients based on number of chronic disabilities. *American Journal of Medicine, 80,* 429–434.

Tinetti, M. E. (1986). Performance oriented assessment of mobility problems in elderly patients. *Journal of the American Geriatrics Society, 34,* 119–126.

Chapter 10

PREVENTING PRESSURE ULCERS AND SKIN TEARS

Elizabeth A. Ayello

EDUCATIONAL OBJECTIVES

On completion of this chapter, the reader should be able to
1. Do a pressure ulcer risk assessment.
2. Identify risk factors associated with pressure ulcer development.
3. Interpret the meaning of an individual's risk assessment score.
4. Develop a comprehensive, holistic plan to prevent pressure ulcers in individuals at risk.
5. Classify skin tears.
6. Identify elders at risk for skin tears.
7. Develop a plan to prevent and treat skin tears.

Preserving skin integrity is an important aspect of nursing care. Florence Nightingale (1859) herself identified a link between skin injury (specifically, pressure ulcers) and nursing. Doing a risk assessment and implementing a consistent prevention protocol may prevent some types of skin injuries. Although pressure ulcers and skin tears may look similar, they are different types of skin injury. It is important therefore to assess the wound and to determine the correct etiology so that the proper treatment plan can be implemented.

PRESSURE ULCERS

Pressure ulcers are a significant health care problem. The National Pressure Ulcer Advisory Panel (NPUAP; "Pressure Ulcers Prevalence," 1989, p. 25) defines these chronic wounds as "localized areas of tissue necrosis that develop when soft tissue is compressed between a bony prominence and an external surface for a prolonged period of time." The primary location for the development of pressure ulcers is on the sacrum, with heels being secondary (Cuddigan, Ayello, & Sussman, 2001). After an extensive data analysis, the NPUAP (2001) concluded that pressure ulcer prevalence in acute care facilities in the United States ranges from 10% to 18% with the best current estimate of pressure ulcer prevalence being 15%. The prevalence of a disease is the number of both old and new cases (of the disease/disorder) in a proportion of a population at any one point in time. Prevalence ranges from 2.3% to 28% in long-term care facilities and 0% to 29% in home care settings. Pressure ulcer incidence in acute care facilities ranges from 0.4% to 38%, with 7% being the current best estimate. Incidence ranges from 2.2% to 23.9% in long-term care and 0% to 17% in home care (Cuddigan et al., 2001). The incidence of a disease is the rate at which new cases occur in a population during a specified period.

Pressure ulcers are associated with complications including cellulitis, osteomyelitis, sepsis, increased length of stays, and financial and emotional costs (Agency for Health Care Policy and Research [AHCPR], 1992). These ulcers occur from a combination of intensity and duration of pressure as well as from tissue tolerance (Bergstrom, Braden, Laguzza, & Holman, 1987; Braden & Bergstrom, 1987, 1989). Immobility as seen in bed-bound or chair-bound patients and those unable to change positions, undernourishment or malnutrition, incontinence, friable skin, impaired cognitive ability, and decreased ability to respond to one's environment are among the identified risk factors for pressure ulcers (Braden, 1998). No one single factor puts a patient at risk for pressure ulcer skin breakdown.

A link between pressure ulcers and nursing was forged by Nightingale (1859). Recent regulatory and government initiatives continue to support the idea of the importance of pressure ulcer prevention in health care. There now is an objective in *Healthy People 2010* to reduce the incidence of pressure ulcers (U.S. Department of Health and Human Services, [USDHHS], 2000). The Centers for Medicare and Medicaid Services (CMS), formerly the Health Care Financing Administration (HCFA), considers the occurrence of a pressure ulcer in a low-risk resident in a long-term care facility to be a sentinel event (HCFA, 2000). Thus, at the beginning of the 21st century, appropriate risk assessment and prevention care take on even more important meaning. Nurses will find the NPUAP competencies for registered nurses on pressure ulcer prevention helpful in guiding their professional practice (see Table 10.1).

The Agency for Health Research and Quality (AHRQ), formerly the AHCPR (AHCPR, 1992) recommends that patients be assessed for pressure ulcer development on admission to a facility, then reassessed periodically. Ayello and Braden (2001, 2002) suggested reassessment intervals based on specific care settings. In acute care, reassess every 48 hours or whenever the patient's condition changes. In long-term care, research has shown that most pressure ulcers occur soon after admission (Bergstrom & Braden, 1992), so reassess these patients weekly for the first 4 weeks, then at least monthly to quarterly or whenever the patient's condition changes. In home care, reassessment for pressure ulcer risk should occur at each nursing visit. Research by Bergstrom and Braden (1992) found no difference in risk assessment scores done by time of day. Thus, in the acute and long-term care setting, risk assessment can be done on either the day or evening shift, depending on which works best for the facility.

RISK ASSESSMENT

The AHRQ Panel Guidelines (AHCPR, 1992) recommend that an assessment for pressure ulcer risk be done using a valid and reliable assessment tool. Although there are several risk assessment scales available, research supports only the reliability and validity of the Norton and Braden scale; therefore, they are the only scales mentioned in the 1992 AHRQ prevention guidelines.

The Braden Scale was created in 1987 as part of a research study (Bergstrom, Braden, Braden, Laguzza, & Holman, 1987). Each of its six factors assesses the etiologic factors in pressure ulcer development.

TABLE 10.1   National Pressure Ulcer Advisory Panel

Purpose:

To prepare registered nurses with the minimum competencies for pressure ulcer prevention.

Competencies:

1. Identify etiologic factors contributing to pressure ulcer occurrence.
2. Identify risk factors for pressure ulcer development.
3. Recognize the presence of factors affecting tissue tolerance.
4. Conduct risk assessment using a valid and reliable tool.
5. Conduct a thorough skin assessment taking into account the individual's uniqueness.
6. Develop and implement an individualized program of skin care.
7. Demonstrate proper positioning to decrease pressure ulcer occurrence.
8. Select and use support surfaces as indicated by risk status.
9. Use nutritional interventions as appropriate to prevent incident pressure ulcers.
10. Accurately document results of risk assessment, skin assessment, and prevention strategies.
11. Apply critical thinking skills to clinical decision making regarding the impact of changes in the individual's condition on pressure ulcer risk.
12. Make referrals to other health care professionals based on client assessment.

Source: National Pressure Ulcer Advisory Panel. (2001). *Pressure ulcer prevention: A competency-based curriculum.* Accessed: www.npuap.org/prevwrr.pdf.

Sensory perception, mobility, and activity address clinical situations that predispose the patient to intense and prolonged pressure. Moisture, nutrition, and friction/shear address factors that alter tissue tolerance for pressure. Each of the six categories is ranked with a numerical score, with 1 representing the lowest possible subscore. The sum of the six subscores is the final Braden score, which can range from 6 to 23. Braden Scale scores are as follows: 1 = highly impaired, 3–4 = moderate to low impairment, total points possible = 23, risk-predicting score = 16 or less.

Low Braden Scale scores indicate that a patient is at risk for pressure ulcers. The risk score for the Braden Scale was originally determined to be 16 (Bergstrom et al., 1987). Further research in the elderly (Bergstrom & Braden, 1992) and in persons with darkly pigmented skin (Lyder et al., 1999, 1998) indicates that a risk score of

18 should be used in patients from these populations. The prevention protocols should be initiated for patients whose Braden Scale score is at or below the risk score.

Use of prevention protocols has shown a 60% drop in pressure ulcer incidence as well as a decrease in severity of ulcers and cost of care (Braden & Bergstrom, 1989). Unfortunately, in another study, the use of an AHRQ prevention protocol shows that the decrease in pressure ulcer incidence and the increase in length of time before a pressure ulcer developed was not sustained over time (Xakellis, Frantz, Lewis, & Harvey, 2001). Frantz and Baranoski (2001) summarized studies from 1990–2000 about the effectiveness of pressure ulcer prevention in various settings. The prevention programs included risk assessment, pressure reduction interventions, and staff education. Pressure ulcer incidence declined in all studies regardless of setting. A decrease in incidence in the four long-term care studies ranged from 3.5% to 24%, which was more variable than the range in the five acute care studies of 11% to 16%. A process for implementing prevention guidelines using a systems approach was suggested by Bryant and Rolstead (2001).

When it comes to severity of pressure ulcers, race may make a difference. Ayello and Lyder (2001) analyzed and summarized the existing data about pressure ulcers across the skin pigmentation spectrum. Lyder (1991, 1996) pioneered research about incidence rates and stage I pressure ulcers in Blacks and Latinos. Blacks have the lowest incidence (19%) of superficial tissue damage classified as stage I pressure ulcers, and Whites have the highest, at 46% (Barczak, Barnett, Childs, & Bosley, 1997). The more severe tissue injury seen in stages II–IV pressure ulcers is higher in persons with darkly pigmented skin (Barczak et al., 1997; Meehan, 1990, 1994). Three national surveys showed that Blacks had 39% (Barczak et al., 1997), 16% (Meehan, 1990), and 41% (Meehan, 1994) higher incidence of stage II pressure ulcers. Subsequent studies by Lyder and colleagues (1998, 1999) continue to support a higher incidence of pressure ulcers in persons with darkly pigmented skin. Therefore, early identification of stage I pressure ulcers in this population is critical.

Lack of sensitivity and specificity by clinicians assessing patients with darkly pigmented skin may contribute to the increased severity and incidence of higher stage pressure ulcers (Barczak et al., 1997; Henderson et al., 1997; Lyder et al., 1998, 1999). Inadequate detection of stage I pressure ulcers in persons with darkly pigmented skin may be because clinicians erroneously believe that dark skin tolerates pressure better than light skin (Bergstrom, Braden, Kemp, Champagne, & Ruby, 1996) or that only color changes (see Table 10.2 on NPUAP stage I definitions) indicate an ulcer (Barczak et al., 1997; Bennett, 1995; Henderson et al., 1997; Lyder, 1996; Lyder et al., 1998, 1999). Bennett (1995, p. 35) defined darkly pigmented skin as "the obvious color of intact dark skin which remains unchanged when pressure is applied over a bony prominence." In 1998, the NPUAP approved a revised definition of a stage I pressure ulcer to include assessment variables other than color, specifically, skin temperature, skin consistency, and sensation (NPUAP, 1998).

Research has begun to validate these assessment characteristics in the new stage I definitions. Lyder and colleagues (2001) reported a higher diagnostic accuracy rate of 78% using the revised definition compared with 58% with the original definition. Sprigle, Linden,

TABLE 10.2 NPUAP Pressure Ulcer Staging System

Stage I

A stage I pressure ulcer is an observable pressure-related alteration of intact skin whose indicators as compared with the adjacent or opposite area on the body may include changes in one or more of the following: skin temperature (warmth or coolness), tissue consistency (firm or boggy feel), and sensation (pain, itching). The ulcer appears as a defined area of persistent redness in lightly pigmented skin, whereas in darker skin tones, the ulcer may appear with persistent red, blue, or purple hues.

Stage II

Partial-thickness skin loss involving epidermis, dermis, or both. The ulcer is superficial and presents clinically as an abrasion, blister, or shallow crater.

Stage III

Full-thickness skin loss involving damage to, or necrosis of, subcutaneous tissue that may extend down to, but not through, underlying fascia. The ulcer presents clinically as a deep crater with or without undermining of adjacent tissue.

Stage IV

Full-thickness skin loss with extensive destruction, tissue necrosis, or damage to muscle, bone, or supporting structures (e.g., tendon, joint capsule). Undermining and sinus tracts also may be associated with stage IV pressure ulcers.

McKenna, Davis, and Riordan (2001) found changes in skin temperature, in particular, that warmth, then coolness, accompanied most stage I pressure ulcers.

Clinicians should pay careful attention to a variety of factors when assessing a client with darkly pigmented skin for stage I pressure ulcers. Differences in skin over bony prominences (e.g., the sacrum and the heels) as compared with surrounding skin may be indicators of a stage I pressure ulcer. The skin should be assessed for alterations in pain or feeling. Also, a change of skin color should be noted by knowing the range of skin pigmentation that is normal for your particular patient (Bennett, 1995; Henderson et al., 1997). The correct lighting source is important to accurately perform this assessment. Use natural or halogen light when performing the assessment (Bennett, 1995). Fluorescent light should be avoided, as it casts a bluish hue to the skin (Bennett, 1995).

Clinicians may find the application of the limited studies and expert opinion helpful in the early detection of skin injury as seen in stage I pressure ulcers in clients across the skin pigment continuum. Box 10.1 presents a nursing standard of practice protocol for pressure ulcer prevention.

SKIN TEARS

Skin tears are traumatic wounds caused by shear and friction (O'Regan, 2002). This skin injury occurs when the epidermis is separated from the dermis (Malone, Rozario, Gavinski, & Goodwin, 1991). Because aging skin has a thinner epidermis, a flatter epidermis and dermis junction, and decreased epidermal ridges, elderly persons are more prone to skin injury from mechanical trauma (Baranoski, 2000; Payne & Martin, 1993; White, Karam, & Cowell, 1994). Therefore, skin tears are common in the elderly, with over 1.5 million occurring annually in institutionalized adults in the United States (Thomas, Goode, LaMaster, Tennyson, & Parnell, 1999). Skin tears are frequently located at areas of age-related purpura (Malone et al., 1991; White, 1994).

ASSESSMENT OF THE PROBLEM

The following areas should be assessed for skin tears: shins, face, dorsal aspect of hands, and plantar aspect of the foot (Malone et al., 1991). Besides elders, others with thinning skin who are at risk for

---

**BOX 10.1   Nursing Standard of Practice Protocol:
Pressure Ulcer Prevention**

I. GOALS
  A. Prevention of pressure ulcers (PU)
  B. Early recognition of PU development/skin changes
II. BACKGROUND/STATEMENT OF PROBLEM
  A. Prevalence: 15%
    1. acute care range: 10% to 18%
    2. long-term care range: 2.3% to 28%
    3. home care range: 0% to 29%
  B. Incidence: 7%
    1. acute care range: 0.4% to 38%
    2. long-term care range: 2.2% to 23.9%
    3. home care range: 0% to 17%
  C. *Healthy People 2010* objective: Reduce the proportion of nursing
     home residents with a current diagnosis of pressure ulcers.
  D. A sentinel event in long-term care (HCFA, 2000)
  E. Definition(s)
    1. PU are "localized areas of tissue necrosis that develop when
       soft tissue is compressed between a bony prominence and an
       external surface for a prolonged period of time" (NPUAP,
       2001, p. 181).
    2. Shear is "mechanical force that acts on a unit area of skin in a
       direction parallel to the body's surface. Shear is affected by
       the amount of pressure exerted, the coefficient of friction
       between the materials contacting each other, and the extent
       to which the body makes contact with the support surface"
       (AHCPR, 1994, p. 117).
    3. Friction is "mechanical forces exerted when skin is dragged
       across a coarse surface such as bed linens" (AHCPR, 1994,
       p. 110).
  F. Etiology and/or Epidemiology
    1. Risk factors (immobility, under or malnutrition, incontinence,
       friable skin, impaired cognitive ability)
    2. Higher incidence stage II and higher in persons with darkly
       pigmented
III. PARAMETERS OF ASSESSMENT
  A. Assess for intrinsic and extrinsic risk factors
  B. Braden Scale risk score
    1. 18 or below for elderly and persons with darkly pigmented
       skin
    2. 16 or below for other adults

BOX 10.1 *(continued)*

IV. NURSING CARE STRATEGIES/INTERVENTIONS
   A. Risk assessment documentation
      1. On admission to a facility
      2. Reassessment intervals whenever the client's condition changes and based on patient care setting:
         • acute care: every 48 hours
         • long-term care: weekly for first 4 weeks, then monthly/quarterly
         • home care: every nursing visit
      3. Use a reliable and standardized tool for doing a risk assessment, such as the Braden Scale (available at http://www.bradenscale.com/braden.PDF)
      4. Document risk assessment scores, and implement prevention protocols based on cutscore.
   B. General care issues and interventions
      1. Culturally sensitive early assessment for stage I pressure ulcers in clients with darkly pigmented skin
         a. Use a halogen light to look for skin color changes—may be purple hues.
         b. Compare skin over bony prominences to surrounding skin—may be boggy or stiff, warm or cooler.
      2. AHCPR (1992) prevention recommendations:
         • Assess skin daily.
         • Clean skin at time of soiling—avoid hot water and irritating cleaning agents.
         • Use moisturizers on dry skin.
         • Do not massage bony prominences.
         • Protect skin of incontinent clients from exposure to moisture.
         • Use lubricants, protective dressings, and proper lifting techniques to avoid skin injury from friction/shear during transferring and turning of clients.
         • Turn and position bed-bound clients every 2 hours if consistent with overall care goals.
         • Use a written schedule for turning and repositioning clients.
         • Use pillows or other devices to keep bony prominences from direct contact with each other.
         • Raise heels of bed-bound clients off the bed; do not use donut-type devices.
         • Use a 30 degree lateral side lying position; do not place clients directly on their trochanter.

(continued)

BOX 10.1   Nursing Standard of Practice Protocol:
Pressure Ulcer Prevention *(continued)*

- Keep head of the bed at lowest height possible.
- Use lifting devices (trapeze, bed linen) to move clients rather than dragging them in bed during transfers and position changes.
- Use pressure-reducing devices (static air, alternating air, gel or water mattresses).
- Reposition chair- or wheelchair-bound clients every hour. In addition, if client is capable, have him or her do small weight shifts every 15 minutes.
- Use a pressure-reducing device (not a donut) for chair-bound clients.

3. Other care issues and interventions
   a. Keep the patient as active as possible; encourage mobilization.
   b. Do not massage reddened bony prominences.
   c. Avoid positioning the patient directly on his or her trochanter.
   d. Avoid using donut-shaped devices.
   e. Avoid drying out the patient's skin; use lotion after bathing.
   f. Avoid hot water and soaps that are drying when bathing elderly.
   g. Teach patient, caregivers, and staff the prevention protocols.
   h. Manage moisture:
      - Manage moisture by determining the cause; use absorbent pad that wicks moisture.
      - Offer a bedpan or urinal in conjunction with turning schedules.
   i. Manage nutrition:
      - Consult a dietitian, and correct nutritional deficiencies by increasing protein and calorie intake and A, C, or E vitamin supplements as needed.
      - Offer a glass of water with turning schedules to keep patient hydrated.
   j. Manage friction and shear:
      - Elevate the head of the bed no more than 30 degrees.
      - Have the patient use a trapeze to lift self up in bed.
      - Staff should use a lift sheet or mechanical lifting device to move patient.
      - Protect high-risk areas such as elbows, heels, sacrum, and back of head from friction injury.

BOX 10.1   *(continued)*

C. Interventions linked to Braden risk scores (Adapted from Ayello
& Braden, 2001)

Prevention protocols linked to Braden risk scores are as follows:

At risk: score of 15–18
- Frequent turning; consider q 2 h schedule; use a written schedule.
- Maximize patient's mobility.
- Protect patient's heels.
- Use a pressure-reducing support surface if patient is bed- or chair-bound.

Moderate risk: score of 13–14
Same as above, but provide foam wedges for 30 degree lateral position.

High risk: score of 10–12
- Same as above, but add the following.
  - Increase the turning frequency.
  - Do small shifts of position.

Very high risk: score of 9 or below
- Same as above, but use a pressure-relieving surface.
- Manage moisture, nutrition, and friction/shear.

V. EVALUATION/EXPECTED OUTCOMES
  A. Patient
    1. Skin will remain intact.
    2. Pressure ulcer will heal.
  B. Provider/nurse
    1. Nurses will accurately perform PU risk assessment using standardized tool.
    2. Nurses will implement PU prevention protocols for clients interpreted as at risk for PU.
    3. Nurses will perform a skin assessment for early detection of pressure ulcers.
  C. Institution
    1. Reduction in development of new pressure ulcers.
    2. Increased number of risk assessments performed.
    3. Cost-effective prevention protocols developed.
VI. FOLLOW-UP MONITORING OF CONDITION
  A. Monitor effectiveness of prevention interventions.
  B. Monitor healing of any existing pressure ulcers.

skin tears are patients on long-term steroid therapy, women with decreased hormone levels, persons with peripheral vascular disease or neuropathy (due to decreased sensation, making them more susceptible to injury), and those with inadequate nutritional intake (O'Regan, 2002).

The three-group risk assessment tool, developed during a research study by White and colleagues (1994), may be employed to assess for risk of skin tears. Within the tool, there are three groups delineated by level of risk: group I, II, and III. Group I refers to a positive history of skin tears within the last 90 days or skin tears that are already present. A positive score in this group requires that the patient be put on a skin tear prevention protocol. Group II includes the following six items: (1) decision-making skills are either impaired or slightly impaired, or extensive assistance/total dependence for activities of daily living (ADLs) is noted; (2) wheelchair assistance needed; (3) loss of balance; (4) bed or chair confined; (5) unsteady gait; and (6) bruises. If a patient has a score of 4 or more items in Group II, then implement a skin tear prevention protocol. Group III includes the following 14 items: (1) physically abusive; (2) resists ADL care; (3) agitation; (4) hearing impaired; (5) decreased tactile stimulation; (6) wheels self; (7) manually/mechanically lifted; (8) contractures of arms, legs, shoulders, and/or hands; (9) hemiplegia/hemiparesis; (10) trunk, partial, or total inability to balance or turn body; (11) pitting edema of legs; (12) open lesions on extremities; (13) three or four senile purpura on extremities; and (14) dry, scaly skin. Positive responses to five or more items in group III requires that the skin tear prevention protocol be implemented. Patients who have a combination of three items in group II and three items in group III also require that a skin tear prevention protocol be utilized.

Several authors have suggested protocols for high-risk patients to prevent skin tears (Baranoski, 2000; Mason, 1997; O'Regan, 2002; White et al., 1994). Box 10.2 gives guidelines for high-risk patients with skin tears.

BOX 10.2   Skin Tear Prevention Protocol

I. GOALS
   A. Prevent skin tears in elderly clients.
   B. Identify clients at risk for skin tears.
   C. Foster healing of skin tears by
      1. Retaining skin flap
      2. Providing a moist, nonadherent dressing
      3. Protecting the site from further injury
II. BACKGROUND/STATEMENT OF PROBLEM
   A. Traumatic wounds from mechanical injury of skin
   B. Need to clearly differentiate etiology of skin tears from pressure ulcers
   C. Common in the elderly, especially over areas of age-related purpura
III. PARAMETERS OF ASSESSMENT
   A. Use the three-group risk assessment tool (White et al., 1994) to assess for skin tear risk.
   B. Use the Payne-Martin (1993) classification system to assess clients for skin tear risk.
      • Category I: a skin tear without tissue loss
      • Category II: a skin tear with partial tissue loss
      • Category III: a skin tear with complete tissue loss, where the epidermal flap is absent
IV. NURSING CARE STRATEGIES/INTERVENTIONS
   A. Preventing skin tears
      1. Provide a safe environment:
         • Do a risk assessment of elderly patients on admission.
         • Implement prevention protocol for patients identified as at risk for skin tears.
         • Have patients wear long sleeves or pants to protect their extremities.
         • Have adequate light to reduce the risk of bumping into furniture or equipment.
         • Provide a safe area for wandering.
      2. Educate staff or family caregivers in the correct way of handling patients to prevent skin tears. Maintain nutrition and hydration:
         • Offer fluids between meals.
         • Use lotion, especially on dry skin on arms and legs, twice daily.
         • Obtain a dietary consultation.

(continued)

BOX 10.2   Skin Tear Prevention Protocol *(continued)*

3. Protect from self-injury or injury during routine care:
   - Use a lift sheet to move and turn patients.
   - Use transfer techniques that prevent friction or shear.
   - Pad bed rails, wheelchair arms, and leg supports.
   - Support dangling arms and legs with pillows or blankets.
   - Use nonadherent dressings on frail skin. If you must use tape, be sure it is made of paper, and remove it gently.
   - Use gauze wraps, stockinettes, or other wraps to secure dressings rather than tape.
   - Use emollient antibacterial soap.

B. Treating skin tears
   - Gently clean the skin tear with normal saline.
   - Let the area air dry or pat dry carefully.
   - Approximate the skin tear flap.
   - Apply petroleum-based ointment, Steri-Strips, or a moist nonadherent wound dressing.
   - Use caution if using film dressings, as skin damage can occur when removing dressings.
   - Consider putting an arrow to indicate the direction of the skin tear on the dressing to minimize any further skin injury during dressing removal.
   - Always assess the size of the skin tear; consider doing a wound tracing.
   - Document assessment and treatment findings.

V. EVALUATION/EXPECTED OUTCOMES
   A. No skin tears will occur in at risk clients.
   B. Skin tears that do occur will heal.

VI. FOLLOW-UP MONITORING OF CONDITION
   A. Continue to reassess for any new skin tears in elderly clients.

INTERVENTION/CARE STRATEGIES

If a skin tear does occur, it is important to correctly identify it and begin an appropriate plan of care. The Payne-Martin (1993) classification system may be used to describe skin tears. The three categories are:

- Category I: a skin tear without tissue loss
- Category II: a skin tear with partial tissue loss
- Category III: a skin tear with complete tissue loss, where the epidermal flap is absent

The usual healing time for skin tears is 3 to 10 days (Krasner, 1991). Although skin tears are prevalent in the elderly, there is no consistent approach to managing these skin injuries (Baranoski, 2000; O'Regan, 2002). One study (Edwards, Gaskill, & Nash, 1998) compared the use of four different types of dressings in treating skin tears in a nursing home: three occlusive (transparent film, hydrocolloid, and polyurethane foam) and one nonocclusive dressing of Steri-strips covered by a nonadhesive cellulose-polyester material. The nonocclusive dressing healed faster than the occlusive dressings. Another study by Thomas and colleagues (1999) found that complete healing of skin tears in elders in three nursing homes occurred better in opaque foam dressings when compared with transparent films.

Goals of care for skin tears include retaining the skin flap if present, providing a moist, nonadherent dressing, and protecting the site from further injury (O'Regan, 2002). A consensus protocol for treating skin tears based on suggested plans of care by several authors (Baranoski, 2000; Edwards et al., 1998; O'Regan, 2002) can be found in Table 10.2

CASE STUDY 1*

Mrs. Katie Wilson is a 78-year-old White widow who has been admitted to your acute care hospital unit with a diagnosis of right lower lobe pneumonia. Prior to admission, she was living alone in a two-bedroom apartment. She has had osteoarthritis for the past 20 years, which has limited her mobility, allowing her to ambulate only in her apartment. She is dependent on her neighbor for her grocery shopping. She does her own personal activities of daily living (bathing, dressing, etc.). She has been taking nonsteroidal anti-inflammatory agents for pain associated with her osteoarthritis. She has a son who lives on the opposite coast and is not available for daily care needs.

ADMISSION DATA

Physical Assessment and Pertinent Admission History

General.   Responds to verbal questioning, but is lethargic and does not communicate her needs. Over the past 4 days has been

___
* From the National Pressure Ulcer Advisory Panel (Available at www.npuap.org).

increasingly fatigued, spending most of her time in bed. Is very weak and unable to change her position independently.

Vital signs.   Temperature = 39.2° C, Respiration = 30 and shallow, Pulse = 112 apical and regular, Blood pressure = 96/56.

Weight = 95 pounds, Height = 5'4"

Abdominal.   Intake has been limited to half bowl of cereal twice a day and piece of toast and tea for lunch for the past 4 days. Last bowel movement was 3 days ago; + bowel sounds.

Cardiovascular.   Normal sinus rhythm (NSR), No S_3S_4 at apex, +1 pedal edema, faintly palpable pedal pulses; capillary refill 3 seconds.

Respiratory.   Crackles over right lower lobe, coughing periodically, productive of yellow mucus.

Renal.   Episodes of urinary incontinence for the past 4 days prior to admission. Now is voiding concentrated urine; occasionally incontinent of urine.

Integumentary.   Skin is warm, dry, translucent; tenting noted.

Laboratory data.   Hg 10, HCT 28, RBC = 3.2, WBC = 21,000 shift to the left. Albumin 3.0 g/dl, K = 3.1, BUN = 32 mg/100 ml

MEDICAL ORDERS

D_5½NS with 10 mEq KCL at 100 cc/hr
Bronchodilator inhaler 2 puffs q4h prn
Cephalosporin 1 g IV q 8 h
2 L oxygen via nasal cannula continuously
Colace 100 mg PO tid
Pulse oximetry monitoring continuously
Metamucil 1 package QD
Bedrest
Multivitamin 1 tablet QD
Respiratory toilet q shift
Tylenol 650 mg PO for temp > 38° C
Daily weights
Regular diet as tolerated

CASE STUDY 2

Mrs. Florence Feldman, 87 years old, presents with a diagnosis of senile dementia of the Alzheimer's type with impaired communication skills. She has a history of congestive heart failure and osteoporosis. Her history includes frequent falls, and she requires two-person assistance for ambulation. Her skin is thin and dry, resembling an onion; each arm and leg has a purpura area as well, with one skin tear category I on her lower right leg. She is 10 pounds below her ideal body weight. Laboratory values are total protein 5.5 g/dL, albumin 2.6 g/dL, BUN 28. She is verbally aggressive to the staff on whom she depends for assistance for ADLs.

Assessment of Mrs. Feldman on admission to your long-term care facility needs to be done. Because she already has a skin tear (right lower leg), she is positive in Category I of the Skin Tear Risk Assessment Tool developed by White and colleagues (1994). Other factors that would put her at risk are her thin, dry skin with four purpura present and poor nutritional status. Her dependence on staff for ADLs and assistance coupled with her dementia predispose her to skin injury during bathing and other ADL activities.

A skin tear prevention protocol needs to be implemented for Mrs. Feldman immediately. In order to achieve a safe environment for her, the staff must know how to approach her with her dementia. To address her nutrition and hydration risk factors, a dietary consultation should be performed. A plan to encourage frequent fluids and assist with eating should be implemented. To protect Mrs. Feldman's skin from additional injury, her family can be asked to bring in a soft fleece jogging suit for her to wear. The purpura areas on her arms and legs should be covered with stockinette or some other soft dressing to further protect these areas. Her bed rails and the arms and legs of her wheelchair should be padded. Staff should use the palm of their hands and a turn sheet when repositioning Mrs. Feldman in bed. Lotion can be applied twice a day to her dry skin.

SUMMARY

Skin is the largest organ, so pay attention to it. By doing so, you can prevent and treat skin integrity problems such as tears and pressure ulcers.

REFERENCES

Agency for Health Care Policy and Research. (1992, May). Panel for the prediction and prevention of pressure ulcers in adults. In *Pressure Ulcers in Adults: Prediction and Prevention* (Clinical Practice Guideline No. 3; AHCPR Pub. No. 92-0047). Rockville, MD: Author.

Ayello, E. A., & Braden, B. (2001). Why is pressure ulcer risk so important? *Nursing 2001, 31*(11), 74–79.

Ayello, E. A., & Braden, B. (2002). How and why to do pressure ulcer risk assessment. *Advances in Skin and Wound Care, 15*(3), 125–131.

Ayello, E. A., & Lyder, C. H. (2001). Pressure ulcers in persons of color: Race and ethnicity. In J. Cuddigan, E. A. Ayello, & C. Sussman (Eds.), *Pressure Ulcers in America: Prevalence, Incidence, and Implications for the Future* (pp. 153-162). Reston, VA: National Pressure Ulcer Advisory Panel.

Baranoski, S. (2000). Skin tears: The enemy of frail skin. *Advances in Skin and Wound Care, 13*(3), 123–126.

Barczak, C. A., Barnett, R. I., Childs, E. J., & Bosley, L. M. (1997). Fourth national pressure ulcer prevalence survey. *Advanced Wound Care, 10*(4), 18–26.

Bennett, M. A. (1995). Report of the task force on the implications for darkly pigmented intact skin in the prediction and prevention of pressure ulcers. *Advances in Wound Care, 8*(6), 34–35.

Bergstrom, N., and the AHCPR Treatment of Pressure Ulcers Guideline Panel. (1994). *Treatment of Pressure Ulcers* (Clinical Practice Guideline No. 15; AHCPR Pub. No. 95-0652). Rockville, MD: U.S. Department of Health and Human Services, Public Health Service, and Agency for Health Care Policy and Research.

Bergstrom, N., & Braden, B. (1992). A prospective study of pressure sore risk among institutionalized elderly. *Journal of the American Geriatrics Society, 40*, 747–758.

Bergstrom, N., Braden, B., Kemp, M., Champagne, M., & Ruby, E. (1996). Multi-site study of incidence of pressure ulcers and the relationship between risk level, demographic characteristics, diagnoses, and prescription of preventive interventions. *Journal of the American Geriatrics Society, 44*(1), 22–30.

Bergstrom, N., Braden, B. J., Laguzza, A., & Holman, V. (1987). The Braden Scale for predicting pressure sore risk. *Nursing Research, 36*, 205–210.

Braden, B. J. (1998). The relationship between stress and pressure sore formation. *Ostomy Wound Management, 44*(Suppl. 3A), 265–265.

Braden, B., & Bergstrom, N. (1987). A conceptual schema for the study of the etiology of pressure sores. *Rehabilitation Nursing, 12*(1), 8–16.

Braden, B., & Bergstrom, N. (1989). Clinical utility of the Braden Scale for predicting pressure sore risk. *Decubitus, 2*(3), 44–51.

Bryant R. A. (Ed.). (2000). *Acute and Chronic Wounds: Nursing Management* (2nd ed.). St. Louis: Mosby.

Bryant, R. A., & Rolstead, B.S. (2001). Utilizing a systems approach to implement pressure ulcer prediction and prevention. *Ostomy/Wound Management, 47*(9), 26–36.

Cuddigan, J., Ayello, E. A., & Sussman, C. (Eds.). (2001). *Pressure Ulcers in America: Prevalence, Incidence, and Implications for the Future.* Reston, VA: National Pressure Ulcer Advisory Panel.

Edwards, H., Gaskill, D., & Nash, R. (1998). Treating skin tears in nursing home residents: A pilot study comparing four types of dressings. *International Journal of Nursing Practice, 4,* 25–32.

Frantz, R. A., & Baranoski, S. (2001). Pressure ulcer prevention programs in various settings: What works? What doesn't. In J. Cuddigan, E. A. Ayello, & C. Sussman (Eds.), *Pressure Ulcers in America: Prevalence, Incidence, and Implications for the Future* (pp. 119–123). Reston, VA: National Pressure Ulcer Advisory Panel.

Health Care Financing Administration. (2000, June). *Investigative Protocol, Guidance to Surveyors—Long Term Care Facilities* (Rev. 274). Washington, DC: U.S. Department of Health and Human Services.

Henderson, C. T., Ayello, E. A., Sussman, C., Leiby, D. M., Bennett, M. A., Dungog, E. F., Sprigle, S., & Woodruff, L. (1997). Draft definition of stage I pressure ulcers: Inclusion of persons with darkly pigmented skin. *Advances in Wound Care, 10*(5), 16–19.

Krasner, D. (1991). An approach to treating skin tears. *Ostomy/Wound Management, 32,* 56–58.

Krasner, D. L., Rodeheaver, G. T., & Sibbald, R. G. (Eds). (2001). *Chronic Wound Care: A Clinical Source Book for Healthcare Professionals* (3rd ed.). Wayne, PA: Health Management Communications.

Lyder, C. H. (1991). Conceptualization of the stage I pressure ulcer. *Journal of Enterostomal Therapy Nursing, 18*(5), 162–165.

Lyder, C. H. (1996). Examining the inclusion of ethnic minorities in pressure ulcer prediction studies. *Journal of Wound Ostomy and Continence Nursing, 23*(5), 257–260.

Lyder, C. H., Preston, J., Grady, J., Scinto, J., Allman, R., Bergstrom, N., et al. (2001). Quality of care for hospitalized Medicare patients at risk for pressure ulcers. *Archives of Internal Medicine, 161,* 1549–1554.

Lyder, C. H., Yu, C., Emerling, J., Mangat, R., Stevenson, D., Empleo-Frazier, O., & McKay, J. (1999). The Braden Scale for pressure ulcer risk: Evaluating the predictive validity in Black and Latino/Hispanic elders. *Applied Nursing Research, 12*(2), 60–68.

Lyder, C. H., Yu, C., Stevenson, D., Mangat, R., Empleo-Frazier, O., Emerling, J., & McKay, J. (1998). Validating the Braden Scale for the prediction of pressure ulcer risk in Blacks and Latino/Hispanic elders: A pilot study. *Ostomy/Wound Management , 44* (Suppl. 3A), 42S–50S.

Maklebust, J., & Sieggreen, M. (2001). *Pressure ulcers: Guidelines for Prevention and Nursing Management* (3rd ed.). Springhouse, PA: Springhouse.

Malone, M. L., Rozario, N., Gavinski, M., & Goodwin, J. (1991). The epidemiology of skin tears in the institutionalized elderly. *Journal of the American Geriatrics Society, 39,* 591–595.

Mason, S. R. (1997). Type of soap and the incidence of skin tears among residents of a long-term care facility. *Ostomy/Wound Management, 43*(8), 26–30.

Meehan, M. (1990). Multisite pressure ulcer prevalence survey. *Decubitus, 3*(4), 14–17.

Meehan, M. (1994). National pressure ulcer prevalence survey. *Advances in Wound Care, 7*(3), 27–30, 34.

Morison, M. J. (Ed.). (2001). *The Prevention and Treatment of Pressure Ulcers.* St. Louis: Mosby.

National Pressure Ulcer Advisory Panel. (1989). Pressure ulcers prevalence, cost, and risk assessment: Consensus development conference statement. *Decubitus, 2*(2), 24–28.

National Pressure Ulcer Advisory Panel. (1998). *NPUAP statement on reverse staging of pressure ulcers.* Retrieved June 22, 2002, from http://www.npuap.org

National Pressure Ulcer Advisory Panel. (2001). *Pressure ulcer prevention: A competency-based curriculum.* Accessed: www.npuap.org/prercurr.pdf

Nightingale, F. (1859). *Notes on Nursing. What It Is and What It Is Not.* Philadelphia: Lippincott.

O'Regan, A. (2002). Skin tears: A review of the literature. *Journal of Wound, Ostomy, and Continence Nursing, 22*(2), 26–31.

Payne, R. L., & Martin, M. C. (1993). Defining and classifying skin tears: Need for common language. *Ostomy/Wound Management, 39*(5), 16–19, 22–24, 26.

Sprigle, S., Linden, M., McKenna, D., Davis, K., & Riordan, B. (2001). Clinical skin temperature measurement to predict incipient pressure ulcers. *Advances in Skin and Wound Care, 14*(3), 133–137.

Thomas, D. R., Goode, P. S., LaMaster, K., Tennyson, T., & Parnell, L. K. S. (1999). A comparison of an opaque foam dressing versus a transparent film dressing in the management of skin tears in institutionalized subjects. *Ostomy/Wound Management, 45*(6), 22–28.

U.S. Department of Health and Human Services. (2000). *Healthy People 2010: Understanding and Improving Health* (2nd ed.). Washington, DC: U.S. Government Printing Office.

White, M. W., Karam, S., & Cowell, B. (1994). Skin tears in frail elders: A practical approach to prevention. *Geriatric Nursing, 15*(2), 95–98.

Xakellis, G. C., Frantz, R. A., Lewis, A., & Harvey, P. (2001). Translating pressure ulcer guidelines into practice: It's harder than it sounds. *Advances in Skin and Wound Care, 14*(5), 249–256, 258.

Chapter 11

DEPRESSION IN OLDER ADULTS

Lenore H. Kurlowicz

EDUCATIONAL OBJECTIVES

On completion of this chapter, the reader should be able to
1. Discuss the consequences of late-life depression.
2. Identify nursing strategies for older adults with depression.
3. Discuss the major risk factors for late-life depression.
4. Identify the core competencies of a systematic nursing assessment for depression with older adults.

Contrary to popular belief, depression is not a normal part of aging. Rather, depression is a medical disorder that causes suffering for patients and their families, interferes with a person's ability to function, exacerbates coexisting medical illnesses, and increases utilization of health services (Lebowitz, 1996). Nearly 5 million of the 31 million Americans age 65 and older have depression (Lebowitz, 1996). A review of several studies by Blazer (2002a) reports prevalence rates of combined major and minor depression in various populations of older adults: community dwelling (13%), medical outpatients (24%), acute care (30%), and nursing homes (43%). Certain populations have higher levels of depressive symptoms, particularly those with more severe or chronic disabling conditions, such as those elders in acute and long-term care settings. Depression also frequently coexists with dementia, specifically Alzheimer's disease, with prevalence rates ranging from 10% to 40% (Pearson, Teri, & Reifler, 1989; Teri & Wagner, 1992). Cognitive impairment may be a secondary symptom of depression, or depression may be the result of dementia (Blazer, 2002b). It should be noted that the prevalence of major depression has been increasing in those born more recently, so that it can be expected that the prevalence of depression in older adults will go up in the years to come.

Late-life depression occurs within a context of medical illnesses, disability, cognitive dysfunction, and psychosocial adversity, frequently impeding timely recognition and treatment of depression, with subsequent unnecessary morbidity and death (Lebowitz, 1996). A substantial number of older patients encountered by nurses will have clinically relevant depressive symptoms. Nurses remain at the frontline in the early recognition of depression and the facilitation of older patients' access to mental health care. This chapter presents an overview of depression in older patients, with an emphasis on age-related assessment considerations, clinical decision-making, and nursing intervention strategies for elders with depression. A standard of practice protocol for use by nurses in practice settings is presented.

WHAT IS DEPRESSION?

In the broadest sense, depression is defined as a syndrome comprised of a constellation of affective, cognitive, and somatic or physiological manifestation (National Institutes of Health [NIH] Consensus Development Panel, 1992). Depression may range in severity from mild symptoms to more severe forms, both of which can persist over longer periods of time with negative consequences for the older patient. Suicidal ideation, psychotic features (especially delusional thinking), and excessive somatic concerns frequently accompany more severe depression (NIH Consensus Development Panel, 1992). Symptoms of anxiety may also coexist with depression in many older adults (Blazer, Hughes, & George, 1987).

The *Diagnostic and Statistical Manual of Mental Disorders* (DSM-IV-TR) (American Psychiatric Association, 2000) lists criteria for the diagnosis of major depressive disorder, the most severe form of depression. These criteria are frequently used as the standard by which older patients' depressive symptoms are assessed in clinical settings (American Psychiatric Association, 2000). Five criteria from a list of nine must be present nearly every day during the same 2-week period and must represent a change from previous functioning: (1) depressed, sad, or irritable mood; (2) anhedonia or diminished pleasure in usually pleasurable people or activities; (3) feelings of worthlessness, self-reproach, or excessive guilt; (4) difficulty with thinking or diminished concentration; (5) suicidal thinking or attempts; (6) fatigue and loss of energy; (7) changes in appetite and weight; (8) disturbed sleep; and (9) psychomotor agitation or retardation. For this diagnosis, at least one of the five symptoms must include either depressed mood, by the patient's subjective account or by observation of others, or markedly diminished pleasure in almost all people or activities. Concurrent medical conditions are frequently present in older patients and should not preclude a diagnosis of depression; indeed, there is a high incidence of medical comorbidity.

Older adults may more readily report somatic or physical symptoms than depressed mood (Blazer, 1989). The somatic or physical symptoms of depression, however, are often difficult to distinguish from somatic or physical symptoms associated with acute or chronic physical illness, especially in the hospitalized older patient, or the somatic symptoms that are part of common aging processes (Kurlowicz, 1994). For instance, disturbed sleep may be associated with chronic lung disease or congestive heart failure. Diminished energy or increased lethargy may be caused by an acute metabolic disturbance or drug response. Therefore, a challenge for nurses in acute care hospitals and other clinical settings is to not overlook or disregard somatic or physical complaints while also "looking beyond" such complaints to assess the full spectrum of depressive symptoms in older patients. In elders with acute medical illnesses, somatic symptoms that persist may indicate a more serious depression, despite treatment of the underlying medical illness or discontinuance of a depressogenic medication (Kurlowicz, 1994). Older patients may link their somatic or physical complaints to a depressed mood or anhedonia. Depression may also be expressed through repetitive verbalizations (e.g., calling out for help) or agitated vocalizations (e.g., screaming, yelling, or shouting), repetitive questions, expressions of unrealistic fears (e.g., fear of abandonment or being left alone), repetitive statements that something bad will happen, repetitive health-related concerns, and verbal and/or physical aggression (Cohen-Mansfield, Werner, & Marx, 1990).

MINOR DEPRESSION

Major depression, as defined by the DSM-IV-TR (American Psychiatric Association, 2000), seems to be as common among older as younger cohorts. Depressive symptoms that do not meet standard criteria for a specific depressive disorder are highly prevalent (15%–25%) in older adults. These symptoms are clinically significant and warrant treatment (Koenig & Blazer, 1996). Such depressive symptoms have been variously referred to in the literature as "minor depression," "subsyndromal depression," "dysthymic depression," "subclinical depression," "elevated depressive symptoms," and "mild depression." The DSM-IV-TR also lists criteria for the diagnosis of "minor depressive disorder" and includes episodes of at least 2 weeks of depressive symptoms but with fewer than the 5 criteria required for major depressive disorder. Minor depression is 2 to 4 times as common as major depression in older adults and is associated with increased risk of subsequent major depression and greater use of health services. It also has a negative impact on physical and social functioning and quality of life (Koenig & Blazer, 1996; Wells et al., 1989).

COURSE OF DEPRESSION

Depression can occur for the first time in late life, or it can be part of a long-standing affective or mood disorder with onset in earlier years. Hospitalized elderly medical patients with depression are also more likely to have had a previous depression or other psychiatric illness, including alcohol abuse (Koenig, Meador, Cohen, & Blazer, 1988). As in younger people, the course of depression in older adults is characterized by exacerbations, remissions, and chronicity (NIH Consensus Development Panel, 1992). Therefore, a wait-and-see approach with regard to treatment is not recommended.

DEPRESSION IN LATE LIFE IS SERIOUS

Depression is associated with serious negative consequences for older adults, especially for frail older patients, such as those recovering from a severe medical illness and those in nursing homes. Consequences of depression include amplification of pain and disability, delayed recovery from medical illness or surgery, worsening of medical symptoms, risk of physical illness, increased health care utilization, alcoholism, cognitive impairment, worsening social impairment, protein-calorie subnutrition, and increased rates of suicide and non-suicide-related death (Katz, 1996). The recent "amplification" hypothesis proposed by Katz, Stieim, and Parmalee (1994) stated that depression can "turn up the volume" on several aspects of physical, psychosocial, and behavioral functioning in older patients, ultimately accelerating the course of medical illness. For older nursing home residents, depression is also associated with poor adjustment to the nursing home, resistance to daily care, treatment refusal, inability to participate in activities, and further social isolation (Parmalee, Katz, & Lawton, 1992). Major depression can amplify cognitive impairment and functional disability in Alzheimer's disease (Pearson et al., 1989).

Mortality by suicide is higher among older persons with depression than among their counterparts without depression and cannot be accounted for by sociodemographic factors or preexisting illness (Conwell, 1994). Although older adults account for 12% of the population, they account for 21% of suicides (Conwell, Caine, & Olsen, 1990). White men over age 80 are at greatest risk and are 6 times more likely to commit suicide than the rest of the population (Conwell, 1994). Suicide among older adults is associated with diagnosable psychopathology, most often major depression, in approximately 80% of the cases (Conwell, 1994). Depression can also influence decision-making capacity and may be the cause of indirect life-threatening behavior such as refusal of food, medications, or other treatments in elderly patients (Conwell et al., 1990). Studies have also shown that more than half of those over age 65 visited a physician within 1 week of their suicide, 75% within 1 month, and 90% within 3 months (Barraclough, Bunch, & Nelson, 1974; Katz et al., 1994; Miller, 1978). Most of the suicidal patients experienced their first episode of major depression, which was only moderately severe, yet the depressive symptoms went unrecognized and untreated. These observations suggest that accurate diagnosis and treatment of depression in older patients may reduce the suicide rate in this population. It is in the clinical setting, therefore, that screening procedures and assessment protocols have the most direct impact.

DEPRESSION IN LATE LIFE
IS MISUNDERSTOOD

Despite its prevalence, associated negative outcomes, and good treatment response, depression in older adults is highly underrecognized, misdiagnosed, and subsequently undertreated. It is estimated that as many as 90% of older adults, particularly those in institutions, who are considered to need mental health care receive no services for primary psychiatric disorders, including depression (Burns & Taub, 1990). Barriers to care for older adults with depression exist at many levels. In particular, some older adults refuse to seek help because of the perceived stigma of mental illness. Others may simply accept their feelings of profound sadness without realizing they are clinically depressed. Recognition of depression also is frequently obscured by anxiety and the various somatic or dementia-like symptoms manifested by older patients. Additionally, patients and caregivers may believe that depression naturally follows life changes such as illness, hospitalization, and relocation to a nursing home. However, depression is not a necessary consequence of life adversity. When depression occurs after an adverse life event, it should be treated.

TREATMENT FOR LATE-LIFE
DEPRESSION WORKS

The goals of treating depression in older patients are to decrease depressive symptoms, reduce relapse and recurrence, improve functioning and quality of life, improve medical health and mortality, and reduce health care costs. Depression in older patients can be effectively treated using pharmacotherapy or psychosocial therapies, or both (Blazer, 2002a). If recognized, the treatment response for depression is good: Sixty percent to 80% of older adults remain relapse-free with medication maintenance for 6 to 18 months (NIH Consensus Development Panel, 1992). Recurrence is a serious problem, with up to 40% experiencing depression chronically, especially after acute illness and hospitalization (Koenig et al., 1996). Therefore, continuation of treatment to prevent early relapse and longer-term maintenance treatment to prevent later occurrences are important (Katz et al., 1994). Even in those patients with depression who have a comorbid medical illness or a dementia, treatment response is good

(Teri & Wagner, 1992). In patients with dementia, treatment of depression has been shown to improve cognitive performance, mood, physical and social functioning, and family well-being (Teri & Wagner, 1992).

CAUSE AND RISK FACTORS

Several biological and psychosocial causes for late-life depression have been proposed. Genetic factors seem to play more of a role when older adults have had depression throughout their life. Additional biological causes proposed for late-life depression include neurotransmitter or "chemical messenger" imbalance and dysregulation of endocrine function (Blazer, 2002). Neuroanatomic correlates, cerebrovascular disease, brain metabolism alterations, gross brain disease, and the presence of apolipoprotein E have also been etiologically linked to late-life depression (Krisham & Gadde, 1996). Possible psychosocial causes for depression in older adults include cognitive distortions, stressful life events (especially loss), chronic stress, and low self-efficacy expectations (Blazer, 2002; Holahan & Holahann, 1987).

The social and demographic risk factors for depression in older adults include female sex, unmarried status (particularly widowed), stressful life events, and the absence of a supportive social network (NIH Consensus Development Panel, 1992). In older adults there is additional emphasis on the co-occurrence of specific physical conditions such as stroke, cancer, dementia, arthritis, hip fracture surgery, myocardial infarction, chronic obstructive pulmonary disease, and Parkinson's disease. Medical comorbidity is the hallmark of depression in older patients, and this factor represents a major difference from depression in younger populations (Lebowitz, 1996). Severe medical illness has repeatedly been shown to be among the most robust and consistent of all correlates of depression among older medical patients (Koenig et al., 1988). Those with functional disabilities, especially those with new functional loss, are also at risk. The more severe the medical illness and associated functional disability, the greater the likelihood of depression in elderly patients (Katz et al., 1994). Subgroups of older persons who are at greater risk for major depression include the chronically ill, the institutionalized, the recently bereaved, and family members caring for chronically ill relatives.

ASSESSMENT OF DEPRESSION IN OLDER ADULTS

Box 11.1 presents a standard of practice protocol for depression in older adults that emphasizes a systematic assessment guide for early recognition of depression by nurses in hospitals and other clinical settings. Early recognition of depression is enhanced by targeting high-risk groups of older adults for assessment methods that are routine, standardized, and systematic and by using both a depression screening tool and an individualized depression assessment or interview (Sheikh & Yesavage, 1986).

DEPRESSION SCREENING TOOL

Nursing assessment of depression in older patients can be facilitated by the use of an assessment tool such as the Geriatric Depression Scale—Short Form (GDS-SF) (Sheikh & Yesavage, 1986). The GDS-SF is a 15-item self-report depression screening tool that is frequently used in a variety of clinical settings. This scale has been validated and used extensively with older adults, including those who are mentally ill, mild to moderately cognitively impaired, or institutionalized. It has a brief yes/no response format and takes approximately 5 minutes to complete. The GDS contains few somatic items that may be potentially confounded with symptoms caused by a medical illness. A GDS-SF score of 11 or greater is almost always indicative of depression, and a score of 6 to 9 indicates possible depression, warranting further evaluation (Sheikh & Yesavage, 1986). The GDS-SF is not a substitute for an individualized assessment or a diagnostic interview by a mental health professional but is a useful screening tool to identify an elderly patient's depression.

INDIVIDUALIZED ASSESSMENT AND INTERVIEW

Central to the individualized depression assessment and interview is a focused assessment of the full spectrum of symptoms for major depression as delineated by the DSM-IV (American Psychiatric Association, 2000). Furthermore, patients should be asked directly and specifically if they have been having suicidal ideation (i.e., thoughts that life is not worth living) or if they have been contemplating or have attempted suicide. The number of symptoms, type, duration, frequency, and patterns of depressive symptoms, as well

**BOX 11.1   Nursing Standard of Practice Protocol:
Depression in Older Adults**

I. BACKGROUND
  A. Depression—both major depressive disorders and minor
     depression—is highly prevalent in community-dwelling, medically
     ill, and institutionalized older adults. Depression is not a natural
     part of aging or a normal reaction to acute illness hospitalization.
  Consequences of depression include amplification of pain and
  disability, delayed recovery from illness and surgery, worsening
  of drug side effects, excess use of health services, cognitive impairment, subnutrition, and increased suicide- and non-suicide-related
  death. Depression tends to be long-lasting and recurrent. Therefore,
  a wait-and-see approach is undesirable, and immediate clinical
  attention is necessary. If recognized, treatment response is good.
  Somatic symptoms may be more prominent than depressed mood
  in late-life depression. Mixed depression and anxiety features may
  be evident among many older adults. Recognition of depression is
  hindered by the coexistence of physical illness and social and
  economic problems common in late life. Early recognition,
  intervention, and referral by nurses can reduce the negative
  effects of depression.
II. ASSESSMENT PARAMETERS
  A. Identify risk factors/high-risk groups:
     1. Current alcohol /substance use disorder
     2. Specific comorbid conditions (dementia, stroke, cancer,
        arthritis, hip fracture, myocardial infarction, chronic
        obstructive pulmonary disease, and Parkinson's disease)
     3. Functional disability (especially new functional loss)
     4. Widows/widowers
     5. Caregivers
     6. Social isolation/absence of social support
  B. Assess all at-risk groups using a standardized depression
     screening tool and documentation score. The GDS-SF is
     recommended because it takes approximately 5 minutes to
     administer, has been validated and extensively used with
     medically ill older adults, and includes few somatic items that
     may be confounded with physical illness.
  C. Perform a focused depression assessment on all at-risk groups
     and document results. Note the number of symptoms; onset; fre-
     quency/patterns; duration (especially 2 weeks); and changes in
     normal mood, behavior, and functioning.

(continued)

**BOX 11.1   Nursing Standard of Practice Protocol:
Depression in Older Adults** *(continued)*

     1. Depressive symptoms:
       a. Depressed or irritable mood; frequent crying
       b. Loss of interest, pleasure (in family, friends, hobbies, sex)
       c. Weight loss or gain (especially loss)
       d. Sleep disturbance (especially insomnia)
       e. Fatigue/loss of energy
       f. Psychomotor slowing/agitation
       g. Diminished concentration
       h. Feelings of worthlessness/guilt
       i. Suicidal thoughts or attempts; hopelessness
     2. Psychosis (i.e., delusional/paranoid thoughts, hallucinations)
     3. History of depression; current substance abuse (especially alcohol); previous coping style
     4. Recent losses or crises (e.g., death of spouse, friend, or pet; retirement; anniversary dates; move to another residence or nursing home); changes in physical health status, relationships, or roles
     5. In elderly persons, frequent somatic (physical) complaints may actually represent an underlying depression.
  D. Obtain/review medical history and physical/neurologic examination.
  E. Assess for depressogenic medications (e.g., steroids, narcotics, sedatives/hypnotics, benzodiazepines, antihypertensives, H$_2$ antagonists, beta blockers, antipsychotics, immunosuppressives, and cytotoxic agents).
  F. Assess for related systematic and metabolic processes (e.g., infection, anemia, hypothyroidism or hyperthyroidism, hyponatremia, hypercalcemia, hypoglycemia, congestive heart failure, and kidney failure).
  G. Assess for cognitive dysfunction.
  H. Assess level of functional disability.
III. CARE PARAMETERS
  A. For severe depression (GDS score 11 or greater, 5 to 9 depressive symptoms [must include depressed mood or loss of pleasure], plus other positive responses on individualized assessment [especially suicidal thoughts or psychosis and comorbid substance abuse]), refer for psychiatric evaluation. Treatment options may include medication or cognitive-behavioral, interpersonal, or brief psychodynamic psychotherapy/counseling (individual, group, or family), hospitalization, or electroconvulsive therapy.

BOX 11.1   *(continued)*

B. For less severe depression (GDS score of 6 to 10, fewer than five depressive symptoms, plus other positive responses on individualized assessment), refer to mental health services for psychotherapy/counseling (see above types), especially for specific issues identified in individualized assessment and to determine whether medication therapy may be warranted. Consider resources such as psychiatric liaison nurses, geropsychiatric advanced practice nurses, social workers, psychologists, and other community and institution-specific mental health services. If suicidal thoughts, psychosis, or comorbid substance abuse is present, a referral for a comprehensive psychiatric evaluation should always be made.

C. For all levels of depression, develop an individualized plan integrating the following nursing interventions:

1. Institute safety precautions for suicide risk as per institutional policy (in outpatient settings, ensure continuous surveillance of the patient while obtaining an emergency psychiatric evaluation and disposition).

2. Remove or control etiologic agents:
   a. Avoid/remove/change depressogenic medications.
   b. Correct/treat metabolic/systemic disturbances.

3. Monitor and promote nutrition, elimination, sleep/rest patterns, and physical comfort (especially pain control).

4. Enhance physical function (i.e., structure regular exercise/activity; refer to physical, occupational, and recreational therapies); develop a daily activity schedule.

5. Enhance social support (i.e., identify/mobilize support person(s) [e.g., family, confidant, friends, hospital resources, support groups, patient visitors]); ascertain need for spiritual support, and contact appropriate clergy.

6. Maximize autonomy/personal control/self-efficacy (e.g., include patient in active participation in making daily schedules and setting short-term goals).

7. Identify and reinforce strengths and capabilities.

8. Structure and encourage daily participation in relaxation therapies, pleasant activities (conduct a pleasant activity inventory), and music therapy.

9. Monitor and document responses to medication and other therapies; readminister depression screening tool.

10. Provide practical assistance; assist with problem solving.

(continued)

**BOX 11.1   Nursing Standard of Practice Protocol:
Depression in Older Adults** *(continued)*

    11. Provide emotional support (i.e., empathic, supportive listening; encourage expression of feelings and hope instillation), support adaptive coping, and encourage pleasant reminiscences.

    12. Provide information about the physical illness and treatment(s) and about depression (i.e., that depression is common, treatable, and not the person's fault).

    13. Educate about the importance of adherence to prescribed treatment regimen for depression (especially medication) to prevent recurrence; educate about specific antidepressant side effects due to personal inadequacies.

    14. Ensure mental health community linkup; consider psychiatric or nursing home care intervention.

IV. EVALUATION OF EXPECTED OUTCOMES

  A. Patient:

    1. Patient safety will be maintained.

    2. Patients with severe depression will be evaluated by psychiatric services.

    3. Patients will report a reduction of symptoms that are indicative of depression. A reduction in the GDS score will be evident, and suicidal thoughts or psychosis will resolve.

    4. Patient's daily functioning will improve.

  B. Health care provider:

    1. Early recognition of patient at risk, referral, interventions for depression, and documentation of outcomes will be improved.

  C. Institution:

    1. The number of patients identified with depression will increase.

    2. The number of in-hospital suicide attempts will not increase.

    3. The number of referrals to mental health services will increase.

    4. The number of referrals to psychiatric nursing home care services will increase.

    5. Staff will receive ongoing education on depression recognition, assessment, and interventions.

V. FOLLOW-UP TO MONITOR CONDITION

  A. Continue to track prevalence and documentation of depression in at-risk groups.

  B. Show evidence of transfer of information to postdischarge mental health service delivery system.

  C. Educate caregivers to continue assessment processes.

as a change from the patient's normal mood or functioning, should be noted. Additional components of the individualized depression assessment include evidence of psychotic thinking, especially delusional thoughts, anniversary dates of previous losses or nodal/stressful events, previous coping style (specifically, alcohol or other substance abuse), relationship changes, physical health changes, a history of depression or other psychiatric illness that required some form of treatment, a general loss and crises inventory, and any concurrent life stressors. Subsequent questioning of the family or caregiver is recommended to obtain further information about the elder's verbal and nonverbal expressions of depression.

DIFFERENTIATION OF MEDICAL OR IATROGENIC CAUSES OF DEPRESSION

Once depressive symptoms are recognized, medical and drug-related causes should be explored. As part of the initial assessment of depression in the older patient, it is important to obtain and review the medical history and physical and/or neurologic examinations. Key laboratory tests also should be obtained and reviewed, including thyroid-stimulating hormone levels, chemistry screen, complete blood count, and medication levels, if needed. An electrocardiogram, urinalysis, and serum folate and serum B_{12} tests should be considered to assess for coexisting medical conditions. These conditions may contribute to depression or might complicate treatment of the depression (Alexopoulos, Katz, Reynolds, Carpenter, & Docherty, 2001). In older patients, who frequently have multiple medical diagnoses and are prescribed multiple medications, these "organic" factors are a major issue in nursing assessment (Dreyfus, 1988). Table 11.1 presents physical illnesses that are associated with depression and Table 11.2 shows medications that may cause depression symptoms. In collaboration with the patient's physician, efforts should be directed toward treatment, correction, or stabilization of associated metabolic or systemic conditions. When medically feasible, depressogenic medications should be eliminated, minimized, or substituted with those that are less depressogenic. Even when an underlying medical condition or medication is contributing to the depression, treatment of that condition or discontinuation or substitution of the offending agent alone is often not sufficient to resolve the depression, and antidepressant medication is often needed.

TABLE 11.1   Physical Illnesses Associated with Depression in Older Patients

Metabolic disturbances
  Dehydration
  Azotemia, uremia
  Acid–base disturbances
  Hypoxia
  Hyponatremia and hypernatremia
  Hypoglycemia and hyperglycemia
  Hypocalcemia and hypercalcemia

Endocrine disorders
  Hypothyroidism and hyperthyroidism
  Hyperparathyroidism
  Diabetes mellitus
  Cushing's disease
  Addison's disease

Infections
  Viral
    Pneumonia
    Encephalitis
  Bacterial
    Pneumonia
    Urinary tract infection
    Meningitis
    Endocarditis
  Other
    Tuberculosis
    Brucellosis
    Fungal meningitis
    Neurosyphilis

Cardiovascular disorders
  Congestive heart failure
  Myocardial infarction, angina

Pulmonary disorders
  Chronic obstructive lung disease
  Malignancy

Gastrointestinal disorders
  Malignancy (especially pancreatic)
  Irritable bowel
  Other organic causes of chronic abdominal pain, peptic ulcer,
    diverticulosis
  Hepatitis

TABLE 11.1   *(continued)*

Genitourinary disorders
   Urinary incontinence

Musculoskeletal disorders
   Degenerative arthritis
   Osteoporosis with vertebral compression or hip fractures
   Polymyalgia rheumatica
   Paget's disease

Neurologic disorders
   Cerebrovascular disease
   Transient ischemic attacks
   Stroke
   Dementia (all types)
   Intracranial mass
   Primary or metastatic tumors
   Parkinson's disease

Other illness
   Anemia (of any cause)
   Vitamin deficiencies
   Hematologic or other systemic malignancy

Immune disorders

CLINICAL DECISION MAKING AND TREATMENT

Regardless of the setting, older patients who exhibit the number of symptoms indicative of a major depression, specifically, suicidal thoughts or psychosis, and who score above the established cutoff for depression on a depression screening tool (e.g., 5 on the GDS-SF) should be referred for a comprehensive psychiatric evaluation. Older patients with less severe depressive symptoms without suicidal thoughts or psychosis but who also score above the cutoff on the depression screening tool (e.g., 5 on the GDS-SF) should be referred to available psychosocial services (i.e., psychiatric liaison nurses, geropsychiatric advanced practice nurses, social workers, psychologists, or clergy) for psychotherapy or other psychosocial therapies, as well as to determine whether medication for depression is warranted.

TABLE 11.2   Drugs Used to Treat Physical Illness That Can Cause Symptoms of Depression

Antihypertensives
  Reserpine
  Methyldopa
  Propranolol
  Clonidine
  Hydralazine
  Guanethidine
  Diuretics*

Analgesics, narcotic
  Morphine
  Codeine
  Meperidine
  Pentazocine
  Propoxyphene

Analgesics, nonnarcotic
  Indomethacin

Antiparkinsonian agents
  L-dopa

Antimicrobials
  Sulfonamides
  Isoniazid

Cardiovascular agents
  Digitalis
  Lidocaine+

Hypoglycemic agents++

Steroids
  Corticosteroids
  Estrogens

Others
  Cimetidine
  Cancer chemotherapeutic agents

* By causing dehydration or electrolyte imbalance
+ Toxicity
++ By causing hypoglycemia

The two major categories of treatment for depression in older adults are biological therapies (e.g., pharmacotherapy and electroconvulsive therapy) and psychosocial therapies (e.g., psychotherapies such as cognitive-behavioral, interpersonal, and brief psychodynamic) in both individual and group formats (NIH Consensus Development Panel, 1992). Marital and family therapy may also be beneficial in treating elders with depression. The type and severity of depressive symptoms influence the type of treatment approach. In general, more severe depression, especially with suicidal thoughts or psychosis, requires intensive psychiatric treatment, including hospitalization, medication with an antidepressant or antipsychotic drug, electroconvulsive therapy, and intensive psychosocial support (Blazer, 2002). Less severe depression without suicidal thoughts or psychosis may require treatment with psychotherapy or medication, often on an outpatient basis.

INDIVIDUALIZED NURSING INTERVENTIONS FOR DEPRESSION

Psychosocial and behavioral nursing interventions can be incorporated into the plan of care, based on the patient's individualized need. Provision of safety precautions for patients with suicidal thinking is a priority. In acute medical settings, patients may require transfer to the psychiatric service when suicidal risk is high and staffing is not adequate to provide continuous observation of the patient. In outpatient settings, continuous surveillance of the patient should be provided while an emergency psychiatric evaluation and disposition is obtained.

The promotion of nutrition, elimination, sleep/rest patterns, physical comfort, and pain control has been recommended specifically for depressed medically ill older patients (Dreyfus, 1988). Relaxation strategies should be offered to relieve anxiety as an adjunct to pain management. Nursing interventions should focus on enhancement of the elder's physical function through structured and regular activity and exercise; referral to physical, occupational, and recreational therapies; and the development of a daily activity schedule. Enhancement of social support is also an important function of the nurse. This may be done by identifying, mobilizing, or designating a support person (or persons) such as family, a confidant, friends, volunteers or other hospital resources, a church member, support groups, patient or peer visitors, and appropriate clergy for spiritual support. Nurses should maximize the elder's autonomy, personal control, self-efficacy, and decision making about clinical care, daily schedules, and personal routines (Parmalee, Katz, & Lawton, 1991). The use of a graded task assignment, in which a larger goal or task is subdivided into several small steps, can be helpful in enhancing function, ensuring successful experiences, and building elderly patients' confidence in their performance of various activities (Dreyfus, 1988). Participation in regular, predictable, pleasant activities can result in more positive mood changes for elderly patients with depression (Koenig, 1991). A pleasant events inventory, elicited from the patient, can be used to incorporate pleasurable activities into the older patient's daily schedule (Koenig, 1991). Music therapy customized to the patient's preference also is recommended to reduce depressive symptoms (Hanser & Thompson, 1994).

Pleasant reminiscences can enhance self-esteem and sometimes alleviate a depressed mood (Osborn, 1989). Nursing interventions to encourage reminiscence include asking patients directly about their past and linking events in history with a patient's life experience. The use of photographs, old magazines, scrapbooks, and other objects can also stimulate discussion. Nurses should provide emotional support to depressed older patients by providing empathetic, supportive listening, encouraging patients to express their feelings in a focused manner on issues such as grief and role transition, offering supportive and adaptive coping strategies, identifying and reinforcing strengths and capabilities, maintaining privacy and respect, and instilling hope.

Older patients should be monitored closely for therapeutic response to and potential side effects of antidepressant medication so as to assess whether dose adjustment of antidepressant medication may be warranted. Although, in general, it is necessary to start antidepressant medication at low doses in older patients, it is also necessary to ensure that elders with persistent depressive symptoms receive adequate treatment (American Association of Geriatric Psychiatry, 1992). In particular, it is important to increase the patient's and the patient's family's awareness of the symptoms of depression.

CASE STUDY

Mrs. M. is a 76-year-old woman who had depression for the first time in late life while experiencing a series of psychosocial stresses, including caring for her husband with Alzheimer's dementia and multiple physical illnesses, relocating from her lifelong home, separating from friends, major surgery and subsequent convalescence, and the eventual death of her husband. Mrs. M. was unable to function in her daily life, no longer enjoyed her pastimes, and had contemplated suicide, but she never thought of herself as being depressed. Recognition of her depressive symptoms by her nurse during an acute care hospitalization, subsequent referral to the geropsychiatric consultation liaison nurse, and psychiatric visiting nurse intervention after discharge helped Mrs. M. see her symptoms as being part of a treatable depression. She agreed to a psychiatric evaluation, and antidepressant therapy was initiated. She also participated in individual psychotherapy, a bereavement support group sponsored by her church, and a senior outreach program provided through a local agency on aging. Mrs. M's therapeutic response to the various interventions was good within 6 to 8 weeks. Her depressive symptoms diminished, she no longer contemplated suicide, and her daily physical and social functioning improved. Several months later, she stated: "I'm not happy, mind you; I'm still mourning the loss of my husband of 55 years, and it's a struggle some days, but I now have hope that things will get better."

SUMMARY

Depression significantly threatens the personal integrity and experience of life of older adults. It is often reversible with prompt and appropriate treatment. Early recognition can be enhanced by the use of a standardized protocol that outlines a systematic method for depression assessment. Early identification of depressed intervention and successful treatment demonstrates that depression is the most treatable mental problem in late life. As Blazer (1989) has stated, when there is depression, hope remains.

REFERENCES

Alexopoulos, G., Katz, I. R., Reynolds, C. F., Carpenter, D., & Docherty, J. P. (2001). Pharmacotherapy of depressive disorders in older patients [Special report]. *Postgraduate Medicine*, 1–87.

American Association of Geriatric Psychiatry. (1992). Position statement: Psychotherapeutic medication in nursing homes. *Journal of the American Geriatrics Society, 40,* 946–949.

American Psychiatric Association. (2000). *Diagnostic and statistical manual of mental disorders* (4th ed., TR). Washington, DC: Author.

Barraclough, B. M., Bunch, J., & Nelson, B. (1974). A hundred cases of suicide: Clinical aspects. *British Journal of Psychiatry, 125,* 355–373.

Blazer, D. G. (1989). Depression in the elderly. *New England Journal of Medicine, 320,* 164–166.

Blazer, D. G. (2002a). *Depression in late life* (3rd ed.). St. Louis: Mosby Year Book.

Blazer, D. G. (2002b). Self-efficacy and depression in late life: A primary prevention proposal. *Aging & Mental Health, 6,* 315–324.

Blazer, D. G., Hughes, D. C., & George, L. K. (1987). The epidemiology of depression in an elderly community population. *Gerontologist, 27,* 281–287.

Burns, B. J., & Taub, C. A. (1990) Mental health services in general medical care and in nursing homes. In B. S. Fogel, A. Furino & G. Gottlieb (Eds.), *Mental Health Policy for Older Americans: Protecting Minds at Risk.* Washington, DC: American Psychiatric Press.

Cohen-Mansfield, J., Werner, P., & Marx, M. S. (1990). Screaming in nursing home residents. *Journal of the American Geriatrics Society, 38,* 785–792.

Conwell, Y. (1994). Suicide in the elderly. In L. S. Schneider, B. D. Reynolds, B. D. Lebowitz, & A. J. Friedhoff, (Eds.), *Diagnosis and treatment of depression in late life: Results of the NIH Consensus Development Conference.* Washington, DC: American Psychiatric Press.

Conwell, Y., Caine, E. D., & Olsen, K. (1990). Suicide and cancer in late life. *Hospital and Community Psychiatry, 41,* 1334–1338.

Dreyfus, J. K. (1988). Depression assessment and interventions with medically ill frail elderly. *Journal of Gerontological Nursing, 14,* 27–36.

Hanser, S. B., & Thompson, L. W. (1994). Effects of music therapy strategy on depressed older adults. *Journal of Gerontology, 49,* P265–P269.

Holahan, C. K., & Holahan, C. J. (1987). Self-efficacy, social support, and depression aging: A longitudinal analysis. *Journal of Gerontology, 42,* 65–68.

Katz, I. R. (1996). On the inseparability of mental and physical health in aged persons: Lessons from depression and medical comorbidity. *American Journal of Geriatric Psychiatry, 4,* 1–16.

Katz, I. R., Stieim, J., & Parmalee, P. (1994). Prevention of depression, recurrences, and complications in late life. *Preventive Medicine, 23,* 743–750.

Keane, S. M., & Sells, S. (1990). Recognizing depression in the elderly. *Journal of Gerontology and Nursing, 16,* 21–25.

Koenig, H. G. (1991). Depressive disorders in older medical inpatients. *American Family Practice, 44,* 1243–1250.

Koenig, H. G., & Blazer, D. G. (1996). Minor depression in late life. *American Journal of Geriatric Psychiatry, 4,* (Suppl. 1), S14–S21.

Koenig, H. G., Meador, K. G., Cohen, H. J., & Blazer, D. G. (1988). Depression in elderly patients with medical illness. *Archives of Internal Medicine, 148,* 1929–1936.

Krishnan, K. R., & Gadde, K. M. (1996). The pathophysiologic basis for late life depression. *American Journal of Geriatric Psychiatry, 4*(Supp. 1), S22–S33.

Kurlowicz, L. H. (1994). Depression in hospitalized medically ill elders: Evolution of the concept. *Archives of Psychiatric Nursing, 8,* 124–126.

Lebowitz, B. D. (1996). Diagnosis and treatment of depression in late life: An overview of the NIH consensus statement. *Journal of the American Geriatrics Society, 4*(Suppl. 1), S3–S6.

Miller, M. (1978). Geriatric suicide: The Arizona study. *Gerontologist, 18,* 488–495.

National Institutes of Health (NIH) Consensus Development Panel. (1992). Diagnosis and treatment of depression in late life. *Journal of the American Medical Association, 268,* 1018–1024.

Osborn, C. (1989). Reminiscence: When the past meets present. *Journal of Gerontology and Nursing, 15,* 6–12.

Parmalee, P. A., Katz, I. R., & Lawton, M. P. (1991). The relation of pain to depression among institutionalized aged. *Journal of Gerontology, 46,* 15–21.

Parmalee, P. A., Katz, I. R., & Lawton, M. P. (1992). Depression and mortality among institutionalized elderly. *Journal of Gerontology, 47,* P3–P10.

Pearson, J. L., Teri, L., & Reifler, B. V. (1989). Functional status and cognitive impairment in Alzheimer's patients with and without depression. *Journal of the American Geriatrics Society, 34,* 1117–1121.

Sheikh, J. I., & Yesavage, J. A. (1986). Geriatric Depression Scale (GDS): Recent evidence and development of a shorter version. *Clinical Gerontologist, 5,* 165–173.

Teri, L., & Wagner, A. (1992). Alzheimer's disease and depression. *Journal of Consulting and Clinical Psychology, 60,* 379–391.

Wells, K. D., Stewart, A., Hays, R. D., Burnam, A., Rogers, W., Daniels, M., et al. (1989). The functioning and well-being of depressed patients results from the medical outcomes study. *Journal of the American Medical Association, 262,* 914–919.

MEDICATION IN OLDER ADULTS

Terry Fulmer, Marquis D. Foreman, and DeAnne Zwicker

EDUCATIONAL OBJECTIVES

On completion of this chapter, the reader should be able to

1. Conduct a comprehensive medication assessment.
2. Specify four classes of medications having a high potential for toxicity in the elderly.
3. Identify three factors that place older adults at risk for medication problems.
4. Plan strategies to counteract some common drug-induced problems in older adults.
5. Develop an individualized plan to promote medication safety in an older adult.

Adults become increasingly susceptible to adverse drug events (ADEs) as they age. Physiologic changes characteristic of aging predispose older adults to experience more ADEs than adults who are younger. Persons over the age of 65 experience medication

---

Adapted from a chapter in the original edition by M. Walker, M. Foreman, and the NICHE faculty. Ensuring medication safety for older adults, pp. 131–144. In Abraham, I., Fulmer, T., & Mezey, Eds. *Geriatric Nursing Protocols for Best Practice*. New York: Springer Publishing Company.

problems for five major reasons: (1) age-related physiologic changes that result in altered pharmacokinetics and pharmacodynamics (inability to clear and excrete medications and alterations in blood–brain barrier integrity that predict central penetration); (2) multiple medication prescriptions (polypharmacy), which are often written by multiple providers; (3) incorrect doses of medications (over or under a therapeutic dosage); (4) medication consumption for the treatment of age-related symptoms that are not disease dependent or specific (self-medication); and (5) problems with medication compliance (Besdine et al., 1998).

Older adults are more likely to be taking multiple medications for various health problems and are the largest consumers of over-the-counter (OTC) drugs (Besdine et al., 1998). The evidence reflects that people age 65 and older consume one third of all prescription drugs and purchase 40% of all OTC medications (DeMaagd, 1995; Falvo, Holland, Brenner, & Benshoff, 1990; Hobson, 1992; Kahl, Blandford, Krueger, & Zwick, 1992; Kohn, Corrigan, & Donaldson, 2000). Older persons' susceptibility to ADEs has been a major issue in the recent literature on iatrogenic events and medication errors (Childs, 2000; Hohl, Dankoff, Colacone, & Afilalo, 2001; Riedinger & Robbins, 1998). The elderly often present to the emergency room due to ADEs (Hohl et al., 2001) and are at significant risk for further ADEs while in the hospital. Additionally, ADEs lead to significant morbidity and mortality and cost the health system billions of dollars annually. Doucet and colleagues (2002) suggest the following to clinicians as a means for minimizing adverse drug reactions: reinforcing drug monitoring and focusing on drug–drug interactions and excess dosages, especially during an acute episode. Acute care nurses are in a pivotal position to make an impact on reducing ADEs in hospitalized elderly patients.

ASSESSMENT OF PROBLEM

There has been a major emphasis on appropriate medications for older adults and the hazards associated with iatrogenesis from medication-related problems (Beers, 1997; Besdine et al., 1998; Fulmer, Kim, Montgomery, & Lyder, 2000; Kohn et al., 2000). Hepler and Strand (1990) delineated the following eight categories as potential areas for medication-related problems: (1) *untreated indications*: when patients have medical problems that require drug therapy but are not receiving the medication; (2) *improper drug selection*: when the patient has a problem but is taking the wrong medication; (3) *subtherapeutic dosages*: when the patient has a problem that is treated with an inadequate dose of the correct medication; (4) *failure to receive drugs*: when the patient has a problem that is the result of not receiving a drug, such as for economic reasons; (5) *overdosage*: when a patient has a problem that has been treated with too much of the correct drug; (6) *adverse drug reaction*: when a patient has a medical problem that is the result of an unintended and detrimental adverse drug effect; (7) *drug interaction*: when the patient has a medical problem that is the result of drug–drug, drug–food, or drug–laboratory interaction; and (8) *drug use without indication*: when a patient is taking a drug without a valid medical reason.

Drug–disease interactions must also be considered when providing medications to the elderly. See Hanlon, Shimp, and Semla (2000) for a table of drug–disease interactions to avoid in the elderly. Interactions with herbal remedies must also be considered, as elderly persons are common consumers of these remedies. The categories of medication-related problems can lead to serious outcomes for the older person and are predictable and thus potentially preventable (Besdine et al., 1998). If the categories are carefully assessed by the professional nurse and brought to the attention of the primary care provider, and changes are initiated in the medication regimen, ADEs may be avoided and ultimately result in improved outcomes and a better quality of life for the elderly.

In the past, there have been articles to suggest that because of homeostatic changes in older adults, age-related alterations in pharmacodynamics develop in a predictable way. We now know that there is extraordinary variability in the way in which people age; therefore, the way in which the pharmacodynamics change with aging are also variable. However, there are patterns related to aging that are important to note:

- Age-related changes in absorption that includes increase gastric pH and decreased gastrointestinal motility in an absorptive surface.
- Drug distribution changes that are caused by aging changes such as decreased cardiac output, reduced total body water (higher serum drug levels result with water soluble drugs), decreased serum albumin (higher unbound drug levels result

with protein-bound drugs, e.g., warfarin), and increased body fat (prolongs half-life in lipid-soluble drugs, e.g., long-acting benzodiazepines and some beta blockers).

- Elimination of drugs from the body that may be slowed due to glomerular filtration, renal tubular secretion, and renal blood flow that naturally decrease with age. (Renal function may be reduced by about 50% by the age of 90. A decrease in glomerular filtration usually is not accompanied by an increase in serum creatinine due to decreasing muscle mass with age. Therefore, serum creatinine is not an accurate measure of renal function in the elderly.)
- Changes in drug metabolism that result from decreased liver blood flow or disease states common in older individuals (thyroid disease, congestive heart failure, and cancer) and changes that come from drug-induced metabolic changes (drug interactions from polypharmacy).

Prescribing principles with older individuals are guided by the adages "Start low and go slow" and "Keep it as simple as possible." When considering best practice for older adults, clinicians are urged to first consider whether or not there is medication that can be removed when a new symptom develops (one that may be causing the new symptom) rather than adding another medication to treat the new symptom. It is important to decide whether or not the medication that is being considered for the particular disorder is the best choice, the most appropriate dose, the best dosage form, and the most efficacious route of administration.

As individuals age, they may have a series of difficulties that decrease their ability to comply with medication regimens (e.g., vision impairment, arthritis, and financial constraints). The body of literature related to medication compliance in older adults is beyond the scope of this chapter, but it is extremely important to note. Medication compliance with older adults is complex and needs careful nursing assessment. Special attention is needed to determine whether or not the older individual is taking the correct medication at the correct time for the appropriate purpose. There are a number of ways to calculate compliance (Fulmer et al., 2000; Rohay, Dunbar-Jacob, Sereika, Kwoh, & Burke, 1996), and there are also several devices that can assist in enhancing compliance behavior (Fulmer et al., 1999).

HIGH-RISK MEDICATIONS

The Beers (1997) criteria are now well accepted in the literature with regard to categories of medications that are likely to create problems in older adults. The Beers publication (1997) presents excellent easy-to-use tables for all providers of care to the elderly. The two user-friendly tables contain information on specific drugs with prescribing concerns in the elderly and effects of drugs related to concomitant underlying diagnosis.

Antihypertensive Agents

Hypertension affects a sizable portion of the elderly population. It appears, however, that elderly persons are less tolerant of the potential side effects of this class of medications than are their nonelderly counterparts. The antihypertensives, as a class, tend to produce a variety of unintended effects, including orthostatic hypotension (diuretics and alpha blockers), sedation (some beta blockers), depressive symptoms, confusion (alpha blockers), impotence, and constipation (verapamil, a calcium channel blocker). These unintended effects occur even in individuals under the age of 65; thus, comprehensive and ongoing assessment for potential adverse effects (e.g., routine checking of orthostatic blood pressure) is key to monitoring drug efficacy.

Because of changes in fat/lean body mass that characterize the aging process, elders generally do not tolerate fat-soluble beta blockers. Dose for dose, water-soluble compounds are more potent in aging persons, whereas fat-soluble drugs can be expected to have an extended half-life. Additionally, changes in central penetration that occur as a result of age-related decreases in integrity of the blood–brain barrier predispose elders to untoward experiences with alpha agonists. Alterations in cognitive status, particularly delirium and dementia-like states, have been reported in elders consuming medications that control hypertension (Nolan & Marcus, 2000).

Orthostatic hypotension is a serious problem affecting elders on sustained antihypertensive therapy. Hypovolemia is a common cause of orthostasis and may result from diuretics (e.g., hydrochlorothiazide and furosemide) used to treat hypertension or may be due to concomitant illness (e.g., infection). The known sequelae of orthostatic hypotension in older adults include falls. Because of increased susceptibility to injury, falls represent true trauma and a medical emergency in physically frail or functionally compromised older adults (see chapter 9). Sequelae of falls, including hip fracture and head trauma, account for almost 60% of drug-related injuries and contribute to 6% of patient deaths in this population (Rebenson-Piano, 1998; Tinetti & Speechly, 1989), notably from problems associated with immobility (e.g. pneumonia, pulmonary embolus).

Psychoactive Drugs

Major psychiatric symptoms and disorders occur in 12% to 25% of persons over the age of 65 (Salzman, 1998; Wanich, Sullivan-Marx, Gottlieb, & Johnson, 1992). Sleep problems are frequent correlates of depressive, psychotic, or demented symptomatology in aging persons. Prevailing clinical norms aside, the use of sedative-hypnotics in elderly persons should be avoided. Oversedation, respiratory depression, confusion, and other alterations in cognitive capacity, as well as falls, are frequent correlates of sedative-hypnotic use. Foreman and Wykle (1995) suggested using regular sleep schedules, avoiding caffeine and alcohol consumption, reducing daytime naps, and avoiding stimulant medications as measures to maximize the ability to sleep (see chapter 4).

Psychoactive medications include antidepressants (tricyclics, SSRIs [selective serotonin reuptake inhibitors]), anxiolytic agents (e.g., diazepam), antipsychotics (neuroleptics), mood-stabilizing compounds (lithium), and psychoactive stimulants, in addition to the sedative-hypnotics. These latter medications are known to have relatively narrow therapeutic windows even in fully functional, nonelderly adults. Psychoactive compounds are most frequently prescribed for sedation of agitated behaviors, stabilization of mood, and pharmacotherapeutic effects in true depressive states. Elders are at risk when consuming these medications because of changes in absorption, metabolism, distribution, and excretion of both parent drug and psychoactive metabolites. Furthermore, many unintended interactions may be predictable because of known age-related changes and require careful surveillance on the part of sensible clinicians.

The half-life of psychoactive drugs are prolonged in aging persons. In general, this class of drugs must be used with extreme caution to avoid inducing delirium, falls, and other traumatic events in elders consuming these drugs. As an example, diazepam (an antianxiety agent) has a known half-life of at least 8 to 12 hours in adults. However, one of its major metabolites is known to have a half-life of

54 hours, even in persons whose hepatic and renal clearance is intact. Circulating levels of parent drug and metabolite are extended in persons over the age of 65; therefore, the dosage of drug administered and the frequency of drug administration become critical considerations when medicating older adults. Furthermore, the risk of ADEs increases exponentially with the numbers of drugs consumed.

Although antianxiety agents, such as the benzodiazepines and sedative-hypnotics, are generally overprescribed in older adults, the antidepressants are generally considered to be underprescribed. It is estimated that almost 15% of older persons living in the community, 5% in primary care, and 15% to 25% in nursing homes have significant depressive symptoms (Spina & Scordo, 2002) (see chapter 11 also).

A major deterrent to antidepressant pharmacotherapy in this population has been the high incidence of anticholinergic side effects that occur with administration of tricyclic antidepressants. Anticholinergic side effects such as dry mouth, blurred vision, urinary retention (particularly in the presence of prostatic enlargement), cognitive alterations, cardiotoxicity, and constipation signal to the vigilant clinician that the antidepressant profile needs to be re-evaluated and likely adjusted. Tricyclic antidepressant medications with low anticholinergic profiles include desipramine, nortriptyline, and trazodone.

The SSRIs, as a class of antidepressants, have a striking difference in side effects from other antidepressants. This class does not cause cardiotoxicity or orthostatic hypotension. Additionally, the SSRIs do not have anticholinergic effects, except for paroxetine, which may have mild anticholinergic effects in some elders (Salzman, 1998). In general, these drugs tend to be a better choice in older adults. The most common side effects are gastrointestinal (GI) (e.g., nausea and anorexia), which may be ameliorated by starting with a low dose (half that for younger adults, e.g., fluoxetine 5 mg) and slowly increasing (to 10 mg) after 1 week.

The antipsychotics are often considered first-line pharmacotherapeutic interventions for persons over the age of 65 presenting with agitation and behavioral problems associated with dementia (Kindermann, Dolder, Bailey, Katz, & Jeste, 2002). Their use, however, has received increasing scientific attention. Currently, many investigators and clinicians believe that these drugs have questionable efficacy in elders. Additionally, these potent drugs must be used with extreme caution in this population, largely because of the potential for development of abnormal, and often irreversible, involuntary movements (extrapyramidal symptoms) associated with administration of neuroleptics (e.g., drug-induced Parkinsonism and tardive dyskinetic movements). Further neuroleptic side effects include sedation and anticholinergic toxicity.

Recent research on older people suggests that the newer antipsychotics present a much lower risk of movement disorders, highlighting their importance for prevention. Unlike conventional neuroleptics, the newer atypical ones (e.g., clozapine, risperidone, olanzapine, and quetiapine) apparently provide several advantages with respect to both efficacy and safety. These drugs are associated with a lower incidence of extrapyramidal symptoms than conventional neuroleptics are. For clozapine, the low risk of tardive dyskinesia is well established (Kane, Woerner, Pollack, Safferman, & Lieberman, 1993).

Anticholinergics

Drugs with high anticholinergic properties need to be used with caution in older adults for several reasons. Anticholinergics may cause many adverse effects, including inability to concentrate, delirium, agitation, hallucinations, blurred vision, slowed GI motility, decreased secretions, and constipation (Tune, 2001). Another common effect is urinary retention that can be a lethal side effect in a male with BPH (benign prostatic hypertrophy) and a history of UTIs (urinary tract infections)—urosepsis and death may result. Catterson, Preskorn, and Martin (1997) discussed the vicious cycle of treatment and side effects that may occur after administering anticholinergics. An example is a demented patient who is given oxycodone for osteoarthritic pain and sustains a secondary fecal impaction from the medication. The fecal impaction then causes agitation (from the discomfort of the impaction), which then leads to treatment of the agitation with antipsychotics (which also have anticholinergic effects) and exacerbates the problem further.

Anticholinergic drugs include not only antidepressant and neuroleptic medications, as previously mentioned, but also antihistamines, intestinal and bladder relaxants, corticosteroids, antiarrythmics and other cardiovascular drugs, antihypertensives, and some antibiotics. (Refer to Tune, 2001, for a complete list of medications with anticholinergic effects.) Additionally, syncopal events and falls are common sequelae of high anticholinergic drug use, again resulting in increased morbidity and mortality in aging persons.

Cardiotonics

Digoxin has been found to be useful in treating congestive heart failure (CHF) due to systolic dysfunction in the elderly; however, it is no longer the recommended treatment for CHF from underlying diastolic dysfunction in elderly patients (Packer et al., 1993; Uretsky et al., 1993). Digoxin toxicity occurs more frequently in the elderly, presents atypically, and may result in death. Classic symptoms of toxicity (nausea, anorexia, and visual disturbance) may occur; however, symptomatic cardiac disturbance and arrhythmias are more common in the elderly. The elderly can experience adverse symptoms even with normal plasma levels of digoxin (Flaherty, 1998; Flaherty, Perry, Lynchard, & Morley, 2000). Many older people will have some reduction in renal function with aging; therefore, monitoring for symptoms of digoxin toxicity and renal function as well as potassium levels is important.

Particular caution is necessary when digoxin is given along with diuretics, which can cause hypokalemia. This combination may exacerbate renal impairment, which can potentiate digoxin toxicity. Because the therapeutic window for digoxin is narrow and because it is water soluble (a smaller volume of distribution and thus higher plasma concentration), dosing of older adults is very difficult. The maximum recommended dose in the elderly is 0.125 mg (Beers, 1997). Many debilitated elderly patients have low serum albumin levels; because digoxin binds to protein, this may result in a higher plasma level.

Angiotensin converting enzyme (ACE) inhibitors are recommended in all patients with heart failure (who have normal renal function) due to left ventricular/systolic dysfunction (Packer et al., 1999); however, monitoring of renal function and serum potassium should continue as the dose is titrated up. ACE inhibitors should be used with caution in patients with a creatinine level greater than 3 mg/dL. Some ACE inhibitors (captopril and enalapril) have been noted to cause a change in mental status (Flaherty, 1998).

Over-the-Counter Medications

In community-dwelling older adults in the United States, those over age 65 take about as many OTC drugs as prescription drugs (Hanlon et al., 2001). It is essential to detail the kinds and amounts of OTC medications commonly consumed by older adults. Among these medications, analgesics, laxatives, and nutritional supplements are utilized most frequently (Hanlon et al., 2001). Salicylates, such as aspirin, are of significant concern in explaining adverse drug reactions in older persons. Alcohol, because of its water solubility, is a potent drug that may lead to worsening of age-related renal insufficiency and chronic salicylate intoxication. Manifestations of alcohol toxicity in the elderly include tachypnea, acid–base disorders, noncardiogenic pulmonary edema, and cerebral edema (Karsh, 1990). Additionally, cold remedies that include alcohol are a significant source of drug potentiation in aging persons. Indeed, alcohol consumption is frequently omitted from histories in elders, although alcohol interacts with OTC and prescription medications in frank and subtle ways to produce unintended drug harm.

NURSING CARE STRATEGIES

COMPREHENSIVE MEDICATION ASSESSMENT

Comprehensive medication assessment, as suggested by Pesznecker, Patsdaughter, Moody, and Albert (1990), begins with a thorough drug history and assessment obtained from the older adult or a reliable informant. Specific questions include the following:

- Ascertain the numbers and types of medications typically consumed, along with some estimate of how long the older adult has been taking the drug. It is recommended that elders collect and bring all medications to a provider to document medication types, instructions for self-administration, dates, and duration. This method allows documentation of multiple prescribing providers and dispensing pharmacies and signals polypharmacy and/or possible substance abuse, particularly with analgesics, anxiolytics, and sedative-hypnotics. Directed questions by the provider should address nicotine and alcohol self-administration, as well as vitamins, herbal preparations, and OTC medications that are included in the medication profile.
- Query whether the older person understands what the drug is to be used for, how often it is to be taken, the circumstances of ingestion (e.g., with food), and other aspects of drug self-administration that signal intelligent drug use. Ask the older adult to tell you about circumstances in which the drug has not been used or has been used differently than prescribed. If the older adult cannot do so, consider removing the drug, if possible,

or provide written instruction for the home (Muir, Sanders, Wilkinson, & Schmader, 2001).

- Ask directly whether the elder believes that the drug is actually doing what it is intended to do. If the medication is not useful or not creating symptom relief, consider removing it.
- Assess beliefs, concerns, and problems related to the medication regimen. This assessment should include an evaluation of technical factors, for example, the ability to read the medication label, to open the medication container, and to consume or self-administer the prescribed medication as intended. Create a care plan to address noted problems, and reevaluate at regular intervals.
- Discuss the impact of medication expenses. Many medications, particularly those that are newly released, are prohibitively expensive, particularly for persons on fixed incomes. Ask about concerns that the older persons may have about the costs and risks of administration. Where economic problems are found, try to prescribe generic drugs, and work with the older adult to ascertain how to manage the issue. Use the opportunity to provide important information in a clear, uncomplicated manner. Provide drug sheets or other written materials when these are available, even when an individual has been using a medication for a long time.
- Ask about OTC and "recreational" drugs, alcohol use, and herbal or other folk remedies; be specific about the actual amount and under what circumstances these substances are used. Accurate information can help explain symptoms that otherwise may not make sense.
- Assess for sensory or functional impairment and the devices used to remedy these alterations. For example, tamper-proof lids are often difficult for elders to remove, particularly if they are experiencing arthritic changes. A simple request to the pharmacist to provide a nonchildproof lid may improve the safe and effective use of prescribed medication.
- Assess cognitive and affective status to ensure that memory problems or vegetative symptoms associated with depression are not interfering with the safe use of prescription drugs (see chapter 7).
- Specifically ask about the circumstances of medication storage and other aspects (such as how drugs are dispensed daily) that signal a true understanding of these aspects of medication safety.

- Consider instrumental issues related to drug use, such as availability of family members or other social supports to facilitate medication compliance, how prescriptions are actually filled and reimbursed, and who monitors medication changes dictated by third-party reimbursement.

CASE STUDY

Mr. GP is a 78-year-old blind, hard-of-hearing male who ambulates with assistance (due to blindness from cataracts, for which he refuses to have surgery). He is admitted from the emergency room to the cardiac care unit for a heart rate of 40, intermittent chest pain at night, and change in mental status. He has a past history of atrial fibrillation, hypertension, congestive heart failure, two incidents of myocardial infarction in the past 2 years with left systolic dysfunction, intermittent angina usually relieved with NTG SL, depression, thyroiditis (amiodarone induced; discontinued recently), BPH with occasional UTIs, and mild dementia. He requires assistance with all activities of daily living and lives with his oldest daughter and her two high school–age children. His current medications include prednisone tapering dose now at 10 mg per day, ranitidine 150 mg q HS (hour of sleep), digoxin 0.25 mg q am, Lasix 40 mg bid, captopril 25 mg bid, labetalol 100 mg bid, NTG (nitroglycerine) 1/150 SL q 15 minutes x 3 prn chest pain, and fluoxetine 10 mg, which was discontinued 1 week ago when he reported a loss of appetite and weight loss. He has had a weight loss of 2.5 pounds in 2 weeks, complains of weakness, and has fallen three times without apparent injury. He has no palpitations, cough, or fever. His nighttime chest pain is relieved with NTG 1/150 x 1 tablet. His family is very involved and care for him at home 24 hours a day. They bring in a list of his medications, his blood pressure and heart rate log, and a list of multiple medical providers.

DISCUSSION

The heart rate of 40, particularly in the presence of anorexia, and the dosage of digoxin (0.25 mg), make one consider digoxin toxicity as the etiology. It is important to note that Mr. GP is on a beta blocker as well, which can slow the heart rate. Of particular concern is that he is on Lasix without a potassium supplement.

Particular caution is necessary when digoxin is given along with diuretics, which can cause hypokalemia. This combination may exacerbate renal impairment, which can lead to digoxin toxicity. Therefore, the serum electrolytes (potassium) should be checked immediately, as well as blood urea nitrogen (BUN) and creatinine (keeping in mind that the creatinine level may not be accurate in the elderly and should be compared to the baseline level). Many older people will have some reduction in renal function with aging; therefore, monitoring for symptoms of digoxin toxicity and renal function as well as potassium levels is important. Additionally, because he has had anorexia, an albumin level should be checked, as a low albumin level may result in increased unbound digoxin in the bloodstream. There are multiple reasons why digoxin toxicity is likely in this patient. In addition, the following tests should be considered to rule out other causes of bradycardia: (1) A complete blood count may reveal systemic infection and/or anemia, both of which may cause the falls, and anemia may lead to hypoxia, causing bradycardia. (2) An electrocardiogram (EKG) for heart rate and rhythm, sinus tachycardia changes, and/or changes from a previous EKG may indicate if a new myocardial infarction has occurred. (3) Urinalysis with culture and sensitivity may reveal a UTI that can also present as falls in the elderly.

There are many potential etiologies for the recurrent falls, which need to be evaluated (see chapter 9). Important considerations for falls etiology that may be related to medications in this patient include the following:

- Diuretics may cause orthostatic hypotension and/or dehydration, as well as weakness and mental status change due to electrolyte imbalance (from non-potassium-sparing diuretics). Ask: Would a potassium-sparing diuretic be better? Is the potassium level being monitored regularly? Also note that UTI in the presence of a history of such and BPH may cause both mental status change and falls.
- Confusion may be related to beta blockers, ranitidine, and captopril in the elderly. Ask: Could the ACE inhibitor be changed to a newer ACE inhibitor? You may want to check which beta blockers are the best choice to use in the elderly. It would be important to obtain a complete drug history to inquire about OTCs, herbal remedies, and alcohol consumption. Question the use of the H_2 blocker ranitidine (questioning the efficacy of its usage in the presence of confusion,

dementia, and the elderly patient). You may want to review with the pharmacist or geriatric specialist if there is another class of medication that is more appropriate.

Follow-up/ongoing nursing monitoring should include the following:

- Monitor for subtle signs of toxicity: symptomatic cardiac disturbance and arrhythmias, as well as classic signs (anorexia, arrhythmia, and visual disturbance).
- Monitor for depression, as fluoxetine is discontinued and prednisone is being tapered (use Geriatric Depression Scale).
- Monitor mental status (use MMSE [Mini-Mental Status Exam]).
- Assess baseline and ongoing monitoring of ADL progress.
- Monitor for potential for GI bleeding because patient is on prednisone.
- Recommend a pharmacy consultation for recommendations on appropriate medications in the elderly (e.g., maximum dose).
- Evaluate dietary intake, fluid intake and output, and hydration status.
- Monitor weight daily.
- Monitor heart rate and orthostatic blood pressure.
- Provide family education regarding medications and potential side effects, subtle (and often early) signs of condition changes in the elderly, and medication-related side effects.

SUMMARY

Medication safety is a major concern in the elderly. Although intending to remedy the signs and symptoms of disease and illness, drugs all too frequently are misused. To ensure the therapeutic effects of pharmacotherapy, we have developed the accompanying protocol for medication safety, which addresses the (1) knowledge and skill necessary for performance of a medication assessment, (2) accurate and comprehensive documentation of the assessment, and (3) development of an individualized plan to promote medication safety in older adults.

BOX 12.1   A Protocol for Promotion of Medication Safety in Older Adults

---

I. GOAL: to prevent/decrease adverse drug events (ADEs) in older adults
II. BACKGROUND/STATEMENT OF PROBLEM: Adverse drug events, whether from overmedication, insufficient medication, or interactions among medications, can lead to serious or potentially fatal outcomes for older adults.
    A. Definitions:
        1. Medication-related problems: encompass unintended drug effects, adverse drug reactions, polypharmacy, drug misuse, and drug abuse
        2. Unintended drug effects: features of drug administration that are known (e.g., orthostatic hypotension) but are not intended in the prescription or administration of the drug
        3. Adverse drug reaction: any noxious or unintended response to a medication
        4. Polypharmacy: the prescription, administration, or use of more medications than is clinically indicated in a given individual
        5. Drug misuse: the inappropriate use of a substance intended for therapeutic purposes
        6. Drug abuse: the nontherapeutic use of any psychoactive substance that in some way adversely affects the user's life
        7. Drug–disease interactions: undesired drug effects that occur in patients with certain disease states (e.g., beta blocker given to patient with bronchospasm)
    B. Epidemiology:
        1. Twenty-five percent to 40% of all medication prescriptions written in the United States are for older persons (13% of U.S. population).
        2. Five percent to 15% of admissions to acute care hospitals are for medication-related problems.
        3. It is estimated that over 106,000 fatal ADEs occur annually in the United States.
        4. On average, community-dwelling elders consume four to six medications daily.
        5. Forty percent to 50% of all over-the-counter medications are consumed by elderly persons.
        6. The cost of medication-related problems across all ages in the United States is estimated at 85 billion annually.

(continued)

BOX 12.1   A Protocol for Promotion of Medication Safety in Older Adults *(continued)*

   C. Etiology of drug-related problems:
      1. Therapeutic failure (e.g., inadequate drug therapy)
      2. Adverse drug reactions
      3. Adverse drug withdrawal events
   D. Risk factors for medication iatrogenesis:
      1. Age-related physiologic changes in older age
      2. Polypharmacy
      3. Problems with medication compliance
      4. Inappropriate prescription writing
      5. Inadequate patient teaching
      6. Medication consumption for age-related symptoms
         (self-medication)
   E. Consequences of medication-related problems:
      1. Hospitalization
      2. Additional physical, cognitive, and affective symptoms
      3. Increased morbidity and mortality
      4. Loss of functional independence
III. HIGH-RISK MEDICATIONS
   A. Antihypertensive agents:
      1. Angiotensin converting enzyme inhibitors (e.g., captopril)
      2. Central alpha agonists (e.g., clonidine, guanabenz,
         guanfacine, and methyldopa)
      3. Beta blockers (e.g., propranolol)
   B. Psychoactive drugs:
      1. Antipsychotic/neuroleptic drugs (e.g., haloperidol,
         phenothiazines)
      2. Sedative-hypnotics (e.g., chloral hydrate, benzodiazepines)
      3. Antidepressant medications (e.g., amitriptyline, doxepin)
      4. Anxiolytic medications (e.g., meprobamate)
   C. Anticholinergic drugs:
      1. Atropine, scopolamine, hyoscyamine, and oxybutynin
      2. Phenothiazines
   E. Cardiotonics:
      1. Digoxin
      2. Quinidine preparations
   F. Over-the-counter medications:
      1. Analgesics
      2. Cold and flu remedies
      3. Nonsteroidal anti-inflammatory drugs
      4. Antacids
      5. Laxatives

BOX 12.1   *(continued)*

G. H$_2$ receptor antagonists:
   1. Cimetidine
   2. Ranitidine
   3. Nizatidine
   4. Famotidine
H. Alcohol
I. Folk, herbal, or other home remedies
IV. NURSING ASSESSMENT
   A. Review all prescription, over-the-counter, and nontraditional medications.
   B. Assess the older person for cognitive capacity and social support.
   C. Determine if there are any pharmacodynamic or pharmacokinetic alterations in the older person, which may be abnormal.
   D. Do a careful evaluation of medication compliance to determine whether the older person is able to take medications correctly.
   E. Do an assessment as to the older person's value systems and understandings of the meaning of the medications and how they might help or hurt the individual.
   F. Assessment parameters:
      1. Medical diagnoses, diseases, or health problems
      2. History of previous adverse drug reaction(s)
      3. Numbers and types of medications
      4. Length of time taking medication
      5. Last time the prescription was reevaluated by a competent health provider
      6. Instructions for administration of medication
      7. Deviations from prescription
      8. Storage of medications
      9. Intended effect(s) of medication
      10. Adverse effects of medications
      11. Functional, sensory, cognitive, affective, and nutritional status
      12. Technical problems with medication use (ability to open bottles and read labels)
      13. Allergies to medications and type of reaction
V. NURSING CARE STRATEGIES
   A. Prevention:
      1. Develop a nursing plan that focuses on appropriate medication regimes for older adults.
      2. Consider alternatives to medications, as well as fewer medications and lower doses.

(continued)

BOX 12.1   A Protocol for Promotion of Medication Safety in Older Adults *(continued)*

---

   3. Refer the older adult to teaching materials such as http://www.merck.com.
   4. Document teaching strategies, and follow-up with patients to determine that education was effective.
   B. Treatment:
   1. Establish regular reviews of medications for the prevention of iatrogenesis.
   2. Partner with the pharmacy department and pharmacologists to improve strategies to prevent iatrogenesis.
   C. Education of patients and/or significant others about
   1. Medication regimen
   2. Medications that interact with other medications, foods, and alcohol
   3. Habit-forming and addictive medications
   4. Methods for keeping track of medications
   5. Signals of medication problems
VI. EVALUATION OF EXPECTED OUTCOMES
   A. Patients will:
   1. Experience fewer iatrogenic outcomes from medications.
   2. Understand their medication regimens.
   B. Health care providers will:
   1. Use a range of interventions to prevent, alleviate, or ameliorate medication problems with older adults.
   2. Document ongoing comprehensive medication assessment.
   3. Increase their knowledge about medication safety in the elderly.
   4. Increase referrals to appropriate practitioners (e.g., geriatrician, geriatric/gerontological or psychiatric clinical nurse specialist, nurse practitioner, or consultation-liaison service).
   C. Institution will:
   1. Provide educational materials related to the Beers (1997) criteria.
   2. See decreased morbidity and mortality due to medication-related problems.
   3. See improved documentation of medication usage.
   4. Consider unit dose packaging to avoid incorrect medications.
   5. Review documentation of iatrogenic medication and other iatrogenic events for CQI improvement.
   6. Provide staff with ongoing education related to safe medication management.

BOX 12.1   *(continued)*

VII. FOLLOW-UP TO MONITOR PROTOCOL EFFECTIVENESS
   A. Assess staff competence in the assessment of medication use.
   B. Ensure consistent and appropriate documentation of medication assessment.
   C. Provide consistent and appropriate care and follow-up in the presence of a medication-related problem.
   D. Evaluate nature and origins of medication-related problems sought in a timely manner.
   E. Provide multiple episodes of teaching to reinforce understanding and follow-through with appropriate medication administration.
   F. Ensure the incidence of medication-related problems decrease.

American Geriatrics Society (2002); Besdine et al. (1998); Hanlon et al. (2000); Hazzard, Bierman, & Blass (1999); Lazarou, Pomeranz, & Corey (1998); Weitzel (2001).

REFERENCES

American Geriatrics Society. (2002). *Geriatrics Review Syllabus 2002–2004.* New York: Blackwell.

Beers, M. H. (1997). Explicit criteria for determining potentially inappropriate medication use by the elderly: An update. *Archives of Internal Medicine, 157*(14), 1531–1536.

Besdine, R., Beers, M., Bootman, J., Fulmer, T., Gerbino, P., Manasse, H., & Wykle, M. (1998). *When Medicine Hurts Instead of Helps: Preventing Medication Problems in Older Persons.* Washington, DC: Alliance for Aging Research.

Catterson, M. L., Preskorn, S. H., & Martin, R. L. (1997). Pharmacodynamic and pharmacokinetic considerations in geriatric psychopharmacology. *Psychiatric Clinics of North America, 20*(1), 205–218.

Childs, N. (2000). IOM report spurs patient safety activity on Capitol Hill. *Provider, 26*(2), 10–11.

DeMaagd, G. (1995). High-risk drugs in the elderly population. *Geriatric Nursing, 16,* 198–207.

Doucet, J., Jego, A., Noel, D., Geffroy, C. E., Capet, C., Coquard, A., Couffin, E., Fauchais, A. L., Chassagne, P., Mouton-Schleifer, D., & Bercoff, E. (2002). Preventable and nonpreventable risk factors for adverse drug events related to hospital admission in the elderly: A prospective study. *Clinical Drug Investigations, 22,* 385–392.

Falvo, D., Holland, P., Brenner, J., & Benshoff, J. (1990). Medication use practices in the ambulatory elderly. *Health Values, 3,* 100–116.

Flaherty, J. H. (1998). Psychotherapeutic agents in older adults: Commonly prescribed and over-the-counter remedies—causes of confusion. *Clinics in Geriatric Medicine, 14*(1), 101–127.

Flaherty, J. H., Perry, H. M. III, Lynchard, G. S., & Morley, J. E. (2000). Polypharmacy and hospitalization among older home care patients. *Journal of Gerontology Series A, Biological Sciences and Medical Sciences, 55,* M554–559.

Foreman, M. D., & Wykle, M. (1995). Nursing standard-of-practice protocol: Sleep disturbances in elderly patients. *Geriatric Nursing, 16,* 238–439.

Fulmer, T., Feldman, P. H., Kim, T. S., Carty, B., Beers, M., Molina, M., & Putnam, M. (1999). An intervention study to enhance medication compliance in community-dwelling elderly individuals. *Journal of Gerontological Nursing, 25*(8), 6–14.

Fulmer, T., Kim, T. S., Montgomery, K., & Lyder, C. (2000). What the literature tells us about the complexity of medication compliance in the elderly. *Generations, 24*(4), 43–48.

Hanlon, J. T., Fillenbaum, G. G., Ruby, C. M., Gray, S., & Bohannon, A. (2001). Epidemiology of over-the-counter drug use in community dwelling elderly: United States perspective. *Drugs and Aging, 18,* 123–131.

Hanlon, J. T., Shimp, L. A., & Semla, T. P. (2000). Recent advances in geriatrics: Drug-related problems in the elderly. *Annals of Pharmacotherapy, 34*(3), 360–365.

Hazzard, W. R., Bierman, E. L., & Blass, J. P. (1999). *Principles of geriatric medicine and gerontology.* New York: McGraw-Hill.

Hepler, C. D., & Strand, L. M. (1990). Opportunities and responsibilities in pharmaceutical care. *American Journal of Hospital Pharmacy, 47,* 533–543.

Hobson, M. (1992). Medications in older patients. *Western Journal of Medicine, 157,* 539–543.

Hohl, C. M., Dankoff, J., Colacone, A., & Afilalo, M. (2001). Polypharmacy, adverse drug-related events, and potential adverse drug interactions in elderly patients presenting to an emergency department. *Annals of Emergency Medicine, 38,* 666–671.

Kahl, A., Blandford, D. H., Krueger, K., & Zwick, D. I. (1992). Geriatric education centers address medication issues affecting older adults. *Public Health Reports, 107*(1), 37–47.

Kane, J. M., Woerner, M. G., Pollack, S., Safferman, A. Z., & Lieberman, J. A. (1993). Does clozapine cause tardive dyskinesia? *Journal of Clinical Psychiatry, 54,* 327–330.

Karsh, J. (1990). Adverse reactions and interactions with aspirin: Considerations in the treatment of the elderly patient. *Drug Safety, 5,* 317–327.

Kindermann, S. S., Dolder, C. R., Bailey, A., Katz, I. R., & Jeste, D. V. (2002). Pharmacological treatment of psychosis and agitation in elderly patients with dementia: Four decades of experience. *Drugs and Aging, 19,* 257–276.

Kohn, L., Corrigan, J., & Donaldson, M. (2000). *To err is human: Building a safer health system.* Washington, DC: National Academy Press.

Lazarou, J., Pomeranz, B., & Corey, P. (1998). Incidence of adverse drug reactions in hospitalized patients: A meta-analysis of prospective studies. *Journal of the American Medical Association, 279,* 1200–1205.

McLeod, P., Huang, A., Tamblyn, R., & Gayton, D. (1997). Defining inappropriate practices in prescribing for elderly people: A national consensus panel. *Canadian Medical Association Journal, 156,* 385–391.

Muir, A. J., Sanders, L. L., Wilkinson, W. E., & Schmader, K. (2001). Reducing medication regimen complexity: A controlled trial. *Journal of General and Internal Medicine, 16,* 77–82.

Nolan, P. E., Jr., & Marcus, F. I. (2000). Cardiovascular drug use in the elderly. *American Journal of Geriatric Cardiology, 9*(3), 127–129.

Packer, M., Gheorghiade, M., Young, J. B., Costantini, P. J., Adams, K. F., Cody, R. J., Smith, L. K., Van Voorhees, L., Gourley, L. A., & Jolly, M. K. (1993). Withdrawal of digoxin from patients with chronic heart failure treated with angiotensin-converting-enzyme inhibitors: RADIANCE Study. *New England Journal of Medicine, 329*(1), 1–7.

Packer, M., Poole-Wilson, P. A., Armstrong, P. W., Cleland, J. G., Horowitz, J. D., Massie, B. M., Ryden, L., Thygesen, K., & Uretsky, B. F. (1999).

Comparative effects of low and high doses of the angiotensin-converting enzyme inhibitor, lisinopril, on morbidity and mortality in chronic heart failure: ATLAS Study Group. *Circulation, 100,* 2312–2318.

Pesznecker, B., Patsdaughter, C., Moody, K., & Albert, M. (1990). Medication regimens and the home care client: A challenge for health care providers. In K. O'Connor (Ed.), *Facilitating self care practices in the elderly* (pp. 9–68). Binghamton, NY: Haworth.

Rebenson-Piano, M. (1998). The physiologic changes that occur with aging. *Critical Care Nurse Quarterly, 12*(1), 1–14.

Riedinger, J. L., & Robbins, L. J. (1998). Prevention of iatrogenic illness: Adverse drug reactions and nosocomial infections in hospitalized older adults. *Clinics of Geriatric Medicine, 14,* 681–698.

Rohay, J., Dunbar-Jacob, J., Sereika, S., Kwoh, K., & Burke, L. E. (1996). The impact of method of calculation of electronically monitored adherence data. *Controlled Clinical Trials, 17*(82S–83S), A76.

Salzman, C. (1998). *Clinical geriatric psychopharmacology.* Baltimore: Williams & Wilkins.

Spina, E., & Scordo, M. G. (2002). Clinically significant drug interactions with antidepressants in the elderly. *Drugs and Aging, 19,* 299–320.

Tinetti, M. E., & Speechly, M. (1989). Prevention of falls among the elderly. *New England Journal of Medicine, 320,* 1055–1059.

Tune, L. E. (2001). Anticholinergic effects of medication in elderly patients. *Journal of Clinical Psychiatry, 62*(Suppl. 21), 11–14.

Uretsky, B. F., Young, J. B., Shahidi, F. E., Yellen, L. G., Harrison, M. C., & Jolly, M. K. (1993). Randomized study assessing the effect of digoxin withdrawal in patients with mild to moderate chronic congestive heart failure: Results of the PROVED trial. *Journal of the American College of Cardiologists, 22,* 955–962.

Wanich, C. K., Sullivan-Marx, E. M., Gottlieb, G. L., & Johnson, J. C. (1992). Functional status outcomes of a nursing intervention in hospitalized elderly. *Image: Journal of Nursing Scholarship, 24,* 201–207.

Weitzel, E. A. (2001). Risk for poisoning: Drug toxicity. In M. Maas, K. Buckwalter, M. Hardy, T. Tripp-Reimer, M. Titler, & J. Specht (Eds.), *Nursing care of older adults: Diagnoses, outcomes, and interventions* (pp. 41–43). St. Louis: Mosby.

Chapter 13

PAIN MANAGEMENT

Ann L. Horgas and Susan M. McLennon

EDUCATIONAL OBJECTIVES

On completion of this chapter, the reader should be able to
1. Discuss the importance of effective pain management for elderly adults.
2. Describe several methods of assessing pain.
3. Discuss pharmacological and nonpharmacological strategies for treating pain.
4. State at least two key points to include in education for patients and families.

Physical pain is a significant problem for many elderly adults. It has been estimated that approximately 50% of community-dwelling elders suffer from pain (Herr, 2002a; Mobily, Herr, Clark, & Wallace, 1994), and that the incidence of pain is twice as high in people age 65 and older as in younger adults (Fulmer, Mion, & Bottrell, 1996). In

Adapted from a chapter in the original edition by Fulmer, T., Mion, L., Bottrell, M., and the NICHE faculty. Pain management, pp. 145–157. In Abraham, I., Fulmer, T., & Mezey, Eds. *Geriatric Nursing Protocols for Best Practice*. New York: Springer Publishing Company.

nursing homes, as many as 85% of residents are reported to experience pain (Davis, 1997; Ferrell, Ferrell, & Osterweil, 1990; Sengstaken & King, 1993).

The high prevalence of pain is primarily related to the high rate of chronic health disorders in advanced age, particularly painful musculoskeletal conditions such as arthritis, gout, and peripheral vascular disease (Feldt, Warne, & Ryden, 1998). In addition, there is a high prevalence of more acute conditions such as cancer, surgical procedures, cardiovascular disease, and other painful medical diseases and syndromes in this age group (Feldt et al., 1998; Ferrell, 1991; Parmelee, 1994). Cancer, in particular, is associated with significant pain for one third of patients with active disease and for two thirds of those with advanced disease (Feldt et al., 1998; Ferrell et al., 1990). Thus, pain among elderly adults is quite common and often complicated by the concomitant presence of different types, locations, and causes of pain.

Why is knowledge about pain in elderly adults so important? There are several key reasons. First, pain has major implications for elders' health, functioning, and quality of life (Luggen, 1998). For instance, pain is associated with depression, withdrawal, sleep disturbances, impaired mobility, decreased activity engagement, and increased health care use (Ferrell, 1995; Herr, 2002a). Other geriatric conditions that can be worsened by pain include falls, deconditioning, malnutrition, gait disturbances, and slowed rehabilitation (Ferrell, Ferrell, & Rivera, 1995; Herr, 2002a). Thus, pain has major implications for physical, functional, and mental health among elderly adults.

Second, nurses have a key role in assessing and managing pain. The promotion of comfort and the relief of pain are fundamental to nursing practice. Given that the prevalence of pain in older adults is substantially higher than among younger adults, this nursing role becomes increasingly important in the elderly population. Nurses must work effectively in an interdisciplinary health care environment to assess and treat pain. In addition, nurses have the primary responsibility to teach the patient and family about pain and how to manage it both pharmacologically and nonpharmacologically. As such, nurses must be knowledgeable about pain management in general, and about managing pain in elderly adults in particular.

Third, the Joint Commission on the Accreditation of Healthcare Organizations (JCAHO) now officially recognizes pain as a major health problem and that patients have the right to appropriate assessment and management of pain (JCAHO, 2001). The new requirements implemented in 2001 consider pain the "fifth vital sign" and require systematic and regular assessment of pain in all hospitalized patients. Thus, health care providers must now be compliant with regulatory guidelines about pain management. Unfortunately, this does not address the pain management needs of the elderly adults who are experiencing significant pain unless they are hospitalized.

DEFINITIONS OF PAIN

Pain is a multidimensional, subjective experience with sensory, cognitive, and emotional dimensions (American Geriatrics Society [AGS], 1998; Melzack & Casey, 1968). For clinical practice, Margo McCaffery's classic definition of pain is perhaps the most relevant. According to McCaffery, pain is whatever the experiencing person says it is, existing whenever he says it does (McCaffery, 1968; McCaffery & Pasero, 1999). This definition serves as a reminder that pain is highly subjective and that patients' self-report and description of pain are very important.

TYPES OF PAIN

There are several different types and classifications of pain. The most basic distinction is whether the pain is acute or chronic. Acute pain results from an injury, surgery, or disease-related tissue damage (Panda & Desbiens, 2001). It is usually associated with autonomic activity, such as tachycardia and diaphoresis. Acute pain is usually relatively brief and subsides with healing. In contrast, chronic pain endures past the normal duration of tissue damage (usually more than 3 to 6 months), and autonomic activity is usually absent (Panda & Desbiens, 2001). Chronic pain can lead to functional loss, reduced quality of life, and mood and behavior changes, especially when it is untreated.

Pain is further classified as either nociceptive or neuropathic, depending on the cause of the pain. Nociceptive pain results from disease processes (e.g., osteoarthritis), soft-tissue injuries (e.g., falls), and medical treatment (e.g., surgery, venipuncture, and other procedures) and is associated with stimulation of specific peripheral or visceral receptors. Nociceptive pain is usually localized and responsive to treatment. Neuropathic pain is caused by pathology in the peripheral or central nervous system. This type of pain is often associated with diabetic neuropathies, phantom-limb pain, postherpetic and trigeminal neuralgias, and cerebrovascular accidents. Neuropathic pain is more diffuse and less responsive to analgesics. It is important to note, however, that these pain types often overlap and are not always clearly differentiated.

PAIN ASSESSMENT STRATEGIES

Despite the prevalence and consequences of pain, evidence suggests that pain is underdetected and poorly managed among elderly adults (Horgas & Tsai, 1998). There are a number of factors that contribute to this situation, including individual-based and caregiver-based factors. Individual factors that may impair pain assessment include the following: (1) a belief that pain is a normal part of aging, (2) concern of being labeled a hypochondriac or complainer, (3) fear of the meaning of the pain in relation to disease progression or prognosis, (4) fear of narcotic addiction and analgesics, (5) worry about health care costs, and (6) a belief that the pain is not important to health care providers (AGS, 1998; Wells, Kaas, & Feldt, 1997). Other factors, such as hearing and speech difficulties, may prevent elderly adults from communicating pain to health care providers (Feldt et al., 1998). In addition, cognitive impairment is an important factor in reducing elders' reporting of pain (Feldt et al., 1998; Parmelee, Smith, & Katz, 1993).

Pain detection and management are also influenced by provider-based factors. Health care providers have been found to share the mistaken belief that pain is a part of the normal aging process and to avoid using opioids because of fear about potential addiction and adverse side effects (Wells et al., 1997). Similarly, cognitive status influences providers' assessment and treatment of pain. For example, it has been found that cognitively impaired nursing home residents were prescribed and administered significantly less analgesic medication than were cognitively intact elders (Horgas & Tsai, 1998). This finding may reflect cognitively impaired elders' inability to recall and report the presence of pain to their health care providers. It may also reflect caregivers' inability to detect pain, especially among frail older adults. In one nursing home study, it was found that patients' and caregivers' reports of pain were congruent in only about one third of cases (Horgas & Dunn, 2001).

Furthermore, it was noted that depression was highest in those residents for whom pain was not perceived by their caregivers. Thus, pain assessment and management can be a complicated clinical issue. Health care providers should face the challenge of pain assessment by first systematically examining their own biases and beliefs about pain, then eliciting and understanding the challenges and beliefs that their patients bring to the situation.

SELF-REPORTED PAIN

There is no objective biological marker or laboratory test for the presence of pain. Thus, the most accurate and reliable measure of pain is the patient's self-report. This is consistent with the definition provided earlier in this chapter by McCaffery—that pain is defined as whatever the experiencing person says it is, existing whenever he [or she] says it does (McCaffery, 1968; McCaffery & Pasero, 1999). Evidence suggests that even patients with mild to moderate cognitive impairment can report their pain when asked simple questions and given sufficient time to respond (Ferrell et al., 1995).

The first principle of pain assessment is to ask about the presence of pain on regular and frequent intervals. It is important to allow the patient sufficient time to consider the question and to formulate an answer. This is especially important when working with cognitively impaired elders. It is also important to explore different words that the patient may use synonymously with pain, such as *discomfort* and *aching*.

The intensity of pain can be measured in many ways. Some commonly used tools include the Visual Analog Scale, the Verbal Descriptor Scale, and the Faces Pain Scale (Herr, 2002a). The Visual Analog Scale (VAS) is widely used, especially in hospital settings. Patients are asked to rate the intensity of their pain on a 0–10 scale. The VAS requires the ability to discriminate subtle differences in pain intensity and may be difficult for some elders to complete. A tool that has been specifically recommended for use with elderly adults is the Verbal Descriptor Scale (Herr, 2002a; Herr & Mobily, 1993). This tool measures pain intensity by asking participants to select a word that best describes their present pain (e.g., no pain to worst pain imaginable). This measure has been found to be a reliable and valid measure of pain intensity and is reported to be the easiest to complete and the most preferred by older adults (Herr, 2002a; Herr & Mobily, 1993). In addition, there are several scales that use pictures of faces to represent pain intensity. This type of measure is often recommended for use with cognitively impaired elders. The *Faces Pain Scale* (FPS) was developed to assess pain intensity in children and consists of seven cartoon facial depictions ranging from the least pain to the most pain possible (Bieri, Reeve, Champion, Addicoat, & Ziegler, 1990). The FPS is considered appropriate for use with elderly adults because the cartoon faces are not age, gender, or race specific (Herr, Mobily, Kohout, & Wagenaar, 1998).

OBSERVED PAIN INDICATORS

The assessment of pain behaviors is often necessary in elders, especially in those who are less able to verbally report their pain because of dementia. Pain behaviors include facial grimacing, rubbing, vocalizations, sighing, complaining, screaming, and body rigidity (Feldt, 2000). There is some evidence to suggest that cognitively impaired elders exhibit more pain behaviors than those who are intact, suggesting that these tools may be good measures of pain in impaired elders (Feldt, 2000; Hadjistavropoulos, LaChapelle, MacLeod, Snider, & Craig, 2000).

Pain assessment is a complicated clinical procedure that can be hampered by many factors. Systematic and thorough assessment, however, is a critical first step in appropriately managing pain in elderly adults. Assessment issues are summarized in the recommended pain management protocol (see Box 13.1). The use of a standardized pain assessment tool is important in measuring pain. It enables health care providers to document their assessment, measure change in pain, evaluate treatment effectiveness, and communicate to other health care providers, the patient, and the family. Comprehensive pain assessment includes measures of self-reported pain and pain behaviors and includes information from patients and families.

PAIN MANAGEMENT STRATEGIES

Managing pain in older adults can be a challenging process. Pain treatment approaches that use a multidimensional approach and that are individualized to the patient, however, are often effective (Gibson, Farrell, Katz, & Helme, 1996). The main goal of pain management in older adults is to maximize function and quality of life (Herr, 2002b). Thus, a combination of pharmacological and non-pharmacological strategies should be used to ease the pain.

BOX 13.1   Nursing Standard of Practice Protocol:
Pain Management in Elderly Adults

Standard: All elderly adults will either be pain free or their pain will be controlled to a level that is acceptable to the patient and allows the elder to maintain the highest level of functioning possible.

Overview: Pain is a common experience for many older adults and is associated with a number of chronic (e.g., osteoarthritis) and acute (e.g., cancer, surgery) conditions. Pain is a subjective experience that is influenced by many cognitive, emotional, medical, and cultural factors. Despite the prevalence of pain, evidence suggests that it is often poorly assessed and poorly managed, especially in older adults. Cognitive impairment due to dementia and/or delirium represents a particular challenge to pain management because elders with these conditions may be unable to verbalize their pain. There are many myths associated with pain management, including fear of medication use and belief that pain is a normal part of aging, that nurses must understand in order to provide optimal care and to educate patients and families about managing pain. Nurses are an integral of the interdisciplinary team that is necessary to meet the challenge of effective pain management in elderly adults.

I. BACKGROUND
  A. Definitions:
    1. *Pain:* Pain is defined as an unpleasant sensory and emotional experience (AGS, 1998; Melzack & Casey, 1968) and also as whatever the experiencing person says it is, existing whenever he says it does (McCaffery, 1968; McCaffery & Pasero, 1999). These definitions highlight the multidimensional and highly subjective nature of pain. Pain is usually characterized according to the duration of pain (e.g., acute vs. chronic) and the cause of pain (e.g., nociceptive vs. neuropathic). These definitions have implications for pain management strategies.
    2. *Acute pain:* Defines pain that results from injury, surgery, or tissue damage. It is usually associated with autonomic activity, such as tachycardia and diaphoresis. Acute pain is usually time-limited and subsides with healing.
    3. *Chronic pain:* Defines pain that endures past the normal duration of tissue damage (usually 3–6 months), and autonomic activity is usually absent. Chronic pain is often associated with functional loss, mood and behavior changes, as well as reduced quality of life.

(continued)

**BOX 13.1 Nursing Standard of Practice Protocol:
Pain Management in Elderly Adults** *(continued)*

   4. *Nociceptive pain:* Refers to pain caused by stimulation of specific peripheral or visceral pain receptors. This type of pain results from disease processes (e.g., osteoarthritis), soft tissue injuries (e.g., falls), and medical treatment (e.g., surgery, venipuncture, and other procedures). It is usually localized and responsive to treatment.
   5. *Neuropathic pain:* Refers to pain caused by damage to the peripheral or central nervous system. This type of pain is associated with diabetic neuropathies, postherpetic and trigeminal neuralgias, and cerebrovascular accidents. It is usually more diffuse and less responsive to analgesic medications.
 B. Epidemiology:
   1. Approximately 50% of community-dwelling elders have pain.
   2. Approximately 85% of nursing home residents experience pain.
   3. The prevalence of pain is twice as high among older adults (those ≥ 60 years) than among younger individuals.
 C. Etiology:
   1. More than 80% of elderly adults have chronic medical conditions that are typically associated with pain, such as osteoarthritis and peripheral vascular disease.
   2. Older adults often have multiple medical conditions, both chronic and acute, and may suffer from multiple types and sources of pain.
 D. Significance:
   1. Pain has major implications for older adults' health, functioning, and quality of life. If unrelieved, pain is associated with
      a. Depression
      b. Sleep disturbances
      c. Withdrawal and decreased socialization
      d. Functional loss and increased dependency
      e. Exacerbation of cognitive impairment
      f. Increased health care utilization and costs
   2. Nurses have a key role in pain management. The promotion of comfort and relief of pain is fundamental to nursing practice. Nurses need to be knowledgeable about pain in late life in order to provide optimal care, to educate patients and families, and to work effectively in interdisciplinary pain management teams.

BOX 13.1   *(continued)*

---

3. The Joint Commission on Accreditation of Healthcare Organizations (JCAHO) now requires regular and systematic assessment of pain in all hospitalized patients. Because older adults constitute a significant portion of the patient population in many acute care settings, nurses need to have the knowledge and skill to address the specific pain needs of elderly adults.

II. ASSESSMENT PARAMETERS
   A. Assumptions:
      1. The majority of hospitalized elderly patients suffer from both acute and chronic pain.
      2. Elderly adults with cognitive impairment experience pain but are often unable to verbalize it.
      3. Both patients and health care providers have personal beliefs, prior experiences, insufficient knowledge, mistaken beliefs about pain and pain management that (a) influence the pain management process and (b) must be acknowledged and addressed before optimal pain relief can be achieved.
      4. Pain assessment must be regular, systematic, and documented in order to accurately evaluate treatment effectiveness.
      5. Self-report is the gold standard for pain assessment.
   B. Strategies for pain assessment:
      1. Review medical history, physical examinations, and laboratory and diagnostic tests in order to understand the sequence of events contributing to pain.
      2. Assess present pain, including intensity, character, frequency, pattern, location, duration, and precipitating and relieving factors.
      3. Review medications, including current and previously used prescription drugs, over-the-counter drugs, and home remedies. Determine what pain control methods have been effective for the patient.
      4. Assess patient's attitudes and beliefs about the use of analgesics, anxiolytics, and nonpharmacological treatments.
      5. Gather information from family members about the patient's pain experiences. Ask about the patient's verbal and nonverbal/behavioral expressions of pain, particularly in demented patients.

(continued)

BOX 13.1   Nursing Standard of Practice Protocol:
Pain Management in Elderly Adults *(continued)*

---

    6. Use a standardized tool to assess self-reported pain. Choose
from published measurement tools, and recall that elders
may have difficulty using 10-point visual analogue scales.
Vertical verbal descriptor scales or faces scales may be more
useful with elders, especially those with some cognitive losses.
    7. Assess pain regularly and frequently, but at least every
4 hours. Monitor pain intensity after giving medications to
evaluate effectiveness.
    8. Observe for nonverbal and behavioral signs of pain, such as
facial grimacing, withdrawal, guarding, rubbing, limping,
shifting of position, aggression, depression, moaning, and
crying. Also watch for changes in behavior from patient's
usual patterns.
III. NURSING CARE STRATEGIES
  A. Prevention of pain:
    1. Assess pain regularly and frequently to facilitate appropriate
treatment.
    2. Anticipate and aggressively treat for pain before,
during, and after painful diagnostic and/or therapeutic
treatments.
    3. Educate patients, families, and other clinicians to use
analgesic medications prophylactically prior to and after
painful procedures.
    4. Educate patients and families about pain medications, their
side effects and adverse effects, and issues of addiction,
dependence, and tolerance.
    5. Educate patients to take medications for pain on a regular
basis and to avoid allowing pain to escalate.
    6. Educate patients, families, and other clinicians to use
nonpharmacological strategies to manage pain, such as
relaxation, massage, and heat/cold.
  B. Treatment guidelines
    1. Pharmacologic:
      a. Elderly adults are at increased risk for adverse drug
reactions and drug–drug interactions.
      b. Monitor medications closely to avoid over- or
undermedication.
      c. Administer pain drugs on a regular basis to maintain
therapeutic levels; avoid prn drugs.
      d. Document treatment plan to maintain consistency
across shifts and with other care providers.

BOX 13.1 *(continued)*

2. Nonpharmacologic:
   a. Investigate elderly patients' attitudes and beliefs about, preference for, and experience with nonpharmacological pain treatment strategies.
   b. A variety of techniques exist, but they must be tailored to the individual.
   c. Cognitive-behavioral strategies focus on changing the person's perception of pain (e.g., relaxation therapy, education, and distraction) and may not be appropriate for cognitively impaired persons.
   d. Physical pain relief strategies focus on promoting comfort and altering physiologic responses to pain (e.g., heat, cold, TENS [transcutaneous electrical nerve stimulation] units).
3. A combination approach is often the best.

IV. EXPECTED OUTCOMES
  A. Patient:
   1. Patient will be either free of pain or pain will be at a level that the patient judges as acceptable.
   2. Patient maintains the highest level of self-care, functional ability, and activity possible.
   3. Patient experiences no iatrogenic complications, such as falls, GI upset/bleed, or altered cognitive status.
  B. Nurse:
   1. Nurse will demonstrate evidence of ongoing and comprehensive pain assessment.
   2. Nurse will document evidence of prompt and effective pain management interventions.
   3. Nurse will document systematic evaluation of intervention effectiveness.
   4. Nurse will demonstrate knowledge of pain management in elderly patients, including assessment strategies, pain medications, nonpharmacological interventions, and patient/family education.
  C. Institution:
   1. Facility/institution will provide evidence of documentation of pain assessment, intervention, and evaluation of treatment effectiveness.
   2. Facility/institution will provide evidence of referral to specialists for specific therapies (e.g., psychiatry, psychology, biofeedback, physical therapy, and pain treatment centers).
   3. Facility/institution will provide evidence of pain management resources for staff (e.g., care planning and pain management references, pain management consultants).

Several excellent pain assessment protocols have been developed for use with elderly adults. For example, the American Geriatrics Society (AGS; 1998) has published clinical practice guidelines for managing chronic pain in older adults. These guidelines provide comprehensive information that is specific to the needs of geriatric patients. In addition, the American Pain Society (2002) has published guidelines for the management of pain in osteoarthritis, rheumatoid arthritis, and juvenile chronic arthritis. These guidelines are disease specific, rather than age group specific, but they provide comprehensive information for managing these chronic pain conditions. The Agency for Health Care Policy and Research (U.S. Department of Health and Human Services, 1994) has also developed clinical guidelines for the management of acute pain, but this protocol is less specific to older adults.

PHARMACOLOGIC PAIN TREATMENT

Pain treatment with medications is a complex decision-making process based on multiple considerations. Ideally, it is a mutual process between the health care provider, the patient, and significant others. It includes a careful discussion of risks versus benefits and the establishment of clear goals of therapy. Often it is a process of trial and error that aims to balance medication effectiveness with management of side effects. Other considerations included in the process are frequency of use, type of pain, duration of treatment, and cost.

The World Health Organization (1990) provided an analgesic ladder that has been successfully used as a guide for treating cancer pain. Choices are made from three drug categories based on pain severity: the nonopioids, opioids, and adjuvant agents. Combinations of drugs are used because two or more drugs can treat different underlying pain mechanisms and different types of pain and allow for smaller doses of each analgesic to be used, thus minimizing side effects. Adjuvant drugs have primary purposes other than pain relief, but they can be used for their analgesic effects in certain painful conditions (AGS, 1998).

AGE-RELATED PHYSIOLOGIC CHANGES

Specific age-related changes influence the pharmacodynamics (the pharmacological effect of the drug on the body) and pharmacokinetics (the concentration of active drug in the body) of medications (see chapter 12). Some changes with advanced age include diminished absorption due to increased gastric pH and decreased intestinal blood flow. Drug distribution is affected by less lean body mass, increased body fat and decreased body water content, increased plasma protein, and changes in nutritional state. Drug metabolism is affected by decreased hepatic function. Drug excretion and elimination is reduced by 10% per decade after age 40 due to declines in renal function (Pasero, Reed, & McCaffery, 1999).

SPECIAL CONSIDERATIONS FOR ADMINISTERING ANALGESICS

Older adults are at higher risk for side effects with drug therapy because of an age-related decline in drug metabolism and elimination. Recommendations for beginning medication treatment include starting at low doses and gradually titrating upward while monitoring and managing side effects. The adage "Start low and go slow" is often used. Titrate doses upward to achieved desired effects using short-acting medications first, then consider using longer duration medications for long-lasting pain. Choose a drug with a short half-life and the fewest side effects, if possible (Pasero, Reed, & McCaffery, 1999).

Multiple drug routes are available for the administration of pain medications. Often the first choice is the oral route because it is the least invasive and is very effective. The onset of action is within 30 minutes to 2 hours. For more immediate pain relief, intravenous administration is recommended. In general, intramuscular injections should be avoided in the elderly because of tissue injury and because they are pain producing. Topical and rectal routes may also be used in pain medication administration. Whenever possible, adopting a preventive approach to pain management is recommended. By treating pain before it occurs, less medication is required than to relieve it (Reisine & Pasternak, 1996). Around-the-clock dosing, dosing prior to a painful treatment or event, and giving the next dose before the previous dose wears off are examples of pain prevention.

PAIN MANAGEMENT IN DEMENTIA

People with dementia are often undertreated and poorly assessed for pain even though they have diagnoses (e.g., osteoarthritis) that are known to cause pain. In situations in which clinicians suspect that a patient may be experiencing pain but where cognitive impairment limits the usefulness of pain assessment instruments or observations, clinicians should initiate a clinical trial of pain medication as well as nonpharmacologic strategies. Continued symptoms, such as vocalizations or agitation after administration of pain medication, should be considered as evidence that the patient's symptoms are due to unrelieved pain, and further treatment should be initiated. The Assessment of Discomfort in Dementia (ADD) protocol has been designed to assess and treat physical pain and affective discomfort in persons with late-stage dementia. Use of the protocol has shown a significant decrease in discomfort in dementia patients (Kovach, Weissman, Griffie, Matson, & Muchka, 1999) and may be employed to improve pain control in this population.

ANALGESIC DRUG TOLERANCE, DEPENDENCY, AND ADDICTION

The use of opioids in treating severe, long-lasting pain or in terminal conditions may lead to drug tolerance and dependency. Fear of developing these conditions, however, does not justify withholding these medications, especially in the terminally ill. Understanding tolerance, dependency, and addiction is important in effectively managing pain in the elderly. Drug tolerance is defined as a decline in drug effectiveness over time due to continual use (Panda & Desbiens, 2001). Increasing the dose can overcome this effect. Drug dependence is identified by uncomfortable symptoms that occur with the abrupt withdrawal of the drug (Panda & Desbiens, 2001). Opioid tapering is recommended when discontinuing use to alleviate this effect. The American Pain Society (1999) defines drug addiction as a psychological condition characterized by compulsive drug use and an uncontrollable craving to obtain effects other than relief of pain. It occurs rarely when opioids are used as medications for pain control and occurs even more rarely in the elderly.

TYPES OF ANALGESIC MEDICATIONS

Medications that are commonly used to treat pain in elderly adults are summarized in Table 13.1. This table also includes recommended dosages and special considerations. Specific information about these types of medications is discussed below.

Nonopioids are often the first line in pharmacologic pain treatment. This group includes acetaminophen, nonsteroidal anti-inflammatory

TABLE 13.1 Common Pain Medications for Use with Elderly Patients

Indication and effects	Type	Medication	Initial dose	Half-life	Maximum daily dose	Special considerations
Mild pain	Nonopioids	Acetaminophen (Tylenol)	325–650 mg PO q4–6h	1–3h	4,000 mg	Caution with hepatic disease; possibly associated with renal dysfunction with prolonged use
		NSAIDs: Ibuprofen (Advil, Motrin)	200–400 mg PO q6–8h	1.8–2.5h	3,200 mg	Gastrointestinal bleeding; caution with hepatic and renal disease; may cause central nervous system symptoms
		COX-2 inhibitors: Rofexicob (Vioxx) Celexicob (Celebrex)	12.5–25 mg/d PO q24h 100–200 mg PO q12–24h	17h 11h	50 mg 400 mg	Fewer GI side effects than NSAIDs; Celexicob contraindicated with sulfa sensitivity
		Tramadol (Ultram) for mild to moderate pain	50–100 mg PO q4-6 hr	5–9h	400 mg (300 mg if age > 75)	Nausea, constipation, sedation, seizure; caution with renal or liver impairment; mixed nonopioid and opioid effects

(continued)

TABLE 13.1 Common Pain Medications for Use with Elderly Patients *(continued)*

Indication and effects	Type	Medication	Initial dose	Half-life	Maximum daily dose	Special considerations
Mild-moderate pain	Opioids	Codeine	30–60 mg PO q4–6 h 15–30 mg IV/SC q4–6h	2–4h	No maximum	Nausea, constipation, sedation, respiratory depression, hypotension, dizziness
		Hydrocodone (Vicodin, Lortab)	5–10 mg	3–4h	No maximum	Same as codeine
		Oxycodone (Percocet, Tylox) (Oxycontin)	5–10 mg PO q4–6 h 10–20 mg PO q12	2–3h 4.5h	No maximum	Same as codeine
Moderate to severe pain		Morphine sulfate (MS Contin)	15–30 mg PO q3–6 h 15–30 mg PO q12h	2–4h	No maximum	Same as codeine
		Fentanyl (Duragesic)	25–50 µg/h q 48–72h	13–24h	No maximum	Same as codeine
		Hydromorphone (Dilaudid)	2–4 mg PO q3–4h	2–3h	No maximum	Same as codeine

GI = gastrointestinal; NSAID = nonsteroidal anti-inflammatory drug

Source: Adapted from American Geriatrics Society Panel on Chronic Pain in Older Adults. (1998). The management of chronic pain in older persons. *Journal of the American Geriatrics Society, 46,* 635–651.

Glen, V. L., & St. Marie, B. (2002). Overview of pharmacology. In B. St. Marie (Ed.), *American Society of Pain Management Nurses: Core Curriculum for Pain Management Nursing* (pp. 181–237). Philadelphia: Saunders.

McCaffery, M., & Portenoy, R. (1999). Nonopioids. In M. McCaffery & C. Pasero (Eds.), *Pain clinical manual* (2nd ed.). St. Louis: Mosby.

drug (NSAIDs), cyclooxygenase-2 (COX-2) inhibitors, and tramadol. They are generally used for a wide variety of painful conditions, both acute and chronic, of mild to moderate severity. Acetaminophen (e.g., Tylenol) is considered the drug of choice for relief of musculoskeletal pain (AGS, 1998) because it has few side effects and is probably the safest non-opioid for most people. However, it should be used with caution in people with underlying hepatic or renal disease. The NSAIDs (e.g., ibuprofen and naproxen sodium) are also effective for mild to moderate pain. NSAIDs and acetaminophen are often used in combination with opioids for moderate to severe pain.

The most common side effect of the NSAIDs is gastric damage that occurs locally as a gastric irritant and systemically through inhibition of prostaglandin synthesis, resulting in increased gastrointestinal (GI) tract susceptibility to injury. The elderly are more likely to develop ulcer disease and have a greater incidence of death from the GI effects of NSAIDs. Renal insufficiency is more likely to occur in the elderly with NSAID use. Other side effects include increased bleeding time, central nervous system effects, hepatic disease, and worsening asthma. When NSAIDs are used as single doses, in low doses, and for short periods of time, side effects are usually less common than with long-term use. Coadministration of misoprostol (Cytotec) has been shown to reduce the GI complications associated with NSAID use (Higa, 1997).

The COX-2 inhibitors celexicob and rofexicob are as effective as NSAIDs for pain relief, are indicated for mild to moderate pain, are associated with a lower risk of gastrointestinal bleeding, but have a similar risk for other side effects. Celexicob should not be used with sulfa sensitivities.

Tramadol (Ultram) has characteristics of both nonopioids and opioids in analgesic properties. It is effective for moderate to severe pain, and its mechanism of action is not completely understood. Nausea and vomiting are common side effects associated with the use of tramadol, along with dizziness, sedation, restlessness, diarrhea or constipation, dyspepsia, weakness, diaphoresis, seizures, and respiratory depression (Glen & St. Marie, 2002). It should not be used in people with a history of codeine allergy and should be used cautiously in hepatic or renal impairment.

Opioid drugs (e.g., codeine and morphine) are effective at treating moderate to severe pain from multiple causes. They are effective in the elderly, although many older adults and health care providers are reluctant to use them because of fears of overdose, side effects, and intolerance. Potential side effects include nausea, constipation, drowsiness, cognitive effects, and respiratory depression. The Agency for Health Care Policy and Research (now known as Agency for Healthcare Research and Quality [AHRQ]) recommends achieving safe administration of opioids to the elderly by reducing the dose to 25% to 50% of the adult dose (U.S. Department of Health and Human Services, 1992). Tolerance to the side effects develops with use over time; therefore, coadministration of stool softeners for relief of constipation is recommended.

Adjuvant drugs, or other nonopioid drugs administered in conjunction with other analgesics, are often administered with nonopioids and opioids to achieve optimal pain control through additive analgesic effects or to enhance response to analgesics. Tricyclic antidepressants (e.g., nortriptyline) are used for neuropathic pain. Antidepressants are also used to treat underlying depression and anxiety associated with chronic pain. Anticonvulsants (e.g., carbamazepine) are often used for trigeminal neuralgia. Local anesthetics such as lidocaine as a patch, gel, or cream can be used as an additional treatment for the pain of postherpetic neuralgia.

Equianalgesia refers to equivalent analgesia. Equianalgesic dosing charts provide lists of drugs and doses of commonly prescribed pain medications that are approximately equal in providing pain relief. They can provide practical information for selecting appropriate starting doses or when changing from one drug to another (Pasero, Portenoy, & McCaffery, 1999).

DRUGS TO AVOID IN ELDERS

Medications to avoid in the elderly include meperidine (Demerol), propoxyphene (Darvon or Darvocet), and pentazocine (Talwin) because of the risk of delirium, seizures, and renal impairment (Wilcox, Himmelstein, & Woolhandler, 1994). Additionally, sedatives, antihistamines, and antiemetics should be avoided or used with caution because of long duration of action, risk of falls, anticholinergic effects, and sedating effects (Pasero, Portenoy, & McCaffery, 1999).

NONPHARMACOLOGICAL PAIN TREATMENT

Whenever possible, pain should be treated with a combination of drug and nondrug therapies (Herr, 2002b). A combination approach may help to provide more effective pain management with less potential for negative side effects due to medications (Ferrell, Grant, Padilla, Vemuri, & Rhiner, 1991). In addition, the use of nondrug approaches can often be taught to patients, families, and caregivers.

Nonpharmacological pain treatment strategies generally fall into two categories: physical pain relief approaches and cognitive-behavioral approaches (Herr, 2002b). Physical strategies are things such as transcutaneous electrical nerve stimulation, use of heat and cold, massage, and mild exercise. Cognitive-behavioral approaches are things that change the person's perception of the pain and improve coping strategies (Rudy, Hanlon, & Markham, 2002). These include strategies such as relaxation, distraction, guided imagery, hypnosis, and biofeedback.

Older adults are generally responsive to the use of nondrug methods of treating pain (Herr, 2002b; Sorkin, Rudy, Hanlon, Turk, & Stieg, 1990). In fact, one study showed that 96% of older adults reported using at least one complementary/alternative therapy modality, and that prayer was the most commonly reported coping strategy (Dunn & Horgas, 2000). It is important to recognize, however, that individuals differ in their preferences for and ability to use nonpharmacologic interventions to manage pain. Spiritual and/or religious coping strategies, for instance, must be consistent with individual values and beliefs. Other strategies, such as imagery or relaxation techniques, may not be feasible for cognitively impaired elders. Thus, it is important for health care providers to consider a broad array of nonpharmacological pain management strategies and to tailor the selections to the individual. It is also important to gain individual and family input about the use of home and folk remedies and to support their use as appropriate.

SUMMARY

Pain is a significant problem for older adults, which has the potential to negatively impact independence, functioning, and quality of life. In order for pain to be managed effectively, it must first be carefully and systematically assessed. Pain assessment in older adults should start with self-reported pain, but it should incorporate assessment of nonverbal pain behaviors and family input about usual pain responses and patterns, particularly in patients unable to communicate that they are in pain. The use of established measurement tools is recommended. Pain treatment in older adults should be tailored to the type and severity of pain. Pain medications can be safely used in elders and may be more effective when combined with non-pharmacological treatment. Elderly patients, their families, and their care providers should be knowledgeable about pain and how to manage it. Thus, education about pain is an important component of the pain management process that cannot be overlooked. Managing pain, including empowering individuals and their caregivers to do so, is a critical nursing role that can not only decrease pain but also improve the quality of life for elderly adults.

REFERENCES

American Geriatrics Society (AGS) Panel on Chronic Pain in Older Persons. (1998). Clinical practice guidelines: The management of chronic pain in older persons. *Journal of the American Geriatrics Society, 46,* 635–651.

American Pain Society. (1999). *Principles of analgesic use in the treatment of acute and cancer pain* (4th ed.). Glenview, IL: Author.

American Pain Society. (2002). *Guideline for the management of pain in osteoarthritis, rheumatoid arthritis, and juvenile chronic arthritis.* Glenview, IL: Author.

Bieri, D., Reeve R. A., Champion G. D., Addicoat L., & Ziegler, J. B. (1990). The Faces Pain Scale for the self-assessment of the severity of pain experienced by children: Development, initial validation, and preliminary investigation for ratio scale properties. *Pain, 41,* 139–150.

Davis, G. C. (1997). Chronic pain management of older adults in residential settings. *Journal of Gerontological Nursing, 23*(6), 16–22.

Dunn, K., & Horgas, A. L. (2000). The prevalence of prayer as a spiritual self-care modality in elders. *Journal of Holistic Nursing, 18,* 337–351.

Feldt, K. S. (2000). The checklist of nonverbal pain indicators (CNPI). *Pain Management Nursing, 1*(1): 13–21.

Feldt, K. S., Warne, M. A., & Ryden, M. B. (1998). Examining pain in aggressive cognitively impaired older adults. *Journal of Gerontological Nursing, 24,* 14–22.

Ferrell, B. A. (1991). Pain management in elderly people. *Journal of the American Geriatrics Society, 39,* 64–73.

Ferrell, B. A. (1995). Pain evaluation and management in the nursing home. *Annals of Internal Medicine, 9,* 681–687.

Ferrell, B. A., Ferrell, B. R., & Osterweil, D. (1990). Pain in the nursing home. *Journal of the American Geriatrics Society, 38,* 409–414.

Ferrell, B. A., Ferrell, B. R., & Rivera, L. (1995). Pain in cognitively impaired nursing home patients. *Journal of Pain and Symptom Management, 10,* 591–598.

Ferrell, B. A., Grant, M., Padilla, G., Vemuri, S., & Rhiner, M. (1991). The experience of pain and perceptions of quality of life: Validation of a conceptual model. *Hospice Journal, 7*(3), 9–24.

Fulmer, T. T., Mion, L. C., & Bottrell, M. M. (1996). Pain management protocol. *Geriatric Nursing, 17,* 222–227.

Gibson, S., Farrell, M., Katz, B., & Helme, R. (1996). Multidisciplinary management of chronic nonmalignant pain in older adults. In B. R. Ferrell &
B. A. Ferrell (Eds.), *Pain in the Elderly* (pp. 91–99). Seattle: IASP Press.

Glen, V. L., & St. Marie, B. (2002). Overview of pharmacology. In B. St. Marie
(Ed.), *American Society of Pain Management Nurses: Core Curriculum for
Pain Management Nursing* (pp. 181–237). Philadelphia: Saunders.

Hadjistavropoulos, T., LaChapelle D. L., MacLeod F. K., Snider B., & Craig, K. D.
(2000). Measuring movement-exacerbated pain in cognitively impaired
frail elders. *Clinical Journal of Pain, 16*(1), 54–63.

Herr, K. (2002a). Chronic pain: Challenges and assessment strategies.
Journal of Gerontological Nursing, 28(1), 20–27.

Herr, K. (2002b). Chronic pain in the older patient: Management strategies.
Journal of Gerontological Nursing, 28(2), 28–34.

Herr, K. A., & Mobily, P. R. (1993). Comparison of selected pain assessment
tools for use with the elderly. *Applied Nursing Research, 6,* 39–46.

Herr, K. A., Mobily, P. R., Kohout, F. J., & Wagenaar, D. (1998). Evaluation of
the Faces Pain Scale for use with the elderly. *Clinical Journal of Pain, 14,*
29–38.

Higa, J. H. (1997). Interventions in nursing home residents receiving NSAIDs:
Preventing GI damage and complications. *Consultant Pharmacist, 12,*
304–306.

Horgas, A. L., & Dunn, K. (2001). Pain in nursing home residents:
Comparison of residents' self-report and nursing assistants' perceptions. *Journal of Gerontological Nursing, 27,* 44–53.

Horgas, A. L., & Tsai, P. F. (1998). Analgesic drug prescription and use in cognitively impaired nursing home residents. *Nursing Research, 47,* 235–242.

Joint Commission on the Accreditation of Healthcare Organizations (JCAHO).
(2001). *Accreditation manual for hospitals.* Oakbrook Terrace, IL: Author.

Kovach, C., Weissman, D., Griffie, J., Matson, S., & Muchka, S. (1999).
Assessment and treatment of discomfort for people with late-stage
dementia. *Journal of Pain and Symptom Management, 18,* 412–419.

Luggen, A. S. (1998). Chronic pain in older adults: A quality of life issue.
Journal of Gerontological Nursing, 24, 48–54.

McCaffery, M. (1968). *Nursing practice theories related to cognition, bodily pain,
and man–environment interaction.* Los Angeles: UCLA Students Store.

McCaffery, M., & Pasero, C. (1999). *Pain: Clinical Manual* (2nd ed.). St. Louis:
Mosby.

McCaffery, M., & Portenoy, R. (1999). Nonopioids. In M. McCaffery & C.
Pasero (Eds.), *Pain clinical manual* (2nd ed.). St. Louis: Mosby.

Melzack, R., & Casey, K. L. (1968). Sensory, motivational, and central con-
trol determinants of pain: A new conceptual model. In D. R. Kenshalo
(Ed.), *The Skin Senses* (pp. 423–443). Springfield, IL: Charles C. Thomas
Press.

Mobily, P. R., Herr, K. A., Clark, M. K., & Wallace, R. B. (1994). An epidemiologic analysis of pain in the elderly: The Iowa 65+ Rural Health Study. *Journal of Aging and Health, 6,* 139–154.

Panda, M., & Desbiens, N. A. (2001). Pain in elderly patients: How to achieve control. *Consultant, 41,* 1597–1604.

Parmelee, P. A. (1994). Assessment of pain in the elderly. In M. P. Lawton & J. A. Teresi (Eds.), *Annual review of gerontology and geriatrics: Focus on assessment techniques* (pp. 281–301). New York: Springer Publishing Co.

Parmelee, P., Smith, B., & Katz, I. (1993). Pain complaints and cognitive status among elderly institution residents. *Journal of the American Geriatrics Society, 41,* 517–522.

Pasero, C., Portenoy, R. K., & McCaffery, M. (1999). Opioid analgesics. In M. McCaffery & C. Pasero (Eds.), *Pain: Clinical Manual* (2nd ed.). St. Louis: Mosby.

Pasero, C., Reed, B., & McCaffery, M. (1999). Pain in the elderly. In M. McCaffery & C. Pasero (Eds.), *Pain: Clinical Manual* (2nd ed., pp. 161–299). St. Louis: Mosby.

Reisine, T., & Pasternak, G. (1996). Opioid analgesics and antagonists. In J. G. Hardman & L. M. Limbird (Eds.), *Goodman and Gilman's the pharmacological basis of therapeutics* (9 th ed., pp. 521–555). New York: McGraw-Hill.

Rudy, T. E., Hanlon, R. B., & Markham, J. R. (2002). Psychosocial issues and cognitive-behavioral therapy. From theory to practice. In D. K. Weiner, K. Herr, & T. E. Rudy (Eds.), *Persistent pain in older adults: An interdisciplinary guide for treatment.* New York: Springer.

Sengstaken, E. A., & King, S. A. (1993). The problems of pain and its detection among geriatric nursing home residents. *Journal of American Geriatrics Society, 41,* 541–544.

Sorkin, B. A., Rudy, T. E., Hanlon, R. B., Turk, D. C., & Stieg, R. L. (1990). Chronic pain in old and young patients: Differences appear less important than similarities. *Journal of Gerontology, 45(2),* P64–68.

U.S. Department of Health and Human Services. (1992). *Acute Pain Management: Operative or Medical Procedures and Trauma* (AHCPR Pub. No. 92-0032). Rockville, MD: Author.

U.S. Department of Health and Human Services. (1994). *Management of Cancer Pain: Clinical Practice Guideline* (AHCPR Pub. No. 94-0592). Rockville, MD: Author.

Wells, N., Kaas, M., & Feldt, K. (1997). Managing pain in the institutionalized elderly: The nursing role. In D. I. Mostofsky & J. Lomranz (Eds.), *Handbook of Pain and Aging* (pp. 129–151). New York: Plenum Press.

Wilcox, S. M., Himmelstein, D. U., & Woolhandler, S. (1994). Inappropriate drug prescribing for the community-dwelling elderly. *Journal of the American Medical Association, 272,* 292–296.

World Health Organization. (1990). *Cancer Pain Relief and Palliative Care* (Tech. Report Series 804). Madison: University of Wisconsin–Comprehensive Cancer Center.

Chapter 14

USE OF PHYSICAL RESTRAINTS IN THE ACUTE CARE SETTING

Anne M. O'Connell and Lorraine C. Mion

EDUCATIONAL OBJECTIVES

On completion of this chapter, the reader should be able to
1. Describe the current use of physical restraint in acute care.
2. Describe the perceived benefits of physical restraint.
3. Discuss the potential harm as a direct or indirect result of physical restraint.
4. Identify the most common reasons nurses cite for use of physical restraint.
5. Plan nonrestraint strategies for dealing with common patient problems: disruption of therapy, agitation and confusion, and falls.

The use of physical restraints in acute care is a controversial and problematic practice. The Centers for Medicare and Medicaid Service (CMS; formerly Health Care Financing Administration, HCFA) defines physical restraint as any physical or mechanical device, material, or

Adapted from a chapter in the original edition by Mion, L., Strumpf, N., and the NICHE faculty (1999). Walker, M. In I. Abraham, T. Fulmer, & M. Mezey, (Eds.), *Geriatric Nursing Protocols for Best Practice.* Springer Publishing Company: New York.

equipment attached or adjacent to the patient's body that the individual cannot remove easily and that restricts freedom of movement or normal access to one's body (HCFA, 1999). Examples of these are wrist or leg restraints, hand mitts, Geri-chairs, and full side rails. The purpose of this chapter is to familiarize the reader with physical restraint use in general and intensive care units, nurses' decision-making processes, and alternative methods of caring for common patient problems.

BACKGROUND

PREVALENCE

Recent studies show an overall decrease in physical restraint use in acute care and a change in practice patterns during the past 2 decades (Minnick, Mion, Leipzig, Lamb, & Palmer, 1998). In the 1980s, the overall prevalence of physical restraint use on general floors ranged from 6% to 13% with higher rates (18%–22%) among elderly patients (Mion, Minnick, Palmer, Kapp, & Lamb, 1996). Nurses on these units cited fall prevention as the primary reason for restraint use (56%–77%). Restraint use in intensive care units (ICUs) was not routinely measured during this time. In the late 1990s, restraint prevalence decreased to 3% to 8% on general units but was as high as 46% in ICUs (Minnick et al., 1998). Although fall risk is still a concern, today's hospital nurses cite prevention of patient therapy disruption as the primary reason for restraint use (48%–61%).

BENEFITS

Physical restraints have been defended on the grounds that they are necessary for patient safety and that they protect the patient from harm (Mion et al., 1996). Nurses and other caregivers perceive that physical restraints will prevent patients from removing medical devices such as intravenous catheters and nasogastric tubes. ICU caregivers believe that restraints are essential to prevent patients from removing life-saving devices, such as balloon pump equipment and endotracheal tubes for mechanical ventilators (Mion et al., 2001). The evidence to support these perceptions, however, is lacking. Studies have demonstrated that patients remove these devices even while restrained. The use of physical restraints among those patients who self-extubated ranged from 41% to 91% (Mion, 1996).

Studies have shown that many patients who self-terminate therapies suffer little or no harm (Mion, 1996; Mion et al., 2001) and that as restraints are reduced, rates of therapy disruption either remain unchanged or decrease (Mion et al., 2001).

If physical restraints were truly beneficial and effective, one would expect that no falls would occur with the use of physical restraints and that falls would increase without the use of physical restraints. In a review of several studies, Mion and colleagues (1996) revealed that 13% to 47% of older patients who fall are physically restrained and that serious injuries from falls are greater with the presence of physical restraints. Conversely, a number of investigators have demonstrated that fall injuries either remain unchanged or decrease as physical restraints are reduced (Braun & Capezuti, 2000; Mion et al., 2001). Thus, the perception that physical restraint promotes or maintains medical therapies and prevents injuries from falls is not based on evidence.

HARM/ADVERSE CONSEQUENCES

Frengley and Mion (1998) report that several studies revealed the harmful consequences that occur, either directly or indirectly, as a result of the use of physical restraints. Short-term complications include hyperthermia, new onset of bladder and bowel incontinence, new pressure ulcers, and increased rate of nosocomial infections. Severe or permanent injuries include brachial plexus nerve injuries from wrist restraints, joint contractures, and hypoxic encephalopathy. The most serious injury is death from strangulation.

Obviously physical damage may occur from physical restraints; less appreciated are the psychosocial complications. Strumpf and Evans (1988) interviewed elderly patients discharged from the hospital and found significant psychological distress with recollections of the restraint experience up to 6 months after discharge. Approximately one-third of physically restrained medical patients exhibited psychological distress manifested as anger, agitation, or depression (Mion, Frengley, Jakovcic, & Marino, 1989). Case reports of sudden death have been linked to severe psychological stress from the physical restraint (Miles, 1993; Robinson, 1995).

Additional adverse events are associated with the use of physical restraints, although these are not necessarily a direct cause of the restraint. For example, studies have shown that restrained patients are significantly more likely to die than are non-restrained patients

(Frengley & Mion, 1986; Mion et al., 1989; Robbins, Boyko, Lane, Cooper, & Jahnigen, 1987). The fact that hospitalized older patients who are restrained are more severely ill and have greater mortality rates calls into question the goals of care and therapy. Clinicians need to weigh the benefits and risks not only of providing therapy but also of administering that therapy in the context of quality care at the end of life.

LEGAL CONCERNS

Nurses and other health care providers have a deep routed fear of litigation if an unrestrained patient suffers harm. This fear often dictates a "defensive medicine" type of practice that can lead to inappropriate restraint use (Francis, 1989). Hospitals have been found liable for both the use of physical restraints and for not using restraints (Kapp, 1994, 1997). Although hospitals have a clear duty to protect patients from harm, they "do not have a duty to restrain" (Kapp, 1997). Interventions and documentation demonstrating attempts at providing a safe environment and monitoring patients are essential from both a patient care and legal standpoint.

STANDARDS AND REGULATIONS

The Joint Commission on Accreditation of Healthcare Organizations (JCAHO) and the CMS have increased scrutiny on physical restraint in acute care settings in the past decade. JCAHO has enacted highly prescriptive standards encompassing everything from organization quality monitoring to frequency of basic nursing interventions (JCAHO, 2001). Patient safety and patient rights are two priority JCAHO standards that often conflict with clinicians' use of physical restraint. There is evidence, by association only, that the attention that JCAHO has brought to bear on the use of physical restraints has resulted in a decrease in their use on general medical and surgical units (Minnick et al., 1998).

NURSES' DECISION TO USE PHYSICAL RESTRAINTS

As was true in the long-term care setting, nurses are the primary decision makers regarding the use of physical restraints in acute care. Until recently, many settings, such as ICUs, used broad physician-approved clinical protocols to decide which patients to restrain. JCAHO mandated in 2001 that all patients, regardless of setting, must have individual patient orders and timely licensed independent practitioner assessment. This was to ensure that the decision to restrain involved an interdisciplinary team and to promote prompt medical assessment. Despite these recent changes, nurses still remain the driving-force for initiating physical restraint.

ALTERNATIVE APPROACHES TO CARE

Given the numerous reasons and variations in practice, guidelines for any use of physical restraints are unquestionably needed. As part of the John A. Hartford Foundation Institute for Geriatric Nursing Nurses Improving Care for Health System Elders (NICHE) Project, a panel of gerontological nurse experts developed a standard of practice for hospital nurses to follow when considering or applying physical restraint in care of patients (Box 14.1). The standard provides background information, assessment parameters, and plan of care, as well as expected outcomes for performance improvement in meeting JCAHO guidelines. Central to the standard of care is the recommendation that restraints be applied only after exhausting all reasonable alternatives. Thus, the standard of practice is nonrestraint, except under exceptional circumstances.

The most important task of the nurse is to identify the underlying reason(s) for the use of restraint. Such determination forms the basis for identifying alternative approaches to care. For example, if the patient is at risk for falling, factors that place the patient at risk for falling must be identified. In this way, an individualized plan of care is tailored to the patient to minimize the risk of falling. A brief discussion of some alternative approaches in caring for common patient problems that frequently precipitate physical restraint use follows. For more detailed information on techniques to reduce the use of physical restraints, excellent references and resources are available for both acute and long-term care.

ALTERNATIVES FOR PROTECTING OR MAINTAINING MEDICAL THERAPY

The most common reason for use of physical restraints in the hospital setting is to maintain therapy. The nurse must always ask, "Is

---

BOX 14.1   Nursing Standard of Practice Protocol:
Use of Physical Restraints with Elderly Patients

I.   GOAL: Minimize use of physical restraint except in emergent and
     critical care situations.
II. BACKGROUND/STATEMENT OF PROBLEM
     A. Definition: Physical restraint is any manual method or physical
        or mechanical device that the patient cannot remove, restricts
        physical activity or normal access to his or her body and that
        (1) is not a usual and customary part of a medical, diagnostic,
        or treatment procedure indicated by the patient's medical
        condition or symptoms and (2) does not serve to promote the
        patient's independent functioning.
     B. Risk factors for physical restraint use:
        1. Severe cognitive impairment and/or physical impairment
        2. Presence of medical devices in cognitively impaired patients
        3. Fall-injury risk
        4. Diagnosis or presence of psychiatric disorder (e.g., alcohol
           withdrawal)
     C. Morbidity and mortality risks associated with physical
        restraints:
        1. Increased agitation or confusion
        2. New-onset pressure ulcers
        3. Pneumonia
        4. Nerve injury
        5. Strangulation/asphyxiation
III. PARAMETERS OF ASSESSMENT
     A. Baseline and current cognitive state, determine if new-onset
        delirium
     B. Physical function: ability to transfer and walk (see chapter 3)
     C. Therapeutic devices: alternative modes of therapy
     D. Identify risk factors for falls and disruption of therapy (e.g., for
        fall risk, assess memory, balance, orthostatic blood pressure,
        vision and hearing, use of sedative-hypnotic drugs or narcotic
        agents)
IV. NURSING CARE STRATEGIES
     A. Prevention:
        1. Develop a nursing plan tailored to the patient's presenting
           problem(s) and risk factors.
        2. Consider alternative interventions.
        3. Refer to occupational and physical therapy for self-care deficits
           or mobility impairment; use adaptive equipment as appropriate.
        4. Document use and effect of alternatives to restraints.

BOX 14.1   *(continued)*

B. Treatment:
  1. Use restraints only after exhausting all reasonable alternatives.
  2. When using restraints:
    a. Choose the least restrictive device.
    b. Reassess the patient's response every hour.
    c. Remove the restraint every 2 hours.
    d. Renew orders every 24 hours after evaluation by licensed independent practitioner.
  3. Modify the care plan to compensate for restrictions imposed by physical restraint use:
    a. Change position frequently, and provide skin care.
    b. Provide adequate range of motion.
    c. Assist with activities of daily living, such as eating and use of toilet.
  4. Continue to address underlying condition(s) that prompted restraint use (e.g., delirium). Refer to geriatric nurse specialist, occupational therapist, and so on, as appropriate.

V. EVALUATION/EXPECTED OUTCOMES
  A. Patient: Physical restraints will be used only under well-documented exceptional circumstances, after all reasonable alternatives have been tried.
  B. Health care provider: Providers will use a range of interventions other than restraints in the care of patients.
  C. Institution
    1. Incidence and/or prevalence of restraint use will decrease.
    2. Use of chemical restraints will not increase.
    3. The number of serious injuries related to falls, agitated behavior, and premature disruption of medical devices will not increase.
    4. Referrals to occupational therapists, physical therapists, psychiatric-liaison services, and so on, will increase, as will availability of adaptive equipment.
    5. Staff will receive ongoing education on the prevention of restraints.

VI. FOLLOW-UP MONITORING OF CONDITION
  A. Document incidence and or prevalence of physical restraint, both house-wide and unit-specific, on an ongoing basis.
  B. Educate caregivers to continue assessment and prevention.
  C. Identify patient characteristics and care problems that continue to be refractory and involve consultants (e.g., geriatric specialists, psychiatric-liaison specialists) in devising an expanded range of alternative approaches.

this device necessary?" MacPherson, Lofgren, Granieri, and Myllen-beck (1990) found that nurses and physicians were most likely to restrain patients with medical devices that they personally had to restart or replace; thus, one must conscientiously examine whether a restraint is in place as a matter of convenience. Second, how life threatening is the removal or disruption of particular medical treatment? Clearly, disruption of an endotracheal tube has a greater harm potential than disruption of an indwelling bladder catheter. Yet both are often treated the same when considering whether to restrain a patient.

The risks and benefits of physical restraint must be weighed in maintaining therapy. Are alternative therapies available that might avoid use of physical restraint altogether? For example, if an intravenous line (IV) is needed only for medication, not for fluid replacement, the IV can be replaced by a saline lock.

Any medical device feels strange to a patient. Simple explanations to the confused patient concerning the device and opportunities for guided exploration are often successful for those with mild confusion. If the treatment device is absolutely necessary, and it appears that the patient will disrupt the therapy, other alternatives to physical restraints should be tried. Strategies for protecting IV lines include use of special gauze or wraps, arm casings, or long hospital gowns or robes to hide or camouflage the insertion site; in addition, IV solution bags need to be kept behind the patient's visual field. For more severely demented patients, the latter technique is usually successful.

Nasogastric tubes used for suction are difficult to maintain in the confused older patient. The tubes cause discomfort and can not be camouflaged. Explain the tube and necessity of the tube to the patient. If the nasogastric tube (NGT) is used for feeding, it may be possible to find alternative routes. It is imperative that a speech or occupational therapist should evaluate the swallowing of a patient with an NGT as soon as possible. The patient's ability to swallow must be assessed periodically throughout the hospital course. If tube feedings are deemed necessary, then use of percutaneous gastrostomy tube should be considered. The patient rarely disrupts the tube, as it can be hidden by clothing and/or abdominal binders.

Patients admitted through the emergency department frequently have indwelling urinary catheters in place. Examination of the need for catheters is essential. Catheters need to be removed as soon as possible because of the morbidity and mortality associated with nososcomial urinary tract infections. If the catheter is truly needed for medical conditions (such as obstruction from benign prostatic hypertrophy), consider whether a regularly scheduled straight catheterization is medically feasible.

Protection of life-saving or life-maintaining devices commonly used in ICUs poses an extreme challenge to the caregiver. The task of identifying and treating the underlying cause of the confusion is never more important than in the complex ICU patient who has delirium, pain, and anxiety. Physician collaboration is essential in deciding appropriate use of analgesic, anxiolytic, and antipscyhotic agents. ICU patients managed with clear medication guidelines or algorithms have decreased use of restraints, fewer incidences of self-extubation, and shorter lengths of stay (Bair, Bobek, Hoffman-Hoff, Mion, & Aruglia, 2000).

MINIMIZING FALL RISK

Nurses fear that older patients who fall are likely to sustain an injury; thus, fall prevention is still a common reason for use of physical restraint in acute care. Falls among hospitalized elders are typically caused by multiple interacting factors that include individual or intrinsic host factors (e.g., unsteady gait), external or extrinsic factors (e.g., furniture with wheels), and situational factors such as a patient reaching forward (Tinneti & Speechley, 1989). Fall programs in hospitals and nursing homes typically focus on risk for falling (e.g., the type or number of risk factors present). Although some interventions may be applied uniformly to all patients (e.g., available staff member monitoring the unit at all times), other interventions, such as adaptive equipment, are applied to specific patients. The patient at risk must be carefully assessed to identify the specific risk factors for falls and a to tailor a plan to minimize that risk.

Patients unable to maintain a sitting posture because of poor trunk muscle strength (e.g., post stroke patients) are sometimes restrained to prevent sliding out of the chair. Most hospital chairs are straight backed with an approximately 90-degree sitting angle. A better choice is a reclining chair with a modified leg lift maintains the patient's center of gravity in the chair seat. Occupational therapists can help with adaptive cushions or materials that promote sitting in an upright position without restraints.

Patients who demonstrate a weakened or impaired gait are sometimes restrained to prevent unaided walking. Many acute medical and surgical conditions may impair or weaken ambulation. For patients who were independent before hospitalization, an aggressive approach to mobilize them as soon as possible is essential to prevent or minimize functional decline. Consultation with physical therapists early in the course of hospitalization is important. A restorative nursing approach is also essential. For example, instead of relying on bedpans, patients should be encouraged and assisted to walk to the bathroom on a routine basis. Attention also must be paid to room furnishing. Bed height should be at a level to allow the patient's feet touch the floor while sitting on the edge of the bed. This is difficult when pressure-reducing devices are placed on the mattress. Replacement with wheels of smaller diameter lowers the bed height (Lund & Sheafor, 1985).

Patients with a weakened or impaired gait, along with impaired cognition, pose additional challenges to the nursing staff. Those with poor judgment or memory are unlikely to call for assistance before attempting to walk. Close, frequent observation is essential and may be accomplished in several ways: moving the patient closer to the nurses station; enlisting family or friends to visit, especially during evening shifts; and use of electronic warning devices. Early warning sounding alarms (i.e. weight sensitive alarms) are needed for those with both physical and cognitive impairments. (For a more detailed discussion of fall prevention strategies in hospitals, refer to chapter 9 in this book).

ALTERNATIVES TO MANAGE AGITATION AND DISRUPTIVE BEHAVIOR

Agitation and disruptive behaviors may occur as a result of delirium, dementia, psychosis, or a combination of these conditions. Depending on the underlying cause, interventions will vary. For example, reality orientation is helpful for treating confusion resulting from delirium and psychosis, but not helpful for confusion resulting from dementia. Consultation from geriatric nurse specialists should be obtained as soon as possible to aid staff nurses in sorting out the underlying reasons for the confusion and devising a plan.

Some general interventions that may be used for all patients with confusion include: consistent staff, presence of loved ones, explanation of all procedures, judicious use of lights especially at night, enhancing natural light source, decreasing noise, and promoting normal sleep-wake cycles. Rearranging or combining procedures and treatments so as not to disturb the patient's sleep (e.g., not waking the patient for vital signs at 1:00 a.m. and then again at 2:00 a.m. for medication) is also important. Psychoactive medications (e.g., haloperidol, lorezepam) should be used cautiously in low doses at early signs of psychosis rather than in large doses at times of crisis. Keep in mind that use of psychotropic drugs for an already agitated out-of-control older patient typically does not work quickly. Thus, the nurse must exercise caution in repeating the doses.

Finding alternatives to use of physical restraints in the critical care setting remains a challenge for the staff nurse. Nevertheless, several interventions are known to diminish delirium and/or agitation among critically ill patients (Frengley & Mion, 1998). Attention to the environment of the critical care unit is as important as in other health settings. Excessive light, noise, and disruption of sleep due to medical treatments and monitoring can all lead to the development of delirium in vulnerable populations. Consistent and available nurses can strongly affect patient outcomes. Lack of communication with the patients by caregivers in the intensive care unit results in distress, anxiety, and confusion. Last, undermedication of delirium or pain has been well documented. Thus, a comprehensive approach that focuses on the environment, organizational culture, communication techniques, and utilization of sedation and analgesic guidelines are likely to diminish the rate of physical restraints in the intensive care unit.

CASE STUDY

Mrs. M. was an 87-year-old women admitted to the general medical service via the emergency department with a diagnosis of heart failure. Other diagnoses included diabetes mellitus, glaucoma, hypertension, and hyperlipidemia. She was married and lived with her spouse of 62 years in the nearby community. They had three children, who all resided out of state. Upon admission to the floor, Mrs. M. was noted to have an unsteady gait and she required minimal assistance with transfers. She was mildly forgetful but easily reoriented. She had a peripheral intravenous line, oxygen mask at 40%, and an indwelling urinary catheter. She was admitted to the general unit at 3:00 a.m. after being in the emergency department for the previous 7 hours. The admitting nurse oriented Mrs. M. to the room and the nurse call system. Her room was farthest from the nurse's station. After assessing Mrs. M. and settling her in the room, the nurse returned to the station to take off the medical orders. Within 10 minutes of leaving the room, the personnel heard a loud crash down the hall. Upon reentering Mrs. M.'s room, the nurse found her lying on the floor, with the IV and the bladder catheter pulled out and the oxygen mask off. The nurse assessed Mrs. M. for injury, transferred her back into the bed, and reoriented her to the hospital. Mrs. M.'s IV and indwelling catheter were reinserted, and she was reminded to leave the mask on. Mrs. M. was able to demonstrate how to call for the nurses. Because she had suffered no harm from the fall, the nurse again left the room and returned to the station. At 6:00 a.m., Mrs. M. again removed her oxygen mask, became confused, and attempted to get up out of bed alone. She fell a second time, and her peripheral IV was again disrupted. At that point, the nurse applied a chest restraint to Mrs. M.

The geriatric clinical nurse specialist (GCNS) saw Mrs. M. in the morning while Mr. M. was visiting. The GCNS noted that the oxygen mask was too large and was pressing up against Mrs. M.'s eyes. When queried on the comfort of the mask, Mrs. M. stated that the mask bothered her. The GCNS called the respiratory therapist to obtain a smaller mask. Mrs. M. was again instructed not to attempt getting up alone. The chest restraint was removed. A personal alarm device was shown and explained to Mrs. M. who agreed to allow the pull chain to be attached to her gown. Her husband recorded a message: "Margaret, stay in bed; wait for the nurse to come." The GCNS pulled on the alarm chain so that Mr. and Mrs. M. could hear the recorded warning and the sound of the alarm. Lastly, Mrs. M. was moved to a room closer to the nurse's station. No further falls occurred during her hospital stay.

DISCUSSION

The oxygen mask was a necessity, as was the peripheral intravenous line and indwelling bladder catheter for the initial management of her heart failure and diuresis. Thus, finding an alternative therapeutic device was not feasible initially. However, the oxygen mask was an irritant, but when it was removed by Mrs. M. she became increasingly confused. This was addressed by finding a better fitting mask. Other interventions targeted to the fall risk were improving surveillance by a personal alarm device and moving her closer to the nurse's station.

SUMMARY

Reducing the use of physical restraints in the hospital setting is a complex task that is best accomplished by increasing the staff's awareness and knowledge of alternative methods of care. Nurses need not and should not feel alone in caring for the multiple, intricate problems presenting in elderly patients. Professionals in other health care disciplines are available and are valuable in assisting nurses with planning and providing appropriate care to hospitalized elders.

REFERENCES

Bair, N., Bobek, M. B., Hoffman-Hogg, L., Mion, L. C., & Arroliga, A. (2000). Introduction of sedation guidelines in an intensive care unit: Physician and nurse adherence. *Critical Care Medicine, 28,* 707–713.

Braun, J. A., & Capezuti, E. (2000). The legal and medical aspects of physical restraints and bed siderails and their relationships to falls and fall-related injuries in nursing homes. *DePaul Journal of Health Care Law, 4*(1), 1–72.

Francis, J. (1989). Using restraints in the elderly because of fear of litigation. *New England Journal of Medicine, 320,* 870–871.

Frengley, J. D., & Mion, L. C. (1986). Incidence of physical restraints on acute general medical wards. *Journal of the American Geriatrics Society, 34,* 565–568.

Frengley, J. D, & Mion, L. C. (1998). Physical restraints in the acute care setting: Issues and future direction. *Clinics in Geriatric Medicine, 14*(4), 727–743.

Health Care Financing Administration (HCFA). (1999, July). Medicare and Medicaid programs, hospital conditions of participation: Patients' rights: Interim final rule (42CFR Part 482). *Federal Register, 64*(127).

Joint Commission on Accreditation of Healthcare Organizations (JCAHO). (2001). *2002 Comprehensive accreditation manual for hospitals. The official handbook.* Oakbrook Terrace, IL: Author.

Kapp, M. B. (1994). Physical restraints in hospitals: Risk management's reduction role. *Journal of Healthcare Risk Management, 14*(1), 3–8.

Kapp, M. B. (1997). Legal issues of physical restraints in hospitals. Paper presented at *Reducing Physical Restraints in Hospitals: Issues and Approaches,* 50th Annual Meeting of the Gerontological Society of America, Cincinnati, OH.

Lund, C., & Sheafor, M. L. (1985). Is your patient about to fall? *Journal of Gerontological Nursing, 11,* 37–41.

MacPherson, D. S., Lofgren, R. P., Granieri, R., Myllenbeck, S. (1990). Deciding to restrain medical patients. *Journal of the American Geriatrics Society, 38,* 516–520.

Miles, S. H. (1993). Restraints and sudden death. *Journal of the American Geriatrics Society, 41,* 1013.

Minnick, A. F., Mion, L. C., Leipzig, R., Lamb, K., & Palmer, R. M. (1998). Prevalence and patterns of physical restraint use in the acute care setting. *Journal of Nursing Administration, 28*(11), 19–24.

Mion, L. C. (1996). Establishing alternatives to physical restraint in the acute care setting: A conceptual framework to assist nurses' decision making. *AACN Clinical Issues, 7*(4), 592–602.

Mion, L. C., Fogel, J., Sandhu, S., Palmer, R. M., Minnick, A. F., Cranston, T., et al. (2001). Outcomes following physical restraint reduction programs in two acute care hospitals. *Joint Commission Journal on Quality Improvement, 27*(11), 605–618.

Mion, L. C., Frengley, J. D, Jakovcic, C. A., & Marino, J. A. (1989). A further exploration of physical restraints in hospitalized patients. *Journal of the American Geriatrics Society, 37,* 949–956.

Mion, L. C., Minnick, A., Palmer R., Kapp, M. B., & Lamb, K. (1996). Physical restraint use in the hospital setting: Unresolved issues and directions for research. *Milbank Quarterly, 74*(3): 411–433.

Robbins, L. J., Boyko, E., Lane, J., Cooper, D., & Jahnigen, D. W. (1987). Binding the elderly: A prospective study of the use of mechanical restraints in an acute care hospital. *Journal of the American Geriatrics Society, 35,* 290–296.

Robinson, B. E. (1995). Death by destruction of will: Lest we forget. *Archives of Internal Medicine, 155,* 2250–2251.

Strumpf N. E., & Evans, L. K. (1988). Physical restraint of hospitalized elderly: Perceptions of the patients and nurses. *Nursing Research, 37,* 132–137.

Tinnetti, M. E., & Speechely, M. (1989). Prevention of falls among the elderly. *New England Journal of Medicine, 320,* 1055–1059.

Chapter 15

ADVANCE DIRECTIVES: PROTECTING PATIENT'S RIGHTS

Gloria Ramsey and Ethel L. Mitty

EDUCATIONAL OBJECTIVES

On completion of this chapter, the reader should be able to
1. Explain and differentiate between a durable power of attorney for health care and a living will.
2. Describe assessment parameters to ensure that all patients receive advance directive information.
3. Identify strategies to ensure good communication about advance directives with patients, families, and health care professionals.
4. Describe measurable outcomes to be expected from implementation of this practice protocol.

One of the most difficult situations health care professionals face when caring for elders and other patients is how to assist patients and families with decision making about whether to start, continue,

Adapted from a chapter in the original edition by M. Mezey, M. Bottrell, G. Ramsey, and the NICHE Faculty. Advanced directives: Nurse helping to protect patients' rights, pp. 173–188. In Abraham, I., Fulmer, T., & Mezey, M., Eds. *Geriatric Nursing Protocols for Best Practice.* New York: Springer Publishing Company.

or stop life-sustaining treatments for critically ill patients and those who cannot communicate their treatment preferences. Of the 2.4 million deaths in the United States in 2001, 1.8 million deceased were 65 years of age or older (USDHHS, 2001; Administration on Aging [AOA], 2002); thus, end-of-life treatment decisions are more prevalent among this group. Yet only 20% to 25% of the adult population in the United States have executed some kind of advance directive, and only 15% of community dwelling elderly are likely to have a directive (Bradley, Wetle, & Horwitz, 1998). Making end-of-life decisions can provoke conflict among nurses, physicians, social workers, and families. Decision making can be especially difficult when care providers barely know the patient, have little knowledge of what treatments a patient would or would not want, or there is no one available to speak for the patient. Anecdotally, it is suggested that approximately 30% of the elderly do not have a relative, friend, or guardian who can make health care decisions for them. Health care professionals, especially nurses, can improve end-of-life decision making for elderly patients by talking about, and encouraging the completion of, advance directives before the individual loses decisional capacity.

This chapter discusses the nurse's role in informing patients about advance directives and in supporting patient's treatment decisions. Following a brief overview of the legal background to advance directives, types of directives and related issues (such as capacity determination, benefit–burden assessment, conflict mediation, ethics committees, and cultural aspects of advance care planning) will be discussed. The chapter concludes with a case study and a protocol that can guide nurses in all practice settings to ensure that patients end-of-life care wishes are followed.

Since the passage of the Patient Self Determination Act in 1991 (PSDA, 1992), virtually all health care professionals have come into contact with advance directives. The PSDA requires all facilities that receive Medicare or Medicaid reimbursement to inform their patients/clients of their right to make health care decisions, including their option to complete an advance directive. Predicated on the Western philosophic tradition of individual freedom and choice (i.e., the principal of autonomy), individuals have the moral right to make decisions about their own treatment. On the other hand, the New Jersey Supreme Court held that competent individuals have a constitutionally based legal right to accept or reject medical treatment under the right of privacy (NJSC, 1976). This well-established opinion was persuasive in the matter of Nancy Cruzan (1990), a case that brought the issue of an incompetent individual's right to terminate unwanted treatment into the public eye.

Typically, an advance directive is used to prospectively refuse certain treatments; however, advance directives are value neutral and can be used to request treatments, as well. State statutes generally outline the conditions under which an advance directive is legally valid and when it should be followed. In spite of the various justifications and legal protections for the individual's right to make decisions about their own care, it is difficult to protect a patient's right to autonomy when the person is unable to communicate due to mental or physical incapacity. Advance directives can be most helpful by

1. Allowing individuals to provide directions about the kind of medical care they do or do not want if they become unable to make decisions or communicate their wishes.
2. Providing guidance for health care professionals and families with regard to health care decisions that reflect the person's wishes should that person be unable to make health care decisions.
3. Providing immunity for health care professionals and families from civil and criminal liability when health care professionals follow the advance directive in good faith.

TYPES OF ADVANCE DIRECTIVES

There are two types of advance directive documents: the durable power of attorney for health care (DPAHC) and the living will. The DPAHC allows an individual to appoint someone, called a health care proxy, agent, attorney-in-fact, or surrogate, to make health care decisions if the individual loses the ability to make decisions or communicate his/her wishes. The person appointed has the legal authority to interpret the patient's wishes on the basis of the medical circumstances of the situation and is not restricted to only deciding if life-sustaining treatment can be withdrawn or withheld. Thus, the proxy can make decisions as the need arises, and such decisions can respond directly to the decision at hand rather than being restricted only to circumstances that were thought of previously. Designating a proxy is preferable to completing a living will because it appoints one person to speak for the patient. Although most states have family consent laws that designate the order in which family members can make decisions for an incapacitated patient who did not complete an advance directive, disputes between family members who bear the same relationship to the patient are not uncommon and often very difficult to resolve. A proxy's decision legally supersedes a family wish or decision, and the Family Consent Law is not applicable in that case. The presumption is that the patient and proxy have discussed the patient's treatment wishes; however, a minority of states require that the proxy sign the directive as an attempt to assure that the proxy is put on notice and has accepted the role as proxy. This is not to say, however, that a proxy's decision is always easy and conflict-free or that the burden is light. It has been suggested that the patient–proxy relationship is a covenant built on trust, relationship, and fidelity (Fins, 1999).

For elderly patients who have no one to appoint as their proxy, completing a living will that outlines their wishes is preferable to not providing any information at all about care preferences. This is equally so for patients who want to provide their proxy with some guidance about their treatment preferences and end-of-life care wishes, including artificial nutrition, ventilator support, and pain management.

A living will (LW) provides specific instructions to health care providers about particular kinds of health care treatment that an individual would or would not want to prolong life. Living wills are often used to declare a wish to refuse, limit, or withhold life-sustaining treatment when an individual is unable to communicate. All but three states (New York, Massachusetts, and Michigan) have detailed statutes recognizing living wills. The usefulness of LWs is limited, however, to those clinical circumstances that were thought of before the person became incapable of making decisions. If a situation occurs that the LW will does not address, providers and families may not know how to proceed and still respect the patient's wishes. Assuming that an individual completes both the LW and DPAHC, the proxy/agent may not be obligated to follow the wishes outlined in the LW; those instructions serve as a guide.

Some state statutes have a combined directive that includes elements of the LW and the DPAHC. The document improves on the standalone LW or DPAHC because if the patient's instructions do not apply to the situation at hand, either because they are too general or too specific, the proxy can provide additional information to

assist in decision making. In some states, a section on organ donation ("anatomical gift") has been added to the advance directive
document that allows the individual to indicate if they wish to
donate an organ(s). However, in New York State, the proxy cannot
effect this wish unless that individual is also the identified decision
maker for organ donation, a distinct statutory authority separate
from a health care proxy's rights and responsibilities.

The LW and DPAHC are the base from which states can create
independent documents for advance care decision making. For
example, two such documents that further the goals of advance care
planning and are accepted in many states are the physician order
for life-sustaining treatment (POLST) and the Five Wishes document.
POLST originated in Oregon in 1995 and is a state-endorsed protocol to honor an individual's wish to die in a setting of his or her
choice without unwanted life-supporting interventions. It contains
four separate categories of physician's orders that are based on
patient–physician discussion about comfort measures, antibiotics,
parenteral feeding, and cardiopulmonary resuscitation. Studies indicate that Oregon nursing home residents with POLST documents
received more intense comfort care, fewer aggressive life-sustaining
interventions, were less likely to be transferred to a hospital to die,
and had more orders for narcotic analgesia at the time of death than
did nursing home residents without POLSTs (Tolle, Tilden, Nelson,
& Dunn, 1998). The Five Wishes document embraces one's values
and builds on the spirit and letter of the advance directive laws. It is
legally valid in all but 15 states; individuals and families should be
encouraged to view this document when making end-of-life decisions. The form is available from the organization Five Wishes
(fivewishes@agingwithdignity.org) at a nominal fee; it might not be
available in physician, lawyer, or state health department offices.
Open-ended statements guide individuals to express their thoughts
and wishes about how they want to be physically and emotionally
supported, the medical treatments they want and do not want, and
the funeral arrangements and eulogy they would like.

Although the courts prefer written advance directives, oral
advance directives are respected, especially in emergency situations,
and can be persuasive in a judicial decision to allow withholding a
life-sustaining treatment. In determining the validity of an oral
advance directive, the court seeks information about whether the
statement was made on serious or solemn occasions, consistently
repeated, made by a mature person who understood the underlying

issues, was consistent with the values demonstrated in other aspects of the patient's life (including the patient's religion), made before the need for the treatment decision, and specifically addressed the actual condition of the patient. What might seem like an occasional comment made by a patient (whether in a practitioner's office or at the bedside) it should be recorded for just such an occasion when "clear and convincing evidence" is required.

DO-NOT-RESUSCITATE ORDERS

Consent to cardiopulmonary resuscitation (CPR) is presumed unless the physician writes a do-not-resuscitate (DNR) order to the contrary. Of all the ethical issues that concern nurses, respecting a patient's DNR order is the most prevalent. Nurses report that patient requests for DNR are frequently ignored. Several studies suggest that CPR should not be instituted when it will not offer a medical benefit or when death is inevitable and expected (Tresch et al., 1994). On the other hand, otherwise healthy elderly hospitalized patients may benefit from CPR and should not be denied this life-saving intervention.

Patients have a right to refuse CPR after they have been informed of the risks and benefits involved and may request a DNR order. If the physician is unwilling to write a DNR order to comply with the patient's request, the physician has a duty to notify the patient or family and assist the patient to obtain another physician. Thus, nurses need to be aware when such dilemmas are present and act to advocate on behalf of the patient. Moreover, nurses need to know which patients have a DNR directive, the law in their state governing the DNR directive, and their institutional policy.

ARTIFICIAL NUTRITION AND HYDRATION

As health care professionals and families grapple with care at the end of life, artificial nutrition and hydration continues to pose challenging ethical and legal questions. Providers are particularly hesitant to approach patients about directives when the issue of stopping or withdrawing treatment is imminent (Solomon, O'Donnell, & Jennings, 1993). Many providers erroneously perceive that there is a legal difference between forgoing and discontinuing artificial nutrition and hydration. Physicians and nurses, for example, are unsure about a patient's legal right to discontinue nutrition and hydration (Olson, 1993). A patient has a legal and ethical right to discontinue nutrition and hydration; however, the legal evidence and procedures required to forgo or discontinue this treatment vary by state. Nurses should be aware of their state law in this regard and should be concerned about the extent to which patients (and proxies) are correctly informed about treatment alternatives, consequences, and the relevant law.

PAIN MANAGEMENT

The adage "There is a moral as well as a professional imperative to relieve pain" applies even in the absence of an advance directive. Compassionate pain relief requires consent because it is grounded in respect for and dignity of the person (i.e., principles of autonomy and beneficence). An individual's constitutionally protected interest in pain relief was made clear in the U.S. Supreme Court ruling in *Quill v. Vacco* (1996). Rejecting the argument that there is a constitutionally protected right to assisted suicide, the court reaffirmed the doctrine of double effect. This principle holds that a single act having two foreseen effects, one good and one bad, is not legally or morally wrong or prohibited if the harmful effect is not intended. For a terminally ill incapacitated patient who lacks a directive or proxy to advocate on behalf of his or her comfort needs, it is ethically and legally appropriate to provide as much medication as necessary to relieve pain, even if the effect hastens death. For the patient with capacity, refusal of pain relief might be a value-based choice between intellectual and emotional awareness versus relief from pain.

The wish to be comfortable at the end of life embraces physical pain as well as spiritual suffering; yet wishes expressed in advance directives typically address, or are assumed to refer only to, physiologic pain. Nursing assessment for pain should try to differentiate between physiological pain and existential suffering. One can experience pain without suffering and conversely, suffer without physical pain. The patient might wish to be relieved from pain but suffering might have vital spiritual importance for him or her; hence, clinicians should not medicate for the wrong thing (see chapter 13).

DECISION-MAKING CAPACITY TO EXECUTE A DIRECTIVE

In thinking about who should be approached about advance directives, several things come to mind: the person's capacity to make decisions about his or her health care, language proficiency, and culture. *Competence* and *capacity* are not the same, yet they are frequently used synonymously and interchangeably. Competency means the ability to understand the nature and significance of a particular action in question (Mezey, Teresi, Ramsey, Mitty, & Bobrowitz, 2002). The law presumes competency unless shown otherwise; only the court can rule that an individual is incompetent. Capacity is a clinical determination and is not determined solely by a medical or psychiatric diagnosis or test (Roth, Meisel, & Lidz, 1977). Inability to make financial decisions or communicate verbally does not preclude the ability to communicate important information about one's treatment preferences. In nursing homes, residents perceived to have the requisite cognitive ability almost always have the opportunity to discuss advance directives, usually with a social worker and sometimes with a nurse or physician. On the other hand, residents perceived by staff to lack capacity are not given the opportunity to discuss them. Of this latter group, unless they are comatose or suffering from advanced dementia, the determination that a resident lacks capacity is often made on the basis of a mental status assessment test, an inappropriate measure of decisional capacity. Thus, there is a grave risk that individuals with communication disorders or those with mild dementia may not have the opportunity to appoint a health care proxy or to execute a living will.

THE RELATIONSHIP BETWEEN DECISIONAL CAPACITY AND INFORMED CONSENT

The steps in determining if a patient has sufficient decisional capacity to create an advance directive are similar to the basic elements of a valid consent and are based on observation of a specific set of abilities. These steps include (1) the patient appreciates and understands that he/she has the right to make a choice; (2) the patient understands the medical situation, prognosis, risks, benefits, and consequences of treatment consent (or refusal); (3) the patient can communicate the decision; and (4) the patient's decision is stable and consistent over a period of time (Roth et al., 1977).

Not all health decisions require the same level of decision-making capacity to make a decision. Decision making capacity is not an all-or-none "on-off" switch. Rather, capacity should be viewed as "task specific." An individual may be able to perform some tasks adequately, may have the ability to make some decisions, but is unable to perform all tasks or make all decisions. The notion of "decision-specific capacity" assumes that an individual has or lacks capacity for a particular decision at a particular time and under a particular set of circumstances (Meisel, 2002; Mezey, Mitty, Rappaport, & Ramsey, 1997). Most people have sufficient cognitive capability to make some, but not all decisions. To that degree, an individual might have the requisite capacity or understanding that he or she can choose someone to make health care decisions for the individual when he or she no longer has the capacity to do so. That same individual may not have the capacity, however, to make treatment choices in advance as would be required for a living will. The determination of decisional capacity becomes more exacting in relationship to the complexity and risk associated with the health care decision (Midwest Bioethics Center, 1996). In short, there is no gold standard or "capacimeter" to assess capacity (Kapp & Mossman, 1996). It is generally agreed among bioethicists, legal scholars, and clinicians that a low level of capacity is needed to create a DPAHC, and there is evidence to support this (Mezey et al., 2002). As such, the informed consent necessary to assure that the individual understands the issues relating to a proxy appointment can be simpler and less rigorous than the process required for decisions of greater risk, such as creating a living will.

Nurses can make a valuable contribution in ensuring that the informed consent process is accurately met. Yet nurses have little training in assessing decision-making capacity and tend to undervalue their participation in discussions with other members of the health care team when determining decisional capacity (Mezey, Mitty, & Ramsey, 1997). Those with the most knowledge of the patient should be asked to contribute meaningful and relevant information about the patient, such as, the patient's ability to express their needs, follow directions, state a preference, and exhibit stability of their choices. When nurses and other health care professionals learn how to objectively assess capacity, two types of mistakes can be avoided. First, mistakenly preventing persons who ought to be considered capacitated from directing the course of their treatment and, second, failing to protect incapacitated persons from the harmful effects of their decisions.

ASSESSMENT AND COMMUNICATION

Advance care planning is not without legal, ethical, communication, and cultural dilemmas. Persuasive argument can be brought to set limits on the treatment preferences expressed by a formerly competent but now demented individual. It has been argued that the person with Alzheimer's disease is a different person than the one who existed prior to the profound mental changes and who stated his or her treatment preferences. The opposing position is that the now incapacitated person is the same person who expressed those treatment preferences and that any decision to disregard the wishes should be based on a judgment about the person's quality of life (as he or she is living it) and on the benefits and burdens associated with a particular treatment decision.

BENEFIT–BURDEN ASSESSMENT

It is unlikely that a patient's proxy will know what and how a benefit–burden analysis can assist them in their decision-making responsibilities. Nurses can be invaluable to proxies simply by taking them through the steps of the analysis. A benefit–burden analysis considers the intended and unintended consequences of a particular treatment, estimates the likelihood that the intended benefit will occur, and weighs the importance of the benefit and burden to the patient. As each treatment or intervention is considered, the benefit (advantage) and burden (disadvantage, risk potential) to the patient is evaluated. The proxy can be helped to infer how the patient would evaluate the benefits and burdens based on knowledge of the patient's values, preferences, and past behavior. The nurse can ask the proxy, "If [the patient] could join this discussion, what would he say?" "Faced with similar situations in the past, how did he decide?"

In those situations where the proxy has scant knowledge about the patient for whom he/she must make health care decisions (or there is no advance directive, proxy appointment, or person who speaks for the patient) a decision is made on what would be in the patient's best interest. Known as the "reasonable person" or "best interest" standard, the decision relies on the notion of what an average person in the patient's particular situation would consider beneficial or burdensome. Questions that could move the process along would ask, "What does [this patient] have to gain or lose as a result of this treatment?" In what ways will [this patient] be better or worse off as a result of this treatment—or not having this treatment?" By fully evaluating the likely positive and negative consequences of various treatment or care options (in terms of the patient's medical condition, prognosis, goals, and wishes) a decision that authentically addresses the patients current and future care can be reached.

CULTURAL PERSPECTIVES ON ADVANCED CARE PLANNING

Autonomy is a Western concept; the notion of informed consent epitomizes the right to self-determination. Yet many people from many cultures and ethnic groups regard an advance directive as a refusal if not a legitimized denial of care. They do not view the DPAHC as a means for someone to advocate for their desired care. In addition, for the close-knit family, an advance directive is viewed as intrusive if not irrelevant. Disinterest in creating an advance directive because of a present-day rather than a future orientation and an unwillingness to write, speak, or plan for one's death are pervasive cultural influences on a decision not to create an advance directive. As well, deference to physician decision making, the family's role in protecting the patient from the burdens of life and death decision making, and spiritual obligations or beliefs, can exert a powerful influence on the decision. We are learning not only what people want and do not want for end-of-life care, but also their willingness to talk about it.

Cultural assimilation as well as cultural diversity makes even a simplistic assumption about why people do and do not create an advance directive extremely hazardous. When patients and health care professionals are from different ethnic backgrounds, the value systems that form the basis for advance directive decision making may conflict, often leading to distinct ethical and interpersonal tensions. The nurses' role in the midst of diverse cultural and religious belief systems is to approach the patient and/or the proxy with awareness, sensitivity, and competency that respects their values. These conversations occur over time; they are not interviews, per se. Discussion is always patient centered, not proxy or provider centered.

CONFLICT MEDIATION

It can be difficult to meet the health care wishes of patients with unstable medical conditions who may not have either decisional capacity or advance directives. Given these circumstances, differing opinions about the kind and intensity of treatments will differ. Describing a difference of opinion as a "conflict" when it is not seen that way by the proxy, the patient's family, or the health care providers, can be unhelpful. A meeting to search for the best outcome for the patient levels the playing field so that all parties can voice their concerns while avoiding power struggles. A key role for nurses could be the calming voice which states that medical uncertainty about diagnosis is a natural part of decision making and yes, it will influence treatment decisions.

The purpose of mediation is to solve problems by identification of the concerned parties and determination of their needs and interests, provision of relevant information, identification of options, and the search for agreement and how to bring it about (Dubler & Marcus, 1994). It bears repeating that sensitivity to the values of all the involved parties—professional, familial, and cultural—will facilitate exploration of alternatives and agreement about the best decisions for the patient. Steps in mediation and their general sequence are collection of information about the patient's medical conditions and nursing needs; discussion of the goals of care and the medical uncertainties; review of the process by which health care decisions were made in the past; and identification of any legal, ethical, cultural, or spiritual issues that exert pressure on the decision. A "principled solution" is one that reflects the fairness of the process and one that was not predetermined by the power status of any one of the parties (Dubler & Marcus, 1994). If this type of informal but focused deliberation is unable to arrive at resolution that reflects the patient's wishes and with which all are in accord, an ethics consultation or meeting of the institution's ethics committee may be the next step.

ETHICS COMMITTEES OR CONSULTANTS

Just as physicians and patients will turn to medical specialists for advice and consultation on questions of medical interventions, patients, families, proxies, and care providers may need to turn to an ethics committee or consultant to discuss treatment dilemmas. An ethics committee should look like members of the health care team: interdisciplinary. If the institution's lawyer or risk manager is a committee member, it is essential that the potential legal risk to the institution does not dominate discussion and trump ethically challenging discussions relevant to health care providers.

An ethics committee can serve several purposes: it may educate itself, the administration, and the staff about medical-ethical issues; participate in policy development (e.g., DNR orders, determination of brain death, weaning off ventilator support); and through consultation may assist in the resolution of bioethical dilemmas and/or offer specific recommendations. In some cases, an ethics committee improves communications between proxy and family, thereby removing some if not all disagreement between two concerned parties. There is no requirement that patient care decisions must change after an ethics consultation. However, by participating in consultation, providers, patients, and families may feel that their concerns have been addressed and they will better understand the rationale for the treatment decision that is being proposed or that emerged from the discussion.

Nurses serving on ethics committees should expect to be respected by colleagues and peers for their clinical judgment and their interpersonal skills. Members must be receptive to different ideas and points of view, be able to deal with emotionally charged issues and interpersonal disagreements/conflicts, and be able to tolerate ambiguity (Lo, 1999). For example, despite widespread agreement that artificial nutrition and hydration are simply another form of life sustaining medical treatment, many people feel strongly that these kinds of treatment are fundamental and owed to all people. Thus, patients and families are extremely resistant to suggestions to terminate them, and the ethics committee may be the best forum to mediate between such perceptions.

Disagreement that stems from uncertainty or miscommunications between patient and family might warrant an ethics consultation or committee meeting. Uncertainty may arise because of the difficulty in determining the effect of various treatment alternatives. Likewise, the patient's failure to explicitly state his or her treatment preferences can create uncertainty. A dilemma may result from miscommunication that fails to convey clear and relevant information about diagnosis, prognosis, and treatment options to the concerned parties. Accordingly, regardless of the source of the disagreement, health care providers should be sensitive to warning signs of a brewing disagreement. In most agencies, any member of the caregiving team can refer a situation to the ethics committee or consultant to request discussion and review of decision making. Rather than being viewed as an intrusion on professional clinical decision-making prerogatives, an ethics conference can clarify and strengthen the relationship between the parties.

Poorly resolved disagreements about the use of life sustaining treatments can also give rise to litigation. The institution's lawyer is well suited to advise and educate the health care team about, for example, decision making in the absence of an HCP, family decision making, life-sustaining treatment decisions, and request for "treatment without medical benefit." In addition, the lawyer might ease some of the fears and dispel some of the misconceptions that health care providers have about the law and litigation and address, as well, the potential liability and immunities for members of the ethics committee.

INTERPRETERS

Under state law and JCAHO standards, patients have the right to have a qualified interpreter translate and transmit discussion between themselves and the health care professional. The interpreter may be the only person who recognizes that patients and their families have a totally different "take" than the health care team on words like "health" and "illness," on what a treatment is supposed to do, and on what dying is and what it is not. If "telling bad news" is prohibited (e.g., Navajo, Greece, Korea, Horn of Africa nations), then it will be difficult to discuss end-of-life planning. It should not be assumed that facility, family or other interpreters are neutral and simply "translate" words. An interpreter is communicating fact and nuance, explanation and rationale, and might be advocating for a particular treatment course simply by the translated words and sentence structure. Nurses are with patients and their families more than any other clinical discipline; thus, any opportunity should be taken to check what the patient or family heard or understands by asking another individual to translate questions and answers.

NURSES' ROLES IN ADVANCE DIRECTIVES

All adult patients, regardless of their sex, religion, socioeconomic status, diagnosis, or prognosis should be approached to discuss advance directives. Evidence suggests that patients from certain demographic groups are less likely to be approached about advance directives or be provided with information about them (Mezey, Leitman, Mitty, Bottrell, & Ramsey, 2000). Advance directive completion is more concentrated among White patients with higher education and income levels than among Black and Hispanic patients at low-income levels and less than a high school education (Mezey et al., 2000). The information and discussions about advance directives should be translated into the patient's preferred language and transmitted in a culturally appropriate manner by health care providers: Understanding is the first element of informed decision making. Failure to take hearing and visual deficits into account can result in the erroneous conclusion that the person lacks the capacity to execute an advance directive.

Nurses have an important role in introducing patients to information about advance directives and helping patients complete them (Kirmse, 1998). Although surveys of the general public report positive attitudes toward advance directives, few patients actually have completed one. Even patients at higher risk of becoming incapable of making decisions and who, therefore, might be more likely to need one are not necessarily more likely to complete a directive.

Evidence suggests that talking with patients about advance directives can make a difference in completion rates. Patients who had regular conversations with their health care provider about advance directives were more likely to complete a directive (Luptak & Bould, 1994). Nurses should not wait for the patient to broach the subject. Patients want to discuss end-of-life care and living wills, but they expect providers to initiate these discussions. Patients often state that they complete advance directives to ease their family's financial and emotional burden and to ease decision making. For patients who find it difficult to initiate such discussions with their families or physicians, the nurse can provide a format for discussions, help ensure that the conversation is comprehensive, and minimize disagreements between patients and their families.

The nurse can begin by helping the patient and/or proxy explore and express what quality of life means for the patient, the importance of preservation of life, and how the patient's illness (and death) will affect others (i.e., emotionally, financially, etc.). Some patients might want to focus on the quality of their living while others, the quality of their dying. Some patients might want to talk about from whom and where they will receive care at the end of life. Some may abhor their coming dependence on others; others may not like or want it, but will accept it. Still others might opt for hospice care out of the home to distance their dependency on family caregivers. Patients and proxies might need or want to talk about what they each fear most and what will be important when dying.

Copies of the completed advance directive(s) should be distributed to the primary health care provider (physician, nurse practitioner), agency or institution, and the proxy. Nurses can take the initiative to review the document with patients annually and in the event of a significant change of condition. While doing so, the nurse or other appropriate person should check whether the proxy is still alive and willing to continue to act in that capacity. If the proxy has died, the nurse should discuss with the patient which person he or she would like to become the surrogate decision maker, follow through that someone has been selected, and check that the new agent is aware of the patient's wishes and preferences regarding care at the end of life. In nursing homes, especially, nurses are sometimes the first if not the only caregivers to know that the proxy died. After discussion among the team, the clinician with whom the nursing home resident has the best relationship should select the best time and place for this kind of discussion; not uncommonly, this would be the nurse.

CREATING A FAVORABLE CLIMATE FOR ADVANCE DIRECTIVE DISCUSSION

An environment that is conducive to meaningful discussions about advance directives and end-of-life care requires an appropriate time and location. An emergency admission is not an appropriate time. Distribution without discussion, commonly done in admissions offices at the time of an elective admission is not an appropriate time either. Patients may be more receptive to read about advance directives if the information is part of a preadmission package or discussed as part of the discharge process when the impact of hospitalization is still fresh but the acute symptoms (and probable anxiety) are no longer present. Information that is provided by the physician or nurse during a regular office visit might also improve the quality of these discussions. It is unlikely that education and information about advance directives will completely counteract the natural discomfort associated with discussing death and dying; this is generally as true for patients and families as it is for care providers. Awareness of the patient and family's spiritual and cultural "surround," as well as the provider's moral biases about life-sustaining treatment, can give rise to sensitive and realistic discussion. If a patient or proxy's treatment choice conflicts with a nurse's beliefs and the nurse cannot offer care in accordance with those wishes, the appropriate person within the facility should be notified, and the nurse should request transfer to another assignment or unit. The overriding concern should be that the patients care wishes are followed.

The right to not complete an advance directive must also be respected. Patients statements related to their decisions, particularly value statements, should be documented so that their wishes and privacy can be respected. It is very important that patients are informed (and, in some cases, reassured) that neither providers nor the facility will abandon them or provide substandard care if the patient elects not to formulate an advance directive.

When health care providers expresses negative feelings about advance directives, it might be that they mistrust the validity of the information contained in the advance directive; they might be concerned that the patient did not fully understand the advance directives' content or purpose (Jacobsen et al., 1994). Although some studies have demonstrated that the ability to predict specific treatment choices, based on the patient's beliefs, is not uniformly congruent for patients and their proxies (Emanuel, Weinberg, Gonin, Hummel, & Emanuel, 1993; Schneiderman, Pearlman, Kaplan, Anderson, & Rosenberg, 1993), other studies report that proxies are more likely than others to approximate the patient's own treatment preferences. In general, patients' decisions are fairly stable over time, especially among patients who have completed advance directives (Danis, Garret, Harris, & Patrick, 1994).

CASE STUDY

Mrs. R. is an 88-year-old female, Jewish, widowed for 22 years and with no next of kin, who lived alone prior to her admission to the nursing home 2 years ago, at which time she consented to a DNR order. She has severe COPD, chronic renal failure (BUN 58), dementia mild/moderate (MMSE 20/30), is mildly depressed (by GDS score), and is below her ideal body weight (–22 pounds). Mrs. R. now requires one person for all personal care; she bruises easily. Her prognosis is poor; goals of care are symptom management with comfort/palliative care. She has had multiple hospitalizations for "pneumonia"; the latest was 10 weeks ago, after which she had further weight loss and developed a grade II pressure ulcer on her right hip. She is receiving the standard medications for COPD, an antianxiety medication, a short-acting sleeping medication, and appetite stimulants. Recent discussion about her quality of life by the interdisciplinary team noted that she no longer attends parties, Sabbath candle lighting, and discussions, all of which she used to enjoy. Mrs. R. seemed unable to make health care decisions as of 6 months ago; her decisional capacity appears to fluctuate in relation to her oxygen saturation. She

created a living will 5 years ago that stipulated "aggressive comfort care, including ventilator support." There are no verbal statements documented that might indicate Mrs. R.'s feelings about
being hospitalized if she has another COPD exacerbation, which is
to be expected given the trajectory of this disease.

Two days ago, Mrs. R. began to have stertorous breathing, a
nonproductive cough, and episodes of diaphoresis. She appears
exhausted; her solid food intake is minimal, and she gets very dys-
pneic when taking small sips of fluid. A chest x-ray was equivocal
and is to be repeated today. At present, her vital signs are: T 100.8,
Pulse Ox (oxygen saturation): 82%; P and BP WNL. The nursing
home has the resources to provide oxygen and IV fluids, including
antibiotics.

DISCUSSION

The difficulty of this case is an advance directive that might not
address what Mrs. R. would want in a projected disease condition,
that is, the current situation. Whose voice will articulate the benefits and burdens of hospitalization or remaining in the nursing
home for palliative/terminal care? The nursing assistants feel she
should be hospitalized; their advocacy is based on 2 years of
knowing her and feelings of great affection for her. The clinical professional staff argue from prognostications about the likely aggressive interventions (e.g., intubation and ventilator support) and
probable multiple skin breakdowns if she is hospitalized. The standard of "substituted judgement" that a proxy uses when deciding
on behalf of a patient whose wishes and preferences are known is
not available to us. One could ask, "What would Mrs. R. choose if
she could join the discussion?" The "best interest" standard of
decision making asks what we think would promote Mrs. R.'s well-
being. Can we bring her back to baseline (the status at which staff
knew and loved her)? At this point, the benefit–burden assessment becomes a critical part of the discussion.

Conflict among the professional and paraprofessional staff has
to be addressed. For the nurses, administering morphine to provide comfort might well hasten Mrs. R.'s death. Are we prolonging
life or prolonging death? Are we treating resident or institutional
anxiety? What are our learning needs? COPD is a disease with no
cure; it progresses inexorably to death. What is meant by quality
of life? It is a personal phenomenon and judgment, not a medical
determination. To what extent can the facility provide a reasonable quality of life, a degree of comfort and safety that might meet

Mrs. R.'s interests at this time? It will be different from the one the staff previously enjoyed with her. What are the contingencies, the "what ifs" for the nursing home? What are the legal and ethical implications of departing from Mrs. R.'s advance directive? Of the doctrine of double effect?

After discussion with an ethics consultant at an interdisciplinary meeting, the decision was made not to hospitalize Mrs. R. The decision was guided by the clinical facts, Mrs. R.'s prior wishes ("aggressive comfort care" as stated in her living will), and focused on the goals of care. Conflict mediation that included education about COPD, fact gathering, values discussion, and reflection about Mrs. R.'s condition after each hospitalization enabled a consensus decision reached by all staff involved in her care. This case teaches us that advance care planning is not a static one-time event. Whether a person's wishes and preferences are stated through an advance directive document or verbally, they must be carefully written down and periodically reviewed upon a person's change of condition, life style, proxy, heart, and mind. The ability to reach consensus through mediation that addressed each person's concerns but kept the discussion resident centered was key to arriving at a medically and ethically appropriate decision.

SUMMARY

Well-informed nurses are reportedly more comfortable, have more discussions, and their patients complete more advance directives than do patients of uneducated providers (Richter, Eisemann, Bauer, & Kribeck, 1998; Robinson, DeHaven, & Kock, 1993). However, education requires more than knowledge of the PSDA and steps in formulating directives. Nurses need to learn how to discuss advance care planning with patients and families, assess decisional capacity to execute an advance directive, identify methods to help patients analyze benefits and burdens of decisions, and resolve conflicts emerging from different values and beliefs about end-of-life treatment. In addition, nurses need to understand the dynamics of decision making and learn how to formulate an ethical dilemma so that it can be appropriately and efficiently discussed between those who advise and those who carry such recommendations to the bedside (Solomon et al., 1993).

A recent study of hospitalized frail nursing home residents found that advance care planning tended to focus on CPR preference and that life-sustaining treatment was gradually limited pursuant to review after an acute illness or hospitalization (Happ et al., 2002). Of the few residents who received hospice services at the end of life, most referrals and palliative care interventions occurred in the week preceding death. In addition, there was little evidence of pain and symptom management. The authors' conclusion, not surprisingly, was that advance care planning had to be more responsive to individual preferences. Clearly, advance care planning should be part of nurses' skill repertoire.

Nurses must have opportunities to critically think and articulate their views and positions on dilemmas that they face as individuals and professionals. Ethics committees, rounds and colloquia, continuing education sessions and conferences all provide forums for nurses, students, faculty, and clinicians to enhance their ethical and legal awareness. The American Nurses Association Center for Ethics and Human Rights is one of a number of rich resources for nurses who seek consultation and ethics information to empower patients and families (see Resources). Nurses ethical responsibilities as set forth in the ANA Code of Ethics (ANA, 2001) and legal and professional responsibilities discussed in this chapter make nurses active participants in end of life decisions. Nurses must advocate to and educate patients and families about the importance of advance directives and planning ahead (Basile, 1998). Gaining ethical and legal competence will empower nurses to fulfill this professional commitment.

**BOX 15.1   Geriatric Nursing Standard of Practice:
Advance Directives Protocol**

Guiding Principles:
1. All people have the right to decide what will be done with their bodies.
2. All individuals are presumed to have decision-making capacity until deemed otherwise.
3. All patients who can participate in a conversation, either verbally or through alternate means of communication, should be approached to discuss advance directives.
4. Health care professionals can improve the end-of-life decision making for elderly patients by encouraging the use of advance directives.
I. BACKGROUND
   A. Decisions about stopping treatment are more prevalent among the elderly.
      1. Patients uniformly state that they want more information about advance directives.
      2. Patients want nurses (and doctors) to approach them about advance directives.
      3. Fewer than 20% of Americans have completed an advance directive.
   B. Advance directives:
      1. Allow individuals to provide directions about the kind of medical care they do or do not want if they become unable to make decisions or communicate their wishes.
      2. Provide guidance for health care professionals and families about health care decision making that reflect the person's wishes.
      3. Provide immunity for health care professionals and families from civil and criminal liability when health care professionals follow the advance directive in good faith.
   C. Two types of advance directives: durable power of attorney for health care (DPAHC) (also called a health care proxy) and Living Will
      1. A *durable power of attorney* allows an individual to appoint someone, called a health care proxy, agent, or surrogate, to make health care decisions for him or her should he or she lose the ability to make decisions or communicate his or her wishes.
      2. A *living will* provides specific instructions to health care providers about particular kinds of health care treatment an individual would or would not want to prolong life. Living wills are often used to declare a wish to refuse, limit, or withhold life-sustaining treatment.

(continued)

BOX 15.1 Geriatric Nursing Standard of Practice:
Advance Directives Protocol *(continued)*

   D. Oral advance directives (verbal directives) are allowed in some states if there is clear and convincing evidence of the patient's wishes. Clear and convincing evidence can include evidence that the patient made the statement consistently and seriously, over time, specifically addressed the actual condition of the patient, and was consistent with the values seen in other areas of the patient's life. Legal rules surrounding oral advance directives vary by state.

II. ASSESSMENT PARAMETERS

   A. All patients (with the exception of patients with persistent vegetative state, severe dementia, or coma) should be asked if they have a living will or if they have designated a proxy.

   B. All patients, regardless of age, gender, religion, socioeconomic status, diagnosis, or prognosis, should be approached to discuss advance directives and advance care planning.

   C. Discussions about advance directives should be conducted in the patient's preferred language to enable information transfer and questions and answers.

   D. Patients who have been determined to lack capacity to make other decisions may still have the capacity to designate a proxy or make health care decisions. Decision-making capacity should be determined for each individual based on whether the patient has the ability to make the specific decision in question.

   E. If a living will has been completed or proxy has been designated:

      1. Is the document readily available on the patient's current chart?

      2. Does the attending physician know the directive exists and has a copy?

      3. Does the designated health care proxy have a copy of the document?

      4. Has the document been recently reviewed by the patient, attending physician/nurse, and proxy to determine if it reflects the patient's current wishes and preferences?

III. CARE STRATEGIES

   A. Nurses can help patients and families trying to deal with end-of-life care issues.

   B. Patients who may be reluctant to discuss their own mortality or begin coping with their current health situation may be willing to discuss these issues with a nurse or clergyman.

BOX 15.1   *(continued)*

C. Race, culture, ethnicity, and religion can influence the health care decision-making process. Nurses should be mindful of these factors but should always treat the patient as an individual, not as a class of persons.
D. Assess each patient's need for and ability to cope with the information provided. Patients from other cultures may not subscribe to Western notions of autonomy, but that does not mean that these patients do not want to talk about advance care planning or advance directives or that they would not have conversations with their families.
E. Respect each person's right not to complete an advance directive.
F. Inform patients that you will not abandon them or provide substandard care if they elect to formulate an advance directive.
G. Know the institution's mechanism for resolving conflicts between family members and the patient or between the patient/family and care providers. This may include consultation with a social worker or the patient advocate or bringing the issue to the hospital ethics committee.
H. Notify the appropriate person if you are unable to provide care should the patient's wishes conflict with your personal beliefs.

IV. EVALUATION OF EXPECTED OUTCOMES
To determine whether implementation of this protocol influenced the nature as well as the number of advance directives created, some changes would be measurable and can contribute to the facility's ongoing quality improvement program.
A. As documented in the record:
 • the percent of patients asked about advance directives
 • whether a patient does or does not have an advance directive
B. Of those patients with an advance directive, the percentage of advance directives included in patient charts
C. The use of interpreters to assist staff discussion of advance directives with patients for whom English is not their primary language
D. Advance directives completed in association with admission to, or receipt of services from, the facility
E. Nurses' referral of patient or staff situations regarding advance directives to the ethics committee

BIOETHICS RESOURCES

American Nurses Association (ANA)
ANA Center for Ethics and Human Rights
600 Maryland Avenue, SW, Suite 100 West
Washington, DC 20024-2571
Phone: (202) 651-7055
www.nursingworld.org
- Code for Nurses with Interpretive Statements
- Position Statements on Assisted Suicide and Active Euthanasia, Do-Not-Resuscitate, Comfort and Relief, Patient Self-Determination Act
- Selected bibliographies on ethical issues such as End-of-Life Decisions, Forgoing Artificial Nutrition and Hydration, Nursing Ethics Committees, and Assisted Suicide and Euthanasia

The American Society of Bioethics and Humanities
4700 West Lake Avenue
Glenview, IL 60025
Phone: (847) 375-4745
www.asbh.org
- *International Journal of Nursing Ethics*

Choice in Dying/Partnership for Caring, Inc.
National Office
1620 Street, NW, Suite 202
Washington, DC 20006
Phone: (202) 296-8071
http://www.choices.org
- Questions and Answers: Advance Directives and End-of-Life Decisions; Medical Treatments and Your Advance Directives; Artificial Nutrition and Hydration and End-of-Life Decision Making; Do-Not-Resuscitate Orders and End-of-Life Decisions
- Video: Who's Death Is It, Anyway? (PBS special)

Hospice and Palliative Nurses Association
Medical Center East, Suite 375
211 North Whitfield St.
Pittsburgh, PA 15206-3031
Phone: (412) 361-2470
- Standards of Hospice Nursing
- Symptom Management
- Algorithms for Palliative Care

The Kennedy Institute of Ethics
Box 571212
Georgetown University
Washington, DC 20057-1212
www.georgetown.edu/research/kie/
• Scope Note series
• Ethics Journal (available electronically)

Last Acts
1620 I Steet, NW, Suite 202
Washington, DC 20006
Phone: (202) 296-8352
www.lastacts.org
• Journal article summaries
• State Initiatives on EOL Care—Focus: Pain Management
• Helping employees deal with EOL issues
• Statement on diversity in EOL care

End-of-Life Nursing Education Consortium (ELNEC)
American Association of Colleges of Nursing
One Dupont Circle, NW, Suite 530
Washington, DC 20036
Phone: (202) 785-8320
www.aacn.nche.edu/elnec

End-of-Life Physician Education Research Center (EPERC)
Medical College of Wisconsin, MEB, Room 3235
8701 Watertown Plank Road
Milwaukee, WI 53226
Phone: (414) 456-4353
www.eperc.mcw.edu

REFERENCES

American Nurses Association (ANA). (2001). *Code of ethics.* Washington, DC: American Nurses Association Center for Ethics and Human Rights.
Administration on Aging (AOA). (2002). Retrieved July 22, 2002, from http://www.aoa.gov/aoa/stats/profile/2001/1.html
Basile, C. M. (1998). Advance directives and advocacy in end of life decisions [Review]. *Nurse Practitioner, 23*(5), 44–46.
Bradley, C. H., Wetle, T., & Horwitz, S. M. (1998). The Patient Self-Determination Act and advance directive completion in nursing homes. *Archives of Family Medicine, 7,* 417–423.

290 Geriatric Nursing Protocols for Best Practice

Cruzan v. Director, 497 U.S. 261, 100 (S. Ct. 1990) 2841, 111 L. Ed. 2d 224.

Danis, M., Garret, J., Harris, R., & Patrick, D. L. (1994). Stability of choices about life-sustaining treatments. *Annals of Internal Medicine, 120,* 567–573.

Dubler, N. N., & Marcus, L. J. (1994). *Mediating bioethical disputes.* New York: United Hspital Fund of New York.

Emanuel, E. J., Weinberg, D. S., Gonin, R. G., Hummel, L. R., & Emanuel, L. L. (1993). How well is the Patient Self-Determination Act working? An early assessment. *American Journal of Medicine, 95*(6), 619–628.

Fins, J. J. (1999). Commentary: From contract to covenant in advance care planning. *Journal of Law, Medicine and Ethics, 27,* 46–51.

Happ, M. B., Capezuti, E., Strumpf, N. E., Wagner, L., Cunningham, S., Evans, L., & Maislin, G. (2002). Advance care planning and end-of-life care for hospitalized nursing home residents. *Journal of the American Geriatrics Society, 50*(5), 829–835.

Jacobsen, J. A., White, B. E., Battin, M. P., Francis, L. P., Green, D. J., & Kansworm, E. S. (1994). Patients' understanding and use of advance directives. *Western Journal of Medicine, 160*(3), 232–236.

Kapp, M. B., & Mossman, D. (1996). Measuring decisional capacity: Cautions on the construction of a capacimeter. *Psychology and Public Policy Law, 2,* 73–95.

Kirmse, J. M. (1998). Aggressive implementation of advance directives. *Critical Care Nursing Quarterly, 21*(1), 83–89.

Lo, B. (1999). The patient–provider relationship: Opportunities as well as problems. *Journal of General Internal Medicine, 14*(Supp. 1), S41–44.

Luptak, M. K., & Bould, C. (1994). A method for increasing elders' use of advance directives. *Gerontologist, 34,* 409–

Meisel, A. (2002). *The right to die* (2 vols.) New York: Aspen Law & Business.

Mezey, M., Mitty, E., & Ramsey, G. (1997). Assessment of decision-making capacity: Nurse's role. *Journal of Gerontological Nursing, 23*(3), 28–35

Mezey, M., Mitty, E., Rappaport, M., & Ramsey, G. (1997). Implementation of the Patient Self-Determination Act in nursing homes in New York City. *Journal of the American Geriatrics Society, 45*(1), 43–49.

Mezey, M., Teresi, J., Ramsey, G., Mitty, E., & Bobrowitz, T. (2002). Determining a resident's capacity to execute a health care proxy. In *Voices of decision in nursing homes: Respecting residents' preferences for end-of-life care* (pp. 28–35). New York: United Hospital Fund of New York.

Mezey, M. D., Leitman, R., Mitty, E. L., Bottrell, M. M., & Ramsey, G. C. (2000). Why hospital patients do and do not execute an advance directive. *Nursing Outlook, 48*(4), 165–171.

Midwest Bioethics Center. (1996). *Ethics Committee Consortium: Guidelines for the determination of decisional incapacity.* Kansas City: Midwest Bioethics Center.

New Jersey Supreme Court (NJSC). (1976). 70 N.J. 10, 335 A.2d 647, cert. den., 429 U.S. 922.

Olson, E. (1993). Ethical issues in the nursing home. *Mt. Sinai Journal of Medicine, 60,* 555–559.

Patient Self-Determination Act (PSDA). Pub. L. No. 101-508 (42 U.S.C.A. 1395cc(f) (1992)).

Quill v. Vacco, 80 F.3d 716 (2nd Cir. 1996).

Robinson, M. K., DeHaven, M. T., & Kock, K. A.(1993). Effects of the patient self-determination act on patient knowledge and behavior. *Journal of Family Practice, 37*(4), 363–368.

Richter, J., Eisemann, M., Bauer, B., & Kribeck, H. (1998). Decisions and attitudes of nurses in the care of chronically ill elderly patients. *Pflege, 11*(2), 96–99.

Roth, L. H., Meisel, A., & Lidz, C. W. (1977). Tests of competency to consent to treatment. *American Journal of Psychiatry, 134,* 279–284.

Schneiderman, U., Pearlman, R. A., Kaplan, R. M., Anderson, J. P., & Rosenberg, E. M. (1992). Relationship of general advance directive instructions to specific life-sustaining treatment preferences in patients with serious illness. *Archives of Internal Medicine, 52,* 2114–2122.

Solomon, M. Z, O'Donnell, L., & Jennings, B. (1993). Decisions near the end of life: Professional views on life-sustaining treatments. *American Journal of Public Health, 83*(1), 14–23.

Tolle, S. W., Tilden, V. P., Nelson, C. A., & Dunn, P. M. (1998). A prospective study of the efficacy of the physician order for life sustaining treatment (1995–1997). *Journal of the American Geriatrics Society, 46*(9), 1097–1102.

Tresch, D., Heudebert, G., Kutty, K., Ohlert, J., VanBeek, K., & Masi, A. (1994). Cardiopulmonary resuscitation in elderly patients hospitalized in the 12990s: A favorable outcome. *Journal of the American Geriatrics Society, 42*(2), 137–141.

U.S. Department of Health and Human Services (USDHHS). (2001). Births, marriages, divorces and deaths: Provisional data for April–June, 2001. *National Vital Statistics Report, 50*(2).

Chapter 16

DISCHARGE PLANNING FOR THE OLDER ADULT

DeAnne Zwicker and Gloria Picariello

EDUCATIONAL OBJECTIVES

On completion of this chapter, the reader should be able to

1. Describe one assessment parameter for discharge planning in each of the following: functional status, cognition, depression, and caregiver support.
2. Describe the elderly most at risk for poor postdischarge outcomes.
3. Define specific care interventions for effective discharge planning.
4. Discuss potential outcome measurements for comprehensive discharge planning.

The elderly account for 36% of all admissions to acute care hospitals, 49% of all the days of hospital care, and 50% of all physician hours (Alliance for Aging Research, 2002). Additionally, the rate of

---

Adapted from a chapter in the original edition by R. Campbell, M. Naylor, and the NICHE faculty. (1999). Discharge planning and home follow-up of elders. In Abraham, I., Fulmer, T., & Mezey, M. (Eds.), *Geriatric Nursing Protocols for Best Practice* (pp. 189–198). New York: Springer Publishing Company.

hospitalizations increases more with advancing age. Those over age 85 have more than twice the rate of hospitalizations than those between the ages of 65 and 74 (Healthcare in U.S., 1999). This is the fastest growing segment of the population in the United States.

Elderly patients are being discharged from the hospital much earlier because of utilization constraints. Nationwide, the average hospital stay is 5.9 days for those between the ages of 65 and 84 and 6.3 days for those over age 85 (HCUPnet, 2002). Shorter hospital stays often result in acute problems that are not completely resolved at the time of discharge. Consequently, the older person is discharged to the home much sicker and is more likely to be readmitted to the hospital. Over one third are readmitted in the first month after discharge, 50% after 3 months, and 80% within 1 year (Inouye et al., 1999).

Elderly persons are particularly vulnerable to adverse outcomes from hospitalization. Those persons with multiple comorbidities, multiple medications, cognitive or functional impairment, and over age 85 are at a particularly high risk for iatrogenic events (Administration on Aging, 2001; Bowles, Naylor, & Foust, 2002; Gorbien, 1992; Naylor, 1999; Rothschild, Bates, & Leape, 2000). Many in this population are also at risk for poor outcomes after discharge from the hospital (Bowles et al., 2002).

Home health reimbursement has declined in the current Medicare and Medicare managed care systems. In fact, since passage of the Balanced Budget Act in 1997, home health reimbursement has declined further and continues to do so annually (CMS, 1999). The increasing numbers of elderly and the high rate of hospital utilization, shortened length of hospital stay, risk for morbidity, and decline in resources for home health reinforce the need for comprehensive discharge planning. Box 16.1 presents a nursing standard of practice protocol for discharge planning for elderly patients discharged from acute care to the home environment.

ASSESSMENT

Discharge planning for the older adult from acute care to home or an alternative setting is a challenging process. The discharge planning process needs to begin at the time of admission and continue throughout the course of hospitalization. This will enable adequate time to develop a multidimensional, comprehensive plan. Information

---

BOX 16.1   Nursing Standard of Practice Protocol:
Discharge Planning for the Older Adult

I. BACKGROUND
   A. The elderly account for 36% of all admissions to acute care
      hospitals, 49% of all the days of hospital care, and 50% of all
      physician hours (Alliance for Aging Research, 2002).
   B. The rate of hospitalizations increases more with advancing age.
      Those over age 85 have more than twice the rate of hospitaliza-
      tions than those between ages 65 and 74, and this is the fastest
      growing segment of the population (Healthcare in the U.S., 1999).
   C. Elderly patients are being discharged much earlier because of
      utilization constraints, which often results in unresolved
      problems at the time of discharge (HCUPnet, 2002).
   D. Elderly persons are particularly vulnerable to adverse outcomes
      from hospitalization, particularly those persons with multiple
      comorbidities, multiple medications, and cognitive or functional
      impairment, and those over age 85.
   E. Elderly persons are at risk for poor outcomes after discharge
      from the hospital.
   F. The elderly population is at high risk for readmission to the
      hospital. Over one third are readmitted within the first month
      after discharge, 50% after 3 months, and 80% within 1 year
      (Inouye et al., 1999).
   G. Home health reimbursement has declined in the current
      Medicare and Medicare managed care systems. In fact, since
      passage of the Balanced Budget Act in 1997, home health
      reimbursement has declined.
   H. The increasing numbers of elderly and high hospital utilization,
      shortened length of hospital stay, high risk for morbidity, and
      decline in resources for home health reinforce the need for
      comprehensive discharge planning.
II. ASSESSMENT
   A. Initiate assessment for discharge planning process at time of
      admission: continue to reassess throughout hospitalization.
   B. Focus on those older adults at high risk for poor postdischarge
      outcomes.
   C. Assessment should include
      1. Functional status (ability to complete IADL and ADL and/or FIM)
      2. Cognitive status (ability to participate in discharge planning
         process and ability to learn new information)
      3. Psychological status of patient, particularly depression
         screening

BOX 16.1 *(continued)*

---

4. Patient's perception of self-care ability
5. Physical and psychological capabilities of family/caregiver
6. Knowledge deficits regarding health care needs postdischarge
7. Environmental factors of postdischarge setting
8. Caregiver formal and informal support needs
9. Nine core caregiving processes that ensure family caregivers can provide care smoothly and effectively
10. Review of medications and simplification of regimen
11. Prior link to community services

III. IMPLEMENTATION OF THE DISCHARGE PLAN
   A. General principles
      1. The discharge plan should be tailored to individual patient and family/caregiver needs.
      2. Assessment findings will guide intervention strategies.
      3. Assessment findings will determine educational and other home health requirements after discharge.
      4. Assessment data may predict potential discharge outcomes.
      5. Discharge planning should begin at admission due to shortened length of stay and complexities of the population.
      6. The discharge plan should be tailored to individual patient and family/caregiver needs.
   B. Strategies to ensure continuity of care (the 4 Cs: communication, coordination, collaboration, and continual reassessment)
      1. Communication:
         a. Communication should occur multidirectionally.
         b. Communication should occur between the multidisciplinary team and the patient and family/caregiver.
         c. Communication with formal and informal prehospital caregivers should be at admission, ongoing, and prior to discharge.
         d. Barriers to communication need to be eliminated.
         e. Communication of medical care needs to continue between hospital and community medical provider.
         f. Written communication should be clear and concise and include the following:
            • Documentation of assessment findings and home care needs on an interdisciplinary record.
            • A summary of the hospital course, particularly the following:

(continued)

BOX 16.1   Nursing Standard of Practice Protocol: Discharge Planning for the Older Adult *(continued)*

- – Include actual or potential sequelae
- – Presentation of unusual symptoms or significant change in status since admission
- – Specific symptom management required (i.e., pain postsurgery and effective management)
- – Medication review and difficulties for patient/family
- – Psychosocial adaptation to stress of illness
- – Anticipated outcomes
- – Advance directive discussions or decisions

  g. Verbal communication of health status and the discharge plan should include the following persons:

- • Patient, family, and/or caregiver.
- • Primary provider who will follow after discharge
- • Multidisciplinary experts
- • Referrals—home health agency, other providers of care

2. Coordination of services/case management:

  a. Case manager or designated team member should coordinate the multidisciplinary team in the discharge planning process.

  b. Case manager will link the person with the most appropriate services postdischarge.

  c. Case manager should ascertain understanding of all communication with patient and family/caregiver.

  d. Communication should be clear between hospital case manager and home health provider and/or any community resources.

3. Collaboration:

  a. Multidisciplinary team members should be used for specialized assessments, recommendations, and case conferences.

  b. Advanced practice nurse or RN expert in geriatrics may collaborate with team and provide home follow-up.

  c. Designate a case manager or nurse expert in geriatrics to coordinate discharge plan.

  d. Family or caregiver can provide information about past experiences, potential barriers, and biopsychosocial needs of the patient.

  e. Referrals should occur in-hospital, when possible, to limit transfers from home environment.

BOX 16.1 *(continued)*

---

4. Continual reassessment:
   a. The discharge planning process is dynamic, not static.
   b. Status of the patient may change rapidly in this population, requiring frequent reassessment.
   c. Change in condition should be communicated to all team members.
   d. Home care needs change as the assessment is clarified and as the patient status changes.
C. The discharge planning process
   1. Develop the plan to meet unique needs of each individual patient and family/caregiver.
   2. Communication with prehospital formal and informal caregivers should be at admission, ongoing, and prior to discharge.
   3. Involve the patient and family throughout discharge planning process.
   4. Yield to patient and family wishes and preferences for optimal outcomes.
   5. Health teaching, guidance, and counseling (potential areas to address):
      a. Gear teaching to specific learning needs of elderly patient.
      b. Describe required care related to presenting problem.
      c. Describe diet restrictions, and discuss patient preferences.
      d. Discuss medication actions and side effects.
      e. Discuss symptom management.
      f. Define when to call for help
      g. Discuss maintenance of hydration and nutritional status.
      h. Delineate signs of a change of condition and who to report to.
      i. Discuss what to report or do in an emergency.
      j. Discuss whom to contact in an emergency.
      k. Clarify activity level and ability, with a focus on safety and mobility.
      l. Discuss and/or clarify advance directives and care wishes of patient.
      m. Verbally review written discharge instructions and follow-up.
   6. Treatments and procedures (potential areas to address):
      a. Special procedures/care: wound care, tube feedings, hydration, etc.
      b. Discuss how and when to administer medications.
      c. Discuss ADL interventions: mobility, transfers, gait training.

(continued)

BOX 16.1   Nursing Standard of Practice Protocol:
Discharge Planning for the Older Adult *(continued)*

---

     7. Surveillance interventions (potential areas to address):
       a. Ensure adequate functional status before DC, or refer for appropriate home care needs.
       b. Evaluate system-specific physical assessment related to problems or potential problems.
       c. Monitor primary problem and potential sequelae.
       d. Offer iatrogenesis prevention during hospital course.
       e. Functional and cognitive status should be continually monitored.
       f. Medication understanding, management capabilities, and side effects should be ascertained.
       g. Transportation access and availability should be ensured.
       h. Family/caregiver abilities should be evaluated continually.
       i. Psychosocial issues that may affect transition need to be assessed.
     8. Case management (potential activities of CM)
       a. Refer to providers as needed preferably while in-hospital.
       b. Address questions/concerns from pt, caregiver, health providers
       c. Provide caregiver with contact numbers of care providers (primary care and HHA, PT/OT).
       d. Provide follow-up care appointments and contact information.
       e. Ascertain access to transportation services.
       f. Provide information on other community resources.
       g. Assess risk for potential poor discharge outcomes (Table 16.1) to ensure that appropriate discharge services are utilized.
       h. Ensure that caregiver support needs are met.
IV. EVALUATION OF OUTCOMES
   A. Patient and/or family caregiver:
     1. Health status will be maintained or improved, including functional and cognitive status, nutrition, emotional status, and physical status.
     2. Iatrogenic events will be avoided, such as falls and secondary infections.
     3. Complications will be minimized, such as decline in function.
     4. Knowledge of self-care will be improved.
     5. Caregiver competence and confidence will be increased.
     6. Patient self-perception of health will improve.

BOX 16.1   *(continued)*

---

    7. Disease-specific outcomes, such as blood glucose within expected range, will improve.
    8. Caregiver and/or patient able to reiterate discharge plan and implement in home.
    9. Follow-up appointments will be maintained, with transportation easily accessible.
  10. The number of new patients that become depressed postdischarge will decrease.

B. Providers:
    1. Acute care nurses can identify discharge assessment needs, intervention strategies, and follow-up of elderly patients.
    2. Acute care nurses will increase knowledge base regarding unique learning needs of the elderly population.
    3. Acute care nurses will accurately identify patients at high risk for poor outcomes, who benefit most from home care referrals, and are referred most often.
    4. Multidisciplinary team members will collaborate on a regularly scheduled basis.
    5. Communication of a change of status will be done among team members.
    6. Primary medical provider and hospitalist will communicate medical care needs with each other.

C. Institution:
    1. Decrease in the number of hospital readmissions and ER visits
    2. Decline in morbidity and mortality rates of patients discharged to home
    3. High rating of caregiver and patient satisfaction with care
    4. Improvement in cost containment

obtained during the initial assessment will serve as a baseline and offer preliminary structure to the design of the discharge plan. It is important for the discharge planning team to keep in mind, however, that this baseline information can change rapidly due to the frailty of the population and the adverse effects of hospitalization.

Hospitalization is associated with acute deconditioning and subsequent functional decline in older persons. Acute deconditioning refers to "changes that occur within days to a few weeks after a sudden decrease in activity" (Siebens et al., 2000, p. 1545). Included among these changes are mood changes, muscle atrophy with decreased muscle strength, and impaired coordination and balance (McComas, 1996). Hirsch and colleagues (cited in Siebens et al., 2000) reported that 80% of a hospitalized group of older adults experienced dependency in mobility within 2 weeks of hospitalization. This is often due to prolonged bed rest, psychotropic medications, and invasive equipment, such as Foley catheters (Inouye et al., 1999). In addition, iatrogenic conditions can contribute to an irreversible decline in the older adult's functionality. Iatrogenic conditions that may add to functional decline include dehydration, malnutrition, impaired skin integrity, and functional incontinence (Creditor, cited in Siebens et al., 2000). Therefore, ongoing assessment is imperative throughout the course of the hospitalization to implement the most appropriate discharge plan.

Particular attention must be paid to those individuals at greatest risk for poor discharge outcomes (Bowles et al., 2002) and unplanned hospital readmission (Anderson, Helms, Hanson, & DeVilder, 1999). Table 16.1 lists characteristics associated with the need for home care, the likelihood of home care referral, and/or poor discharge outcomes, as reviewed by Bowles and colleagues (2002).

Discharge planning for a frail older adult is multifaceted; therefore, other members of the health care team may be required to provide specialized assessments of the elderly. Other experts of the health care team may include a medical social worker, a physical or occupational therapist, a mental health provider, an advanced practice geriatric nurse, and a nutritionist. A geriatric pharmacist may be consulted to recommend strategies to simplify the medication regimen. Assessment data can be used to project postdischarge needs.

Arenth and colleagues (as cited in Bowles et al., 2002) concluded that acute care nurses overestimate the abilities of patients, the home environment, the patient's self-care ability, and the skill and

TABLE 16.1   Characteristics Associated with the Need for Home Care, the Likelihood of Home Care Referral, and/or Poor Discharge Outcomes

Aged 70 or older

Educational level < 12 years

Activity of daily living impairment

Two or more chronic conditions

Fair or poor subjective health rating

Cognitive impairment

Prior home care use

Homebound

Lives alone

Long length of hospital stay

Toileting problems

Multiple readmissions (≥ 2 in past 6 months)

Suspected nonadherence to diet or medications

Multiple medications or treatments

Less social support

Depression or psychiatric history

Need for skilled nursing care

Complications

Hospital admission in past 30 days

Surgery during the acute stay

History of falls

Readiness for self-care

Source: Adapted from K. Bowles, M. Naylor, & J. Foust (2002). Patient characteristics at hospital discharge and a comparison of home care referral decisions, *Journal of American Geriatrics Society,* © 2002 by Blackwell Science, LTD. Reprinted by permission of Malcolm Allison, Rights Assistant.

availability of caregivers. Additionally, they concluded that functional ability is often underestimated and understanding of treatment plan overestimated. Inaccurate assessments by acute care nurses can result in poor outcomes and underreferral for home health services.

The assessment process should focus on the following areas in the older adult:

- Physical and problem assessment
- Functional status
- Cognitive abilities
- Depression screening
- Formal and informal support systems
- Knowledge deficits regarding health care needs
- Home environment
- Patient and family psychological, socioeconomic, and cultural factors

FUNCTIONAL STATUS

Assessing functional status of the older adult as part of discharge planning helps identify the type and amount of assistance required postdischarge, including community services. Baseline assessment of both activities of daily living (ADL) and instrumental activities of daily living (IADL) is essential. The Functional Independence Measure (FIM™) can be used to assess the rehabilitation needs as well as functional capacity (see Figure 16.1, pp. 304–305). Functional status needs to be reassessed throughout the course of the hospitalization as it may change unexpectedly (Kresevic & Mezey, 1999). Finally, the patient's perception of self-care is important, as he or she may think that no assistance is required when a deficit actually exists.

COGNITIVE STATUS AND DEPRESSION

Cognitive status needs to be evaluated at admission and continually throughout the hospital course. A change in cognition may be the first indication of an acute medical problem and may go unrecognized. The Mini-Mental Status Exam (MMSE) is the most commonly used and tested mental status tool. Assessment for depression is also important. The short-form Geriatric Depression Scale (GDS-SF) is a quick method to perform screening for depression. Major depression can increase the risk of mortality and readmission (Jiang et al., 2001). Assessment for cognitive status and depression will help to determine the older adult's ability to learn and to participate in the discharge plan (Foreman, Fletcher, Mion, & Trygstad, 1999). A significant degree of cognitive impairment will have a major impact on the entire discharge plan, including the setting to which the patient is discharged. Standardized assessment tools that have been shown to be reliable and valid can be used to appreciate small changes in status over time. (Refer to chapters 3, 7, and 11 in this book for further information on assessment of function, cognition, and depression, respectively.)

CAREGIVER SUPPORT

The older adult may have ongoing health care needs once discharged. These needs may be met through professional home care services. However, since implementation of the Prospective Payment System (PPS) in 1983, the reimbursement for professional home health services has declined. Consequently, the majority of care administered to the elderly at home is provided by family caregivers. Families provide an estimated 80% to 90% of long-term care in the community (National Caregiver Alliance, 1997). Therefore, to avoid caregiver burnout and hospital readmission, it is important to evaluate the needs of caregivers.

The needs of caregivers generally fall into a few categories: support, knowledge of the aging process, knowledge of resources, respite, and financial assistance. Table 16.2 presents a tool designed by George and Gwyther (1986) to aid in determining the need for formal and informal support. Table 16.3 outlines nine core caregiving processes that help to ensure that family caregivers can provide care smoothly and effectively (Schumacher, Stewart, Archbold, Dodd, & Dibble, 2000).

Elderly spouses often have special needs. In particular, elderly women may find themselves unable to meet the physical demands of care once they return home. The elderly caregiver may end up being captive in his or her own home. Respite and support from others must be evaluated closely in this group. Proactive assessment of the caregiver's physical and psychological readiness to assume care before a discharge plan is finalized may prevent readmission or other adverse outcomes.

Information regarding the older adult's prior link to community resources should be ascertained. This information may simplify the discharge planning process. These services may have included Meals-on-Wheels, adult medical day care, home attendants, or community transportation. It is important, however, to assess whether these services are still appropriate after the index hospitalization. Because families are the major providers of home care, an intensified review of the informal support systems is imperative.

Assessment of the patient and family/caregiver's knowledge regarding needs after discharge is an integral part of the discharge

L E V E L S

NO HELPER

7 Complete Independence (Timely, Safely)
6 Modified Independence (Device)

HELPER

Modified Dependence
5 Supervision (Subject = 100%+)
4 Minimal Assist (Subject = 75%+)
3 Moderate Assist (Subject = 50%+)

Complete Dependence
2 Maximal Assist (Subject =25%+)
1 Total Assist (Subject = less than 25%)

	ADMISSION	DISCHARGE	FOLLOW-UP
Self-Care			
A. Eating			
B Grooming			
C. Bathing			
D. Dressing - Upper Body			
E. Dressing - Lower Body			
F. Toileting			
Sphincter Control			
G. Bladder Management			
H. Bowel Management			

Transfers

I. Bed, Chair, Wheelchair
J. Toilet
K. Tub, Shower

Locomotion

L. Walk/Wheelchair
M. Stairs

Motor Subtotal Score

Communication

N. Comprehension
O. Expression

Social Cognition

P. Social Interaction
Q. Problem Solving
R. Memory

Cognitive Subtotal Score

TOTAL FIM Score

NOTE: Leave no blanks. Enter 1 if patient not testable due to risk

W Walk / C Wheelchair / B Both

A Auditory / V Visual / B Both

V Vocal / N Nonvocal / B Both

FIGURE 16.1 FIM™ instrument.

FIM™ Instrument. Copyright © 1997 Uniform Data System for Medical Rehabilitation, a division of U B Foundation Activities, Inc. Reprinted with the permission of UDSmr, University at Buffalo, 232 Parker Hall, 3435 Main Street, Buffalo, NY 14214.

TABLE 16.2 Support for Caregivers

For each of the questions below, please indicate how often your family or friends give you each type of help by writing the corresponding number for each question. Then write in the relationship of the person who helps you the most with that task (e.g., sister, daughter, friend Joe, etc.).

Who helps you? _____

Do your family or friends:	How often do you receive help?				
	1 Never	2 Rarely	3 Only if I ask	4 Now and then	5 Regularly
1. Help you out when you are sick?					
2. Shop or run errands for you?					
3. Help you out with money or bills?					
4. Fix things around your house?					
5. Keep house for you or do household chores?					
6. Give you advice on business or finances?					
7. Provide companionship for you?					
8. Provide transportation for you or your confused relative?					
9. Prepare or provide meals?					
10. Stay with your relative while you are away?					
11. Provide personal grooming services for your relative?					
12. Do you wish that your family and friends would help with these kinds of things? a. Yes b. No					

Source: George, L. K., & Gwyther, L. P. (1983). Duke University caregiver well-being survey: Durham, NC, Duke University Study on Aging and Human Development. *Gerontologist, 26,* 253. Reprinted by permission.

TABLE 16.3   Nine Core Family Caregiver Processes Needed for Effective Caregiving

- Monitoring: keeping an eye on things
- Interpreting: making sense of what is observed
- Making decisions: choosing a course of action
- Taking action: carrying out caregiving instructions
- Providing hands-on care: carrying out medical and nursing procedures attending to both safety and comfort
- Making adjustments: finding the "right" strategy
- Accessing resources
- Working together with the ill person sensitivity to personhood of care receiver and caregiver
- Negotiating the health system.

Source: K. Schumacher, B. J. Stewart, P. G. Archbold, M. J. Dodd, & S. L. Dibble (2000). Family caregiving skill: Development of the concept. *Research in Nursing & Health, 23,* 191–203. Adapted with permission.

plan. Potential barriers to learning also need to be identified. These barriers may include limited formal education, age-related visual and auditory changes, and short-term memory impairment. In addition, assessment of the patient and family readiness to learn must to be determined (Dellasega, 1995).

HOME ENVIRONMENT

Information regarding the physical and environmental setting to which the patient will be discharged should be obtained during the assessment phase. This will help to formulate a realistic discharge plan. The following are questions that might be asked in this domain:

- Does the patient reside in a private home, senior housing, or assisted living residence?
- How many stairs are in and outside the residence?
- Where is the location of bathroom facilities and sleeping quarters?
- Is there a need for assistive devices, such as grab bars, shower seat, raised toilet seat, bedside commode, or a personal emergency response system (PERS)?

IMPLEMENTATION OF THE
DISCHARGE PLAN

The "four C's" (coordination, communication, collaboration, and continual reassessment) should be kept in mind throughout the discharge planning process. Discharge planning to the home environment requires a coordinated approach among the discharge team, the patient and family/caregiver, and the home health provider. The planning process needs to begin at the time of admission because of the shortened length of stay and the complexity of needs of this population. The discharge plan should be tailored to the individual patient and caregiver needs (Naylor et al., 1999). Assessment data should be used to project postdischarge service needs (Bowles, 2001; Bowles et al., 2002). The health status may change quickly in this vulnerable population; therefore, the discharge plan must be reassessed throughout the hospital course.

A gap in continuity of care from home to hospital and conversely is a common reason for hospital readmission and increased morbidity in this vulnerable population. The focus of the discharge plan should be on maintaining continuity throughout the care continuum. Communication should occur multidirectionally, including from home to hospital and back. Effective communication among and with caregivers and primary providers should also be ensured. Continuity of medical care can be improved by communication between the hospitalist and the primary medical provider following the patient after discharge.

Collaboration of a multidisciplinary team will provide the most comprehensive perspective to meet the complex needs of this population. The members of the team may include the following: primary physician (hospitalist, geriatrician, or primary provider), advanced practice geriatric nurse, dietitian, medical social worker, primary nurse, physical therapist, occupational therapist, speech therapist, chaplain, regular nursing assistant, mental health professional, and home care agency representative. The patient and family/caregiver should be actively involved in all patient care planning conferences. The family or caregiver can provide a wealth of knowledge about past experiences, biopsychosocial needs of the patient and family, and barriers that may present after discharge.

The members of the multidisciplinary team can meet in a formal care conference setting or make care rounds with the primary medical provider and primary nurse. A designated coordinator of the team is crucial to ensure continuity and smooth implementation of the plan. Many hospitals use a case manager as the coordinator of the discharge plan. This person should be experienced with the complexities of this population. Another option may be to involve a geriatric advanced practice nurse (APN) that will also follow the patient at home. The APN can work with the discharge planning team and patient/family during the hospitalization. This will enhance continuity by allowing the APN to get to know the patient and his or her family prior to discharge. This has been shown to be an effective means of maintaining continuity and preventing adverse outcomes in a number of studies (Naylor, 2000; Naylor et al., 1994, 1999).

Communication with formal and informal prehospital caregivers is the most important first step in the discharge planning process in order to ensure continuity. Communication with prehospital providers and those who will provide follow-up care should be a continual process throughout the hospital course. Any barriers to an effective communication process should be eliminated. Continuity of care, patient satisfaction, and improved outcomes depend on good communication of the status of patient problems (Bowles, 2001).

Patient and family/caregiver teaching, guidance, and counseling are some of the most important areas of communication in the discharge process. Elements of an effective teaching process should be geared for the unique learning needs of this population. Information obtained during the assessment will help to structure the content and design of the teaching plan. Older adult learners are most receptive to problem-centered learning; therefore, the key elements of teaching need to focus on what is most important to the patient. Compensation must be made for age-related changes in hearing and vision. For example, background noises need to be eliminated, and the health care professional must speak slowly and clearly while teaching the older adult. Printed materials must be appropriate to compensate for decreased vision. The older adult learner may also need more time to process information. Therefore, it is important to allow time for questions and to summarize information frequently.

Certain care interventions should occur prior to discharge. Of particular importance is simplification of the medication regimen. This process enables the acute care staff to evaluate the effects of the change prior to discharge and ultimately reduces the risk associated with complex regimens at home. Adequate functional status for the home environment must be ascertained prior to discharge. The caregiver needs to understand the patient's abilities and limitations and how to assist in maintaining safe mobility.

Case managers are critical in facilitating integration of services. A primary objective of case management is to link the person with the most appropriate service. An important case management strategy is arranging for the home care referral. The referral should be initiated prior to discharge in order to avoid poor outcomes, particularly for those patients at high risk (Bowles et al., 2002; Naylor, 2000). Case managers may want to reassess the family/caregiver's understanding, capability, and willingness to proceed with the home care plan prior to discharge. Involvement of the patient and his or her family throughout the discharge planning process and yielding to their wishes and preferences are more likely to result in an optimal outcome (Wu et al., 2002).

Once the discharge is imminent, a summary of the discharge plan should be put in writing and provided to the primary physician, patient and family/caregiver, home care team, and other pertinent providers, such as referrals. Verbal communication among care providers and with the family/caregiver regarding the discharge plan and patient status will aid in clarifying any issues or concerns.

The written summary should highlight the hospital course, current medications, anticipated family or patient limitations, and psychosocial issues. Any decision or discussion about advanced directives should be clearly documented to ensure that the patient's wishes are followed. It should be noted if there has been any significant change since admission, particularly any deterioration in status.

Follow-up care should include the name and telephone number of care providers, such as the primary medical provider, home health service, physical therapy group, referrals, and case manager. A schedule of follow-up appointments should be delineated and reviewed and include addresses and phone numbers. Additionally, access to transportation for follow-up appointments must be ensured. Difficulties in transportation may lead to inappropriate use of emergency service, missed appointments, and lack of appropriate surveillance and monitoring (Campbell & Naylor, 1999).

Implementation of preventive strategies during hospitalization (Counsell et al., 2000; Inouye et al., 1999; Siebens et al., 2000), multi-disciplinary discharge review, and improved follow-up after discharge have reduced readmission rates and must be employed in the discharge planning process (Bean & Waldren, 1995; Benbassat & Taragin, 2000; Lasater, 1996; Naylor et al., 1999). Coordination, collaboration, communication, and continual reassessment will ensure continuity during transitions of care and ensure an effective comprehensive discharge plan.

EVALUATION OF OUTCOMES

An evaluation of access, quality, and cost effectiveness should be included in the evaluation of outcomes of discharge planning. Information given about resource availability, discharge service options, and financial implications of choices are parameters that should be evaluated (Campbell & Naylor, 1999). Access to resources and follow-up should also be reviewed.

Outcome measurements have been reviewed and evaluated in multiple randomized controlled trials (Anderson et al., 1999; Naylor, 2000; Naylor et al., 1999, 1994). Outcomes should be evaluated for the patient and his or her family, the hospital care providers, and the institution providing care. Patient outcomes may include evaluation of health status, self-perception of health, iatrogenic events, and disease-specific clinical outcomes. Care provider outcomes include appropriateness of the discharge plan and patient and family satisfaction with care. Institutional evaluation of outcomes includes cost effectiveness of care (total days when rehospitalized and readmission charges), number of emergency room visits, hospital readmissions, unplanned long-term care placement, and cost for postdischarge health services (Anderson et al., 1999; Naylor, 2000; Naylor et al., 1994, 1999).

CASE STUDY

Mr. J. is an 82-year-old male with a past history of hypertension, BPH, diabetes type 2, and depression. He was discharged home after a CVA with left hemiparesis involving primarily the left lower extremity. Swallowing function was intact. Vision is impaired due to cataracts, and hearing is also impaired. He has been hospitalized twice in the past 6 months for unstable angina. Medications include paroxetine 10 mg q:d, captopril 12.5 mg tid, metropolol 100 mg bid, Glipizide 5 mg bid, Glucophage 500 mg bid, ASA 80 mg q:d, and NTG 0.4 mg SL prn chest pain x 3 tabs maximum. Prior to admission, Mr. J. was functionally independent in all ADLs and had an MMSE of 30/30. IADL function is intact except that Mr. J. no longer drives due to impaired vision. Mr. J.'s daughter drives him and his wife to appointments and shopping, or they take a bus. Mrs. J. is functionally impaired due to OA of the knees and is status post a total knee replacement 1 year ago; otherwise, she is in good health and cognitively intact. Mrs. J. uses a cane for mobility and cannot climb stairs. The couple live in a two-story colonial home.

DISCUSSION

Comprehensive discharge planning for Mr. J. should begin with a detailed assessment of his ability to perform ADLs and IADLs because there is new onset of weakness of the lower extremity. A physical and occupational therapy evaluation will provide recommendations for any further rehabilitation needs or assistive devices postdischarge. The home environment will also affect the discharge plan, for example, the location of the bathroom and bedroom, as well as the number of stairs the patient will have to navigate.

Assessment of the patient's present cognitive abilities and level of depression are essential before initiating discharge. Depression and cognitive function should be assessed prior to teaching as both may affect receptive abilities. Mr. J. has a history of depression (80% of patients become depressed after a new CVA). Therefore, there is a likelihood of an exacerbation postdischarge. Additionally, information regarding his past history of depression and prior coping ability after his last admission would be helpful. Evaluation of other medical problems should occur while the patient is in the hospital, particularly of the unstable angina that resulted in repeat admissions. It would be important to ascertain that the patient is, at minimum, being followed closely as an outpatient for this problem. The likelihood of readmission for cardiovascular disease is quite high.

Attention to family member's capabilities to assume caregiving responsibilities is necessary. Caregivers also need to have a clear understanding of the new functional limitations and the impact it will have at home. Finally, the assessment for an effective discharge plan should acknowledge Mr. J.'s current perception of his health care status and needs.

The teaching plan for Mr. J. should compensate for his decreased auditory and visual acuity and any other limitations discovered during the assessment process, such as education level. Health teaching should address learning needs associated with Mr. J.'s chronic conditions, namely, diabetes and heart disease, and preventive strategies to avoid recurrent cerebrovascular disease. Most importantly, teaching should address Mr. J.'s and his wife's learning concerns.

Names and phone numbers of the primary care provider, medical specialists, and community resources, such as Meals-on-Wheels, senior transportation, and home attendant services, should also be provided in a written discharge plan. To maintain continuity of care, a postdischarge medication regimen should be carefully reviewed, as well as scheduled appointments for follow-up care. Transportation to appointments must be ascertained prior to discharge. Referral to a community "stroke support " group may be beneficial to the patient and his family. Lastly, caregiver support must be evaluated, particularly because Mrs. J. has functional limitations as well. A case manager may be able to provide the best linkage to the required services. Assessment findings that are ascertained during hospitalization will guide many other interventions that can be tailored to this patient and his family's individual needs.

SUMMARY

Older adults utilize more acute care services than any other age group, and this population is at greatest risk for iatrogenic events during hospitalization. As the length of stay for hospitalizations become increasingly short, elderly persons are at high risk for poor outcomes, including hospital readmission. Therefore, comprehensive discharge planning is essential for this vulnerable population.

Discharge planning should begin at the time of admission, and reassessment of discharge needs must be ongoing. A multidisciplinary team should assess predischarge status and design the discharge plan. A teaching plan allows the patient and/or family member to address health care issues following discharge. Communication between the discharge planning team, patient, family members, and relevant community services is critical.

Outcomes demonstrating the effectiveness of discharge planning can be measured from the patient/family perspective, the care provider prospective, or the acute care institution, as well as by a decrease in hospital readmissions and postdischarge emergency room visits. Another area that may be evaluated is the patient's ability to adequately address his or her own health care needs postdischarge.

Interventions proven effective need to be disseminated among gerontology experts and funded to improve the quality of life of this vulnerable population. Proactive planning and innovative approaches will need to be developed to meet cost constraints. The growing demographics of the elderly population will provide a huge challenge for family and community resources as the century moves forward.

REFERENCES

Administration on Aging, Department of Health and Human Services. (2001). *Profile of older Americans: 2001.* Retrieved February 24, 2002, from http://www.aoa.dhhs.gov/aoa/stats/profile

Alliance for Aging Research. (2002). Medical never-never land: Ten reasons why America is not ready for the coming age boom. Accessed April 16, 2002 at www.agingresearch.org/brochures/nevernever/welcome.html

Anderson, M. A., & Helm, L. B. (2000). Talking about patients: Communication and continuity of care. *Journal of Cardiovascular Nursing, 14,* 15–28.

Anderson, M. A., Helms, L. B., Hanson, K. S., & DeVilder, N. W. (1999). Unplanned hospital readmissions: A home care perspective. *Nursing Research, 48,* 299–307.

Bean, P., & Waldron, K. (1995). Readmission study leads to continuum of care. *Nursing Management, 26,* 65, 67–68.

Benbassat, J., & Taragin, M. (2000). Hospital readmission as a measure of quality health care. *Archives of Internal Medicine, 160,* 1074–1081.

Bixby, M. B., Konick-McMahon, J., & MeKenna, C. G. (2000, April). Applying the transitional care model to elderly patients with heart failure. *Journal of Cardiovascular Nursing, 14,* 53–63.

Bowles, K. H. (2001). Patient problems and nurse interventions during acute care and discharge planning. *Journal of Cardiovascular Nursing, 14,* 29–41.

Bowles, K. H., Naylor, M. D., & Foust, J. B. (2002). Patient characteristics at hospital discharge and a comparison of home care referral decisions. *Journal of the American Geriatrics Society, 50,* 336–342.

Bull, M., Hansen, H., & Gross, C. (2000). Predictors of elder and family caregiver satisfaction with discharge planning. *Journal of Cardiovascular Nursing, 14,* 76–87.

Campbell, R., & Naylor, M. (1999). Discharge planning and home follow-up of elders. In I. Abraham, T. Fulmer, & M. Mezey (Eds.), *Geriatric nursing protocols for best practice* (pp. 189–198). New York: Springer Publishing Co.

Center for Medicare and Medicaid Services (CMS), Office of Strategic Planning. (1999). *Profile of Medicare spending.* Retrieved February 24, 2002, from http://www.hcfa.gov/stats/publications/chartbook.html

Counsell, S., Holder, C., Liebenauer, L., Palmer, R., Fortinsky, R., Kresevic, D. M., Quinn, L. M., et al. (2000). Effects of a multi-component intervention on functional outcomes and process of care in hospitalized older patients. *Journal of the American Geriatrics Society, 48,* 1572–1581.

Creditor, M. (1993). Hazards of hospitalization. *Annals of Internal Medicine, 188*, 219–223.

Dellasega, C., Clark, D., McCreary, D., Helmuth, A., & Schan, P. (1994). Nursing process: Teaching elderly clients. *Journal of Gerontological Nursing, 20*, 31–38.

Foreman, M. D., Fletcher, K., Mion, L., Trygstad, L., and the NICHE Faculty. (1999). Assessing cognitive function. In I. Abraham et al. (Eds.), *Geriatric nursing protocols for best practice* (pp. 51–61). New York: Springer Publishing Co.

George, L., & Gwyther, L. (1986). Caregiver well-being: A multidimensional examination of family caregivers of demented adults. *Gerontologist, 26*, 253–259.

Gorbien, M., Bishop J., Beers M., Norman D., Osterweil, D., & Rubenstein, L. Z. (1992). Iatrogenic illness in hospitalized elderly people. *Journal of the American Geriatrics Society, 40*, 1031–1042.

HCUPnet, Healthcare Cost and Utilization Project, Agency for Healthcare Research and Quality. (2002). *Outcomes by patient and hospital characteristics for all discharges* [on-line]. Accessed March 25, 2002: http://www.ahrq.gov/data/hcup/hcupnet.htm

Healthcare in the U.S. (1999). *Health and Aging Chartbook* (PHS# 991232). Retrieved March 25, 2002, at http://www.cdc.gov/nchs/releases/99news/hus.99.htm

Inouye, S., Bogardus, S., Charpentier, P., Leo-Summers, L., Acampora, D., Holford, T., & Cooney, L. (1999). A multi-component intervention to prevent delirium in hospitalized older patient. *New England Journal of Medicine, 340*, 669–676.

Jiang, W., Alexander, J., Christopher, E., Kuchibhatla, M., Gauleden, N. P., Cuffe, M. S., et al. (2001). Relationship of depression to increased risk of mortality and rehospitalization in patients with congestive heart failure. *Archives of Internal Medicine, 161*, 1849–1856.

Kresevic, D., Mezey, M., and the NICHE Faculty. (1999). Assessment of function: Critically important to acute care of elders. In I. Abraham et al. (Eds.), *Geriatric nursing protocols for best practice* (pp. 1–12). New York: Springer Publishing Co.

Lasater, M. (1996). The effect of a nurse-managed CHF clinic on patient readmission and length of stay. *Archives of Internal Medicine, 12*, 351–356.

Maljanian, R., Effken, J., & Kaerhle, P. (2000). *Design and implementation of an outcomes management model.* Retrieved March 2, 2002, from http://www.nursingcenter.com.

McComas, A. (1996). *Disuse in muscular skeletal form and function* (pp. 287–298). Champaign, IL: Human Kinetics.

National Caregiver Alliance. (1997). *Family caregiving in the U.S.: Findings from a national survey.* Retrieved March 20, 2002, from http://www.caregiver.org/factsheets/selected_caregiver_statistics.html

National Center for Health Statistics. (1999). *Health of the elderly, United States, 1999.* Hyattsville, MD: Public Health Service. Retrieved 3/13/02 at http://www.cdc.gov/nchs/faststats/elderly. html

Naylor, M. (2000). A decade of transitional care research with vulnerable elders. *Journal of Cardiovascular Nursing, 14,* 1–14.

Naylor, M., Brooten, D., Campbell, R., Jacobsen, B., Mezey, M., Pauly, M., & Schwartz, J. (1999). Comprehensive discharge planning and home follow-up of hospitalized elders. *Journal of the American Medical Association, 281,* 613–620.

Naylor, M., Brooten, D., Jones, R., Lavizzo-Mourney, R., Mezey, M., & Pauly, M. (1994). Comprehensive discharge planning for the hospitalized elderly: A randomized clinical trial. *Annals of Internal Medicine, 120*(12), 999–1006.

Rothschild, J., Bates, D., & Leape, L. (2000). Preventable medical injuries in older persons. *Archives of Internal Medicine, 160,* 2717–2728.

Schumacher, K. L., Stewart, B. J., Archbold, P. G., Dodd, M. J., & Dibble, S. L. (2000). Family caregiving skill: Development of the concept. *Research in Nursing & Health, 23,* 191–203.

Siebens, H., Aronow, H., Edwards, D., & Hghasemit, Z. (2000). A randomized controlled trial of exercise to improve outcomes of acute hospitalization in older adults. *Journal of the American Geriatrics Society, 48,* 1545–1552.

Stewart, S., Pearson, S., & Horowitz, J. (1998). Effects of home-based intervention among patents with congestive heart failure discharged from acute hospital care. *Archives of Internal Medicine, 158,* 1067–1072.

Wu, A., Young, Y., Dawson, N., Bryant, L., Galanos, A., Broste, J., et al. (2002). Estimated of future physical functioning by seriously ill hospitalized patients, their families, and their physicians. *Journal of the American Geriatrics Society, 50,* 230–237.

Chapter 17

CLINICAL PRACTICE PROTOCOLS: TRANSLATING KNOWLEDGE INTO PRACTICE

Deborah C. Francis and Melissa M. Bottrell

EDUCATIONAL OBJECTIVES

On completion of this chapter the reader should be able to:
1. Discuss factors that influence protocol adaptation.
2. Delineate concepts of behavior change that provide a conceptual framework for guideline dissemination and implementation.
3. Discuss the four-step approach to recognizing problems in implementation.
4. Describe implmentation strategies for successful implementation of a protocol.

Improving geriatric nursing care depends not only on the development of evidence-based clinical protocols but also on their widespread application. However, much of the effort in the protocol movement has focused on protocol development with only recent attention paid to the critical aspects of dissemination, implementation, and use (Mittman, Tonesk, & Jacobson, 1992). Lack of attention to the process of implementation can undermine protocol adoption and derail desired changes in behavior and practice patterns. This chapter seeks to help practitioners and institutions recognize that successful protocol adoption and sustained change in provider behavior depend on a coordinated and comprehensive implementation process. The chapter will highlight those forces that influence clinician behavior and examine strategies that can effectively motivate clinicians to adopt innovative nursing practices, using the case example of the Nurses Improving Care for Health System Elders (NICHE) and its elder-focused clinical practice protocols.

CLINICAL PRACTICE PROTOCOLS DEFINED

Clinical practice protocols, like the widely disseminated clinical practice guidelines from the Agency for Healthcare Research and Quality (AHRQ) and the Cochrane Collaborative, are examples of tools that are used to define how scientifically valid and reliable standards of care should be implemented. In 1973, the American Nurses Association (ANA) developed the first *Standards of Nursing Practice* designed to "assess the quality of nursing care and to determine nursing competency" (Schumacher, 1996). Over time, these standards acquired a patient-oriented focus emphasizing the goals of patient care. The standards now underpin performance improvement programs (Mize, Bentley, & Hubbard, 1991) and emphasize the improvement of patient outcomes through research-based interventions (Schumacher, 1996). Clinical practice protocols, practice guidelines, algorithms, and, more recently, critical pathways and care maps have emerged as tools to guide evidenced-based clinical nursing practice (Dracup, 1996). See Table 17.1. These systematically developed statements reduce practice variation, improve patient outcomes, and lead to more effective and efficient use of scarce medical resources.

WHY CARE ABOUT IMPLEMENTATION?

Developed by nationally recognized experts in geriatric nursing care, the NICHE protocols focus on assessment, prevention, and management of common geriatric syndromes that contribute to functional decline in the elderly. These guidelines address the specific needs of older adults and emphasize nurse-driven care approaches.

TABLE 17.1   A Protocol by Any Other Name

Procedure—set of action steps describing how to complete a clinical function

Protocols—precise guidelines with a structured and logical approach to a closely specified clinical problem (Jenkins, 1991)

Standards of care describe a "competent level of nursing care provided to all clients as demonstrated by the nursing process" (American Nurses Association, 1991)

Algorithms—set of steps that approximates the decision process of an expert clinician

Clinical practice guidelines—systematically developed statements that aid in patient decisions for appropriate health care for specific clinical circumstances (Institute of Medicine, 1992)

Critical pathway—multidisciplinary approach that guides the nurse in what to do and when

Unfortunately, recognition of a concept does not guarantee that it will be integrated into new practice patterns. Like the standards of nursing care that collect dust in hospital policy and procedure manuals between accreditation and regulatory visits, practice protocols have had limited success in changing nursing practice or improving patient outcomes (Oxman, Thomson, Davis, & Haynes, 1995). This lack of effectiveness is due in part to the overreliance on traditional lecture-based in-services or continuing education programs and the dissemination of written materials. These interventions are largely unsuccessful in changing provider behavior when used in isolation (Davis, Thomson, Oxman, & Haynes, 1995; Gross et al., 2001; Lee, Chang, & Mackenzie, 2002; Lomas et al., 1989; Oxman et al., 1995; Weingarten et al., 1995).

A FRAMEWORK FOR THE IMPLEMENTATION PROCESS

To be successful, strategies for protocol implementation must consider theories of behavioral change that address social influences and models of clinical decision making (Mittman et al., 1992) while incorporating an understanding of how innovative practice is diffused within a group. *Social influence theory* postulates that the behavior of one individual affects and may change how another person responds, feels, or thinks about something (Zimbardo & Leippe, 1991). This theory argues that decisions and actions are strongly guided by prevailing practice, social norms, economic pressures, and the habits, customs, assumptions, beliefs, and values held by peers (Mittman et al., 1992). As such, a colleague's judgment and beliefs about new information significantly influence how an individual nurse evaluates and uses that information.

The *transtheoretical model* of behavior change, also referred to as the readiness to change model, identifies five stages through which an individual moves in a continual process of molding new behaviors. Each stage warrants a different approach to influence behavior change. The first two stages, *precontemplation* and *contemplation,* involve knowledge and attitude change. When the individual moves into the *preparation* and *action* phases, attention should be paid to addressing emotional processes and developing positive beliefs about self-efficacy and the necessary skills to initiate the change process. Finally, the practitioner who has adopted the behavior moves into the *maintenance* phase, at which point sustaining the behavior requires attention to the environment and requires social support and reward systems.

However, the person who implements the protocol cannot capitalize on the value of social influence or individual behavior change without understanding how change is communicated within a social group over time (Rogers, 1995). *Diffusion of innovation* theory posits that change occurs when a small group of one or more "innovators" conceives an idea for change. In a hospital, innovators may be advanced practice nurses or clinical experts who believe that adoption of a protocol will improve patient care. The new "change idea" is passed from the innovator to "early adopters." Typically, the early adopters are well-respected and credible opinion leaders within a peer group. The idea "takes off" when the early adopters act as role models and communicate best practice patterns to peers. This information sharing makes diffusion of the innovations a social process that occurs naturally as clinicians learn about the protocol, are persuaded to use it, subsequently integrate it into practice, and evaluate it for future use. Although early adopters may be easily convinced to take on a new practice, the majority of the group usually resists change until overwhelming evidence and peer pressure demonstrate that change is the only appropriate option (Rogers, 1995).

Together, these theories provide not only a useful explanation of how change occurs within an individual and is communicated within a social group over time but offer a valuable framework to design a more effective implementation process.

FACTORS INFLUENCING PROTOCOL ADOPTION

Successful change requires recognition of the factors that can both encourage and inhibit initial and sustained protocol adoption. These factors include the qualities of the protocol, the characteristics of the health care professional, the practice setting, incentives for adoption, regulatory requirements, and the patient (Davis & Taylor-Vaisey, 1997). Moreover, assessing the change environment must include a focus on both the needs of the individual clinician and the specific organizational and group barriers to change (Grol & Grimshaw, 1999). Although some of these factors are not amenable to change by those responsible for protocol implementation, highlighting and publicizing those factors that support adoption of the protocol can significantly facilitate the implementation process.

Critical attributes of a protocol that will enhance its adoption and ultimate success include its perceived advantages, complexity, compatibility with existing practices, and ease of testing and evaluating (Rogers, 1995). Providers must first perceive a benefit to changing practice, or the protocol will be ignored. Bolman, de Vries, and Mesters (2002) demonstrated that perceived advantage and simplicity of the protocol are most predictive of a nurses' continued use of a smoking cessation protocol. Using reliable data to highlight specific problem areas and articulating the significance of the problem to target staff and administrators are key steps in establishing the need for a new protocol. For instance, if staff do not recognize that a large percentage of older patients on their unit are at risk for nosocomial infection resulting from urinary catheters, then the staff is unlikely to accept the necessity of an incontinence protocol.

The protocol must be concise, containing only the most salient points, and be readily available to the practitioner. Grilli and Lomas (1994) found that relatively uncomplicated protocols that could be observed or tried by the clinician tended to be adopted more readily. Placing the protocol in an easily accessible location on the unit or on pocket cards with bullet points or checklists, as opposed to placement in a manual behind a desk, will encourage its use. Additionally, computer-based triggers can offer readily available interventions or reminders tied to the protocol (Shiffman, Liaw, Brandt, & Corb, 1999). Computer-based approaches, however, can require complex programming, as well as time and resources to develop and maintain them (Greenes et al., 2001; Shiffman et al., 1999).

The protocol must be compatible with either an individual's previous experience or to existing beliefs and values. If a practitioner does not believe that using a behavioral approach or environmental modifications will calm an agitated patient, chemical or physical restraints will most likely remain the treatment of choice. A good protocol must be easy to implement and must readily demonstrate improvement in patient care. A protocol that facilitates identification of a clinical problem and directs appropriate changes in the patient's treatment plan is more likely to remain in use than one that requires a call to other providers or whose impact is difficult to assess. Geriatric-specific nursing assessments via trigger cards, such as the various SPICES mnemonics (Fulmer, 1991; Guthrie, Edinger, & Schumacher, 2002; Lee & Fletcher, 2002) that initiate nurse-driven patient interventions, are examples of screening and intervention strategies used in NICHE sites. Finally, the ability of the provider to observe the protocol in practice and interact with other providers who have incorporated the new approach, such as in patient care conferences, may facilitate its acceptance.

Uncertainty about the validity or usefulness of the protocol will directly affect how much an individual will rely on the opinions of peers before forming a personal opinion about the protocol (Bandura, 1986). Thus, attempts to implement a protocol could be hampered by an opinion leader, such as a nurse manager or credible staff person, who does not believe in or support the use of the protocol. Prior to implementation, canvassing the opinions of influential staff may identify opposition or indifference to the protocol. When lack of support is identified, a preimplementation phase may be required to obtain the cooperation of opinion leaders through marketing, promise of rewards, or if necessary, organizational coercion. Table 17.2 provides a format for assessing protocol adoption.

Even with the availability of excellent protocols, modifying a health practitioner's behavior to conform to clinical guidelines has proven to be a difficult task that usually requires significant behavioral interventions (Backer, 1995). Factors unrelated to the protocol are far less easy to control and will influence the ability to change

TABLE 17.2   Factors to Assess Protocol Adoption

Advantage—What benefit does the protocol provide in comparison to current practice?

Complexity—How easily can the protocol be introduced into regular practice?

Compatibility—How well does the new practice fit with the practitioner's previous experience, values, and existing beliefs?

Trialability—How easily can the practitioner try the protocol on one patient?

Observability—Are the improvements in practice or changes readily or easily visible to the practitioner?

practice patterns. Clinician-specific characteristics that may affect implementation include age, country and source of training, and knowledge of the domain addressed by the protocol. In addition, a variety of irrational forces, such as fear of change or anxiety about modifying routines, even when change is perceived as desirable, can produce formidable barriers to protocol adoption. Resistance to change also can arise from an individual's psychology and life experiences, feelings of competition and jealousy, need for rewards, sense of autonomy, and ownership of any change out of egotism (Backer, 1995). The degree of a clinician's readiness to change is highly associated with his or her personal beliefs about self-efficacy, as well as having reservations about guidelines in general. Perceptions that guidelines are inherently too rigid to meet the care needs of an increasingly diverse patient population, are not compatible with the individualized nature of patient care, or undermine the way nurse's perceive they work best with patients all will affect protocol adoption (Mulhall, Alexander, & Le May, 1997).

Social and organizational characteristics of the health care setting may hinder adoption of a practice innovation. These include insufficient administrative support and local constraints, such as limited resources and personnel. Commitment by nursing administration has been found to be pivotal to the use of evidence-based practice (Champion & Leach, 1989). Without the commitment and support of both mid-level and top-level managers, clinicians will be less apt to integrate evidence-based protocols into their practice. In a study of nurses' perceived barriers to using research findings in practice Funk, Tornquist, and Champagne (1995) determined that 8 of the top 10 barriers were related to the work environment and organizational process. These barriers are directly influenced by management and include the lack of authority to change practice, little support from other staff and physicians, management refusal to allow implementation, and insufficient time.

The prevailing institutional culture, with its customs, attitudes, and beliefs, must actively support the protocol adoption and implementation process. This includes allowing the extra time required for the implementation process, providing access to expert consultants, and having documentation systems and communication processes that support the new standard of care. The organizational culture must encourage the active involvement of clinicians in the process, particularly in the critical protocol review and modification process. Finally, once the protocol is adopted, a line of accountability must be established. Nurse managers must be accountable to nursing administration, and in turn, nursing staff must be accountable to their nurse managers.

Some target groups may require more formalized, if not coercive approaches, in order to adopt and sustain practice change. Financial or professional incentives (acknowledgment on performance appraisals, advancement on a clinical ladder, or provision of merit pay increases) can encourage adoption of the protocols and may be an excellent way to demonstrate institutional support for protocol use. The priority nurse managers give to protocols that address issues mandated by regulatory agencies or that are tied to the nurse manager's budget may facilitate their adoption. Similarly, protocols dictated by readily observable clinical problems, such as a sentinel event or outbreaks of methicillin-resistant *staphyllococcus aureus* (MRSA), may achieve rapid adoption because of the obvious seriousness of the problem and its impact on nursing care. It is no surprise that a restraint reduction protocol has been somewhat easier to implement in NICHE pilot sites (due, in part, to regulatory mandates) than efforts to decrease the incidence of urinary incontinence or sleep disorders, which have no regulatory implications.

Adopting change through institutional policy or procedure has several advantages: Institutional policy carries the weight of a local standard of care, providing legal liability as well as disciplinary action from the institution as incentives to comply. Institutional policies usually require fastidious documentation of compliance, while supporting the education and supervision of personnel who are involved in carrying out the protocol. However, protocols that appear created for the convenience or financial interests of the institution, rather than explicitly providing ways to meet an accepted standard of care, could be met with resistance by clinicians, if they feel caught between legal liability if they adhere to the policy and disciplinary action if they do not (Murphy, 1997).

DESIGNING A THEORETICAL FRAMEWORK FOR PROTOCOL IMPLEMENTATION

A systematic review of five theories of behavior change identified nine concepts that provide a conceptual framework for guideline dissemination and implementation (Moulding, Silagy, & Weller, 1999):

- Behavior change is an ongoing process through which practitioners progress with the aid of specific interventions that encourage movement from one stage to the next.
- The agents of change must identify with the clinicians and their concerns.
- Preassessment of the clinicians' readiness to change and the specific nature of individual and organizational barriers to change is essential.
- Multiple change strategies are always more effective than single interventions.
- Educational strategies must be participatory and interactive.
- Clinician education needs to focus not only on knowledge and attitudes but also on specific skill development.
- Social influence theory can be used to substantially facilitate or inhibit behavior change.
- There must be support in the work environment for the implementation and maintenance of the behavior change.

Adoption of an innovative clinical practice will require the consideration of the foregoing concepts, while focusing on improvement of processes rather than individual performance (James, 1993). Established procedures for quality assurance (known by such names as *continuous quality improvement, total quality management,* and *workplace reengineering*) can foster protocol implementation (Kaluzny, Konrad, & McLaughlin, 1995). Such quality efforts have the added advantage of more effectively building organizational support for institutionalization of the protocol and promoting a sustained change in behavior. The PDCA ("Plan, Do, Check, Act") performance improvement model organizes and plans the change process, implements the improvement on a small group of patients or a single unit, quickly evaluates the outcomes, and acts immediately to modify or sustain the change process on an institutional level (Dianis & Cummings, 1998; Redick, 1999). Another model is the 10-step process to monitor and evaluate patient care developed by the JCAHO (Walker & Claflin, 1991). Reengineering moves beyond clinical quality indicators (CQI) to examine and dramatically change an organization's core work processes in order to build the innovation into care routines. Such efforts should be considered to promote change in those institutions where change historically has been difficult to accomplish (Kaluzny et al, 1995).

IMPLEMENTATION: RECOGNITION AND IDENTIFICATION OF THE PROBLEMS

Regardless of the model chosen to drive the implementation of a protocol, several basic steps need to be accomplished. Kibbe, Kaluzny, and McLaughlin (1994) suggested that institutions take a four-step approach, in which the institution first recognizes that a problem exists, identifies that the practice protocol is the solution, then implements and institutionalizes the solution. If a change in nursing practice is to be adopted, the initial, essential step is to recognize that there is a discrepancy between how the institution is currently performing and how it could or should be performing (Kaluzny et al., 1992). Adequate time and energy must be invested in developing awareness of a perceived performance gap and identifying, defining, and refining the specific clinical problem. The type and magnitude of the performance gap can be gleaned from analyzing internal data such as utilization review, financial performance, and consumer feedback, as well as external data from regulatory agencies like the JCAHO.

Once it is recognized that the standard of care should be improved, the search for an appropriate intervention begins (the so-called identification phase). This process will involve

- Gathering and synthesizing information about the institution and from the target audience, as well as from other institutions' experience with similar problems

- Identifying factors within the organizational culture that will facilitate as well as impede the desired change
- Developing group consensus and strategies to overcome institutional barriers
- Iterative drafting, critiquing, and revising the protocol

Information gathering should involve a "diagnostic analysis" of the target audience and setting. This step has been described as the most important factor in successfully implemented programs (Grol, 2001). The assessment should focus not only on the needs of the individual clinician but also on specific organizational and group barriers to change, including the social arena within which care is provided (Grol & Grimshaw, 1999). Assessing the clinicians' baseline knowledge and attitudes and identifying specific concerns related to caring for the target patient population will more readily clarify the problem and facilitate organizational buy-in. Clinicians' readiness for change must be evaluated. These efforts can be accomplished with surveys, such as the NICHE Geriatric Institutional Assessment Profile (GIAP) or focus groups. One-on-one discussions with individual clinicians can be tried when their number is small. Convening study groups of individuals from a single discipline to examine and address a specific quality issue fosters a sense of ownership that makes group members more apt to effectively influence one another and develop new behavioral norms.

Based on the information gathered in the surveys, focus groups, or interviews, advocates for change ("organizational champions") need to be identified at the administrative level, and sympathetic opinion leaders need to be recruited among the target groups of clinicians. Gilmore (1988) refers to this process as "stakeholder mapping," in which all key stakeholders are identified and ranked according to (1) whether they are in favor of or opposed to the project and (2) their power within the organization to influence the outcome of the protocol identified. Identification of those most opposed to the change process is essential, as interventions will need to be tailored and targeted to stave off their influence.

A team approach is recommended. The team may be convened at either the recognition or the identification phase. The successful team will acquire a sense of group ownership over the protocol and will show cohesiveness among its members. Successful teams usually are multidisciplinary and include key clinical and administrative staff. The team must include the right individuals for the job: those who will remain committed enough to invest the time and energy needed to maintain the momentum and complete the effort despite bureaucratic obstacles. The number and type of individuals are not as important as their skills, expertise, experience, and interest. Staff nurses should to be involved in the implementation of elder-focused protocols, because it is they who have to live with the results of the change. The organization must also provide team members with adequate support in terms of time, access to resources, reward systems, and specialized training required to accomplish the task.

Active participation of bedside clinicians from the onset will promote a sense of ownership that has been found to be critical to achieving quality outcomes (Harvey & Kitson, 1996). Participatory guideline development is a social influence process that involves unit-based staff to develop or critically review and modify the desired protocol. When staff identify and understand the need for practice change and participate in designing and implementing the remedy, they are more likely to develop consensus and a sense of ownership and to adopt and sustain practice changes. In examining how well clinical staff accepted change at the clinical level in an evaluation of implementation strategies of various nursing quality systems, Harvey and Kitson (1996) concluded that the most important factors were ownership of quality by all staff and support from the top for action and change.

Although involvement of the staff in the implementation process is the key to effective implementation, it has been found that participation, in and of itself, is insufficient to successfully change practice patterns (Mittman et al., 1992). The methods used to disseminate the findings of the work group and the use of multiple intervention strategies will be more likely to enhance the effectiveness of the protocol implementation.

Important tasks at this juncture will be to review and modify relevant institutional policies and to adapt the implementation process to meet specific local practice needs and situations. This process must also include identifying and documenting the specific key steps that are necessary to get the job done and sharing this process with others for feedback (Gates, 1995). It is during this phase that a guiding philosophy of geriatric care is developed and adopted by the institution and organizational commitment is solidified.

Protocols must be credible in the minds of the end user. As such, it is essential to invest time and energy in ensuring that the protocol is evidence-based, as exemplified by the NICHE protocols. Besides the literature review and involving local experts, many important Internet resources are available to those trying to keep up to date on important clinical areas. The Cochrane Collaboration (http://www.update-software.com/Cochrane/default.HTM) conducts and makes available systematic evidence-based reviews of the effects of health care interventions.

Protocol development is an iterative process. As drafts are prepared, it is important to obtain feedback from end-user staff to ascertain what it is they like or do not like about the protocol. Because the protocols are considered guidelines that need to be individualized to each patient rather than mandated standards of care, it is important to consider how to document those specific interventions implemented and the patient's response to them.

As part of the diagnostic analysis, implementers should clarify whether the identified clinical problem is due to impaired decision making on the part of the providers and/or a result of organizational systems and process problems (Kibbe et al., 1994). If the problem is considered to be primarily a lack of awareness, interventions would naturally focus on identifying and articulating problem areas through the use of performance improvement data, a staff awareness campaign, and introducing the use of automated reminders whenever possible. Knowledge deficits are best addressed through creative educational programs and unit-based social influence strategies. In settings where resistance to change is perceived to be a barrier, it is important to utilize behavioral approaches designed to identify and win the support of those most resistant, provide reminders, and concurrent feedback and, because nursing time is often perceived to be an issue, introduce time-management strategies. When problems exist with organizational systems and processes, it may be more important to focus on developing and implementing a screening process to identify appropriate patients, modifying or developing documentation forms, optimizing teamwork, leadership, and communication processes, and creating reminder systems.

THE IMPLEMENTATION AND INSTITUTIONALIZATION STAGES

Systematic reviews of implementation strategies demonstrate that the most crucial factor is the use of a multifaceted strategy rather than a single intervention (Kaluzny et al., 1995; Moulding et al., 1999;

Oxman et al., 1995; Solberg et al., 2000). For example, a major challenge during this phase may be persuading administrators that a committee decision to adopt the protocol is just the beginning of the process—that merely placing the protocols in a unit binder will not positively impact patient care. The effort must not be done in isolation but be part of a broader organizational strategy in which a consistent infrastructure is created and utilized in the implementation process. Enlist the efforts of institutional committees and councils, such as quality improvement and peer review groups to support the protocol adoption process. Their involvement lends credibility to the change process and helps the clinical champions and potentially discourages adversaries (Kaluzny et al., 1995).

The implementation strategy most effective in producing a change in behavior will vary according to the desired behavior changes, the type of practitioner, the technologies involved, and the settings in which the change will occur (Kibbe et al., 1994). Mittman and colleagues (1992) studied the effectiveness of social influence strategies to implement guidelines in each type of health care setting. In moderate-sized target groups characterized by closely interacting providers, such as hospital nursing unit, social influence strategies are far more effective in implementing and adopting change. These strategies, all of which have been used to varying degrees with relative success at the various NICHE sites, include the use of opinion leaders, performance improvement, study groups, patient care rounds, and participatory guideline development. It is in this type of setting where the NICHE protocols are more apt to be implemented by nursing staff and where appropriately addressing group norms and culture is crucial.

It has been suggested that communication with peers is critical in influencing behavior in persuasion settings, and Rogers (1995) concluded that increased peer communication is the most important strategy to promote the adoption of guidelines. In promoting the adoption of a NICHE protocol, opinion leaders attempt to convince colleagues that the proposed change in practice represents state-of-the-art, research-based interventions that are superior to current practice

The experience of the NICHE sites demonstrated that involvement of nursing opinion leaders, including outside experts, significantly enhances protocol implementation. The support of staff members known to be excellent clinicians or a respected local nursing expert, such as advanced practice nurses or nursing school faculty members, can build both excitement about practice improvements and momentum in the implementation process. In the geriatric resource nurse (GRN) model of care, resource nurses play a crucial role as clinical opinion leaders who educate peers, model appropriate behavior, and ultimately influence changes in clinical practice (Fulmer, 1991).

Depending on the local environment, social influence strategies need to be considered to more successfully disseminate both printed and verbal information, educate staff, modify the medical record and information systems, develop incentives and reminders, provide concurrent feedback, and evaluate the success of the protocol. Consider using multiple dissemination media to ensure that protocols are seen more easily and managed by staff, such as written information in newsletters and on bulletin boards, laminated pocket cards, posters, and algorithms printed on the nurses' charting forms. Printed guidelines serve best as reference material for those already acculturated to the change process, although they also can provide interim education to new personnel as they await formal instruction in the use of protocols. Promote compliance with creative rewards and incentives that encourage active participation and friendly competition between nursing units.

The information should be discussed routinely at every opportunity, including during staff meetings, one-on-one discussions, patient care conferences, and shift reports. Interdisciplinary patient care rounds offer an excellent opportunity to use social influence processes to regularly and effectively educate staff, model best practice, encourage group participation, and influence behavior. Patient care rounds are an integral component of the GRN and Acute Care for the Elderly (ACE) models of care and are being used at numerous NICHE sites to better manage frail older patients.

It is important to individually tailor the educational program to the target group, by addressing not only knowledge deficits and attitudes but also the development of necessary skills. For example, a fall prevention protocol that expects the nursing staff to assess fall risk will be useless unless they are confident in their ability to perform simple gait and balance assessment. Use adult learning theory and, most importantly, creative learning strategies including sensitivity training, small group discussions, case presentations, and a variety of media that encourage active participation. Consider developing the initial training for the opinion leaders and clinical champions, who will then be able to role model appropriate behavior when training for all staff commences.

Educating the consumer through public relations is important to sustain the behavior change. Knowledge of best practice empowers the consumer to make choices that are more informed and may provide a framework by which patients can evaluate the appropriateness of care.

A final, but critical, component of the implementation phase is the evaluation, which needs to be designed from the outset and is used to drive the process. Consider quality improvement and utilization-review data in developing the evaluation plan. Outcome measures must address the purpose and goals of the protocol and should include both patient outcomes and staff compliance. Meaningful, timely, and constructive feedback must be provided not only to the target nursing staff, but to all staff, including other disciplines, as well as nonprofessional and temporary staff (Harvey & Kitson, 1996).

With completion of these steps, the protocol is ready to be institutionalized or integrated into the day-to-day operations of the organization. Educating new team members about the protocol and the justification for use, continuing to evaluate the outcomes, and modifying the process design will need to be considered if the protocol is to be fully integrated into nursing practice. Attention must be paid to integrating the protocol into the orientation for all newly hired, float and traveler nurses, since transfer of information occurs during the socialization process when an individual first encounters the new social setting (Mittman et al., 1992). It is important to include critical protocols such as falls, restraint management and management of difficult behaviors into annual competency training for all staff to further reinforce the information and help to sustain the behavior change. Titler and colleagues (Titler, Mentes, Rakel, Abbott, & Baumler, 1999) encourage the "reinfusion" of evidenced-based practice by developing a plan for systematically reintroducing the protocol and monitoring its ongoing use.

SUMMARY

Elder-focused clinical practice protocols have the potential to dramatically improve patient care by fostering clinical decision making based on best practice geriatric nursing standards. However, without an administrative commitment and a comprehensive organizational strategy, they may be perceived as unnecessary additional work for the already overburdened staff. It is critical for the organization to pay close attention to both the how and the what of protocols and develop highly specific, localized, and targeted efforts at developing, disseminating, assimilating, evaluating, and adopting geriatric patient standards of care. Be proactive and highly visible in your endeavor. Recognize the importance of small successes in winning over additional support, publicize the attainment of small goals early on, and provide ongoing and timely feedback to both the decision makers and those involved in the change process. Implementation of any practice change is a huge endeavor but one that is certainly worth the effort.

REFERENCES

American Nurses Association. (1991). *Standards of clinical nursing practice.* Kansas City, MO: Author.

Backer, T. E. (1995). Integrating behavioral and systems strategies to change clinical practice. *Joint Commission Journal of Quality Improvement, 21,* 351–353.

Bandura, A. (1986). *Social foundations of thought and action: A social cognitive theory.* Englewood Cliffs, NJ: Prentice-Hall.

Bolman, C., de Vries, H., & Mesters, I. (2002). Factors determining cardiac nurses' intentions to continue using a smoking cessation protocol. *Heart Lung, 31*(1), 15–24.

Champion, V. L., & Leach, A. (1989). Variables related to research utilization in nursing: An empirical investigation. *Journal of Advanced Nursing, 14,* 705–710.

Davis, D. A., & Taylor-Vaisey, A. (1997). Translating guidelines into practice. A systematic review of theoretic concepts, practical experience and research evidence in the adoption of clinical practice guidelines. *Canadian Medical Association Journal, 157,* 408–416.

Davis, D. A., Thomson, M. A., Oxman, A. D., & Haynes, R. B. (1995). Changing physician performance: A systematic review of the effect of continuing medical education strategies. *Journal of the American Medical Association, 274,* 700–705.

Dianis, N. L., & Cummings, C. (1998). An interdisciplinary approach to process performance improvement. *Journal of Nursing Care Quality, 12,* 49–59.

Dracup, K. (1996). Putting clinical practice guidelines to work. *Nursing, 26*(2), 41–44, 46–47.

Fulmer, T. T. (1991). Grow your own experts in hospital elder care. *Geriatric Nursing, 12*(2), 64–66.

Funk, S. G., Tornquist, E. M., & Champagne, M. T. (1995). Barriers and facilitators of research utilization. An integrative review. *Nursing Clinics of North America, 30,* 395–407.

Gates, P. E. (1995). Think globally, act locally: An approach to implementation of clinical practice guidelines. *The Joint Commission Journal of Quality Improvement, 21*(2), 71–84.

Gilmore, T. (1988). *Making a leadership change: How organizations and leaders can handle leadership change successfully.* San Francisco: Jossey-Bass.

Greenes, R. A., Peleg, M., Boxwala, A., Tu, S., Patel, V., & Shortliffe, E. H. (2001). Sharable computer-based clinical practice guidelines: Rationale, obstacles, approaches, and prospects. *Medinfo, 10*(Pt. 1), 201–205.

Grilli, R., & Lomas, J. (1994). Evaluating the message: The relationship between compliance rate and the subject of a practice guideline. *Medical Care, 32,* 202–213.

Grol, R. (2001). Successes and failures in the implementation of evidence-based guidelines for clinical practice. *Medical Care, 39*(8, Suppl. 2), II46–54.

Grol, R., & Grimshaw, J. (1999). Evidence-based implementation of evidence-based medicine. *The Joint Commission Journal of Quality Improvement, 25*(10), 503–513.

Gross, P. A., Greenfield, S., Cretin, S., Ferguson, J., Grimshaw, J., Grol, R., Klazinga, N., Lorenz, W., Meyer, G. S., Riccobono, C., Schoenbaum, S. C., Schyve, P., & Shaw, C. (2001). Optimal methods for guideline implementation: Conclusions from Leeds Castle meeting. *Medical Care, 39*(8, Suppl. 2), II85–92.

Guthrie, P. F., Edinger, G., & Schumacher, S. (2002). TWICE: A NICHE program at North Memorial Health Care. *Geriatric Nursing, 23*(3), 133–139.

Harvey, G., & Kitson, A. (1996). Achieving improvement through quality: An evaluation of key factors in the implementation process. *Journal of Advanced Nursing, 24*(1), 185–195.

Institute of Medicine. (1992). *Guidelines for clinical practice: From development to use.* Washington, DC: National Academy Press.

James, B. C. (1993). Implementing practice guidelines through clinical quality improvement. *Frontiers of Health Service Management, 10*(1), 3–37.

Jenkins, D. (1991). Investigations: How to get from guidelines to protocols. *British Medical Journal, 303,* 323–324.

Kaluzny, A. D., Konrad, T. R., & McLaughlin, C. P. (1995). Organizational strategies for implementing clinical guidelines. *The Joint Commission Journal of Quality Improvement, 21,* 347–351.

Kaluzny, A., McLaughlin, C., & Kibbe, D. (1992). Continuous quality improvement in the clinical setting: Enhancing adoption. *Quality Management in Health Care, 1*(1), 37–44.

Kibbe, D. C., Kaluzny, A. D., & McLaughlin, C. P. (1994). Integrating guidelines with continuous quality improvement: Doing the right thing the right way to achieve the right goals. *The Joint Commission Journal of Quality Improvement, 20,* 181–191.

Lee, F. K., Chang, A. M., & Mackenzie, A. E. (2002). A pilot project to evaluate implementation of clinical guidelines. *Journal of Nursing Care Quality, 16*(2), 50–59.

Lee, V. K., & Fletcher, K. R. (2002). Sustaining the geriatric resource nurse model at the University of Virginia. *Geriatric Nursimg, 23,* 128–132.

Lomas, J., Anderson, G. M., Domnick-Pierre, K., Vayda, E., Enkin, M. W., & Hannah, W. J. (1989). Do practice guidelines guide practice? The effect of a consensus statement on the practice of physicians. *New England Journal of Medicine, 321*(19), 1306–1311.

Mittman, B. S., Tonesk, X., & Jacobson, P. D. (1992). Implementing clinical practice guidelines: Social influence strategies and practitioner behavior change. *Quality Review Bulletin, 18,* 413–422.

Mize, C. P., Bentley, G., & Hubbard, S. (1991). Standards of care: Integrating nursing care plans and quality assurance activities. *AACN Clinical Issues in Critical Care Nursing, 2*(1), 63–68.

Moulding, N. T., Silagy, C. A., & Weller, D. P. (1999). A framework for effective management of change in clinical practice: Dissemination and implementation of clinical practice guidelines. *Quality Health Care, 8,* 177–183.

Mulhall, A., Alexander, C., & Le May, A. (1997). Prescriptive care? Guidelines and protocols. *Nursing Standards, 11*(18), 43–46.

Murphy, R. N. (1997). Legal and practical impact of clinical practice guidelines on nursing and medical practice. *Nurse Practitioners, 22,* 138, 147–138.

Oxman, A. D., Thomson, M. A., Davis, D. A., & Haynes, R. B. (1995). No magic bullets: A systematic review of 102 trials of interventions to improve professional practice. *Canadian Medical Association Journal, 153,* 1423–1431.

Redick, E. L. (1999). Applying FOCUS-PDCA to solve clinical problems. *Dimensions in Critical Care Nursing, 18*(6), 30–34.

Rogers, E. M. (1995). Lessons for guidelines from the diffusion of innovations. *The Joint Commission Journal of Quality Improvement, 21,* 324–328.

Schumacher, S. B. (1996). Integrating guidelines into nursing practice. *Medical Surgical Nursing, 5,* 374–377.

Shiffman, R. N., Liaw, Y., Brandt, C. A., & Corb, G. J. (1999). Computer-based guideline implementation systems: A systematic review of functionality and effectiveness. *Journal of the American Medical Informatics Association, 6,* 104–114.

Solberg, L. I., Brekke, M. L., Fazio, C. J., Fowles, J., Jacobsen, D. N., Kottke, T. E., Mosser, G., O'Connor, P. J., Ohnsorg, K. A., & Rolnick, S. J. (2000). Lessons from experienced guideline implementers: Attend to many factors and use multiple strategies. *Joint Commission Journal of Quality Improvement, 26,* 171–188.

Titler, M. G., Mentes, J. C., Rakel, B. A., Abbott, L., & Baumler, S. (1999). From book to bedside: Putting evidence to use in the care of the elderly. *Joint Commission Journal of Quality Improvement, 25,* 545–556.

Walker, J., & Claflin, N. (1991). Standards of care and practice: A vital link in quality assurance. *AACN Clinical Issues in Critical Care Nursing, 2*(1), 90–95.

Weingarten, S., Stone, E., Hayward, R., Tunis, S., Pelter, M., Huang, H., & Kristopaitis, R. (1995). The adoption of preventive care practice guidelines by primary care physicians: Do actions match intentions? *Journal of General and Internal Medicine, 10,* 138–144.

Zimbardo, P. G., & Leippe, M. R. (1991). *The psychology of attitude change and social influence.* Philadelphia: Temple University Press.

APPENDIX

NATIONAL GERIATRIC WEB SITES

LINKS TO AGING INSTITUTIONS AND ASSOCIATIONS

The John A. Hartford Foundation	http://www.jhartford.org
Administration on Aging	http://www.www.aoa.org
Alzheimer's Association	http://www.alz.org
American Association of Homes and Services for the Aging	http://www.aahsa.org
American Association of Retired Persons	http://www.aarp.org
American Geriatrics Society	http://www.ags.org
American Healthcare Association	http://www.ahca.org
The American Society of Consultant Pharmacists (ASCP)	http://www.ascp.com/public/pr/geriatrics/
American Society on Aging	http://www.asaging.org
Elder Web	http://www.elderweb.com
Caregiver resources	http://www.state.il.us/aging/1caregivers/caregiver_links.htm
Gerontological Society of America	http://www.geron.org
Hospice and Palliative Nurses Association	http://www.hpna.org
Centers for Medicare & Medicaid Services (HCFA)	http://cms.hhs.gov/
Hospice and Palliative Nurses Association	http://www.hpna.org
National Association of Geriatric Education Centers	http://www.hcoa.org/nagec/
National Citizen's Coalition for Nursing Home Reform	http://www.nccnhr.org
National Chronic Care Consortium	http://www.ncconline.org/

National Conference of Gerontological   http://www.ncgnp.org
  Nurse Practitioners

National Council on Aging   http://www.www.ncoa.org

National Gerontological   http://www.ngna.org
  Nursing Association

National Institute on Aging   http://www.nih.gov/nia/

On-line Resources for Geriatric   http://www.geriatricvideo.com/
  Healthcare Providers

Curriculum Guides

Long-Term Care Nursing Leadership   http://ltcnurseleader.umn.edu/
  and Management

GeroNet Health & Aging Resources   http://www.ph.ucla.edu
  for Higher Education

Teaching Gerontology Newsletter   http://www.brookdale.org

Gerontology Centers/Education Centers

Andrus Gerontology Center   http:/www.usc.edu/dept/gero/

Brookdale Center on Aging   http://brookdale.org

Gerontological Nursing Interventions   http://www.nursing.uiowa.edu/
  Research Center   centers/gnirc

Iowa Geriatric Education Center   http://www.medicine.uiowa.edu/
                                         igec/igec/index.html

Reynolds Center on Aging   http://www.uams.edu/main.asp

Texas Consortium of Geriatric   http://www.bcm.tmc.edu/hcoa/
  Education Centers   links/.tcgec.html

Wayne State University Institute   http://www.iog.wayne.edu
  of Gerontology

Wisconsin Geriatric Education Center   http://www.marquette.edu/wgec/

Listservs

AGING-DD (Aging and developmental   mailto:listserv@lsv.uky.edu
  disabilities)

GERINNE (Gerontological Nursing   mailto:listserv@ubvm.cc.buffalo.
  Issues)   eduGERO-NURSE (Listserve for
                                         the Research Develpment and
                                         Dissemination Core-University of
                                         Iowa Gerontological Nursing
                                         Intervention Project). mailto:
                                         gero-nurse-list@list.uiowa.edu

INDEX

Springer Publishing Company

Geriatric Interdisciplinary Team Training

Eugenia L. Siegler, MD, FACP, Kathryn Hyer, DrPA, MPP, Terry Fulmer, RN, PhD, FAAN, and Mathy Mezey, RN, EdD, FAAN

"This book provides a robust analysis of the critical issues relevant to the next phase of geriatric interdisciplinary team training in the United States. It is a critical resource...."
–from the Foreword by John W. Rowe, MD

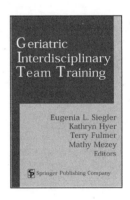

The authors describe their experience as participants in the ground-breaking Hartford Foundation initiative to create replicable new models for geriatric interdisciplinary team training (GITT).

Partial Contents:

- The John A. Hartford Foundation GITT Program
- A Perspective on Health Care Teams and Team Training
- Recruiting Students for GITT
- Selecting and Preparing Team Training Educators
- Using Existing and Emerging Technologies to Promote GITT
- Evaluating the Effects of GITT
- Geriatric Team Training in Managed Care Organizations
- Turning the Clinical Agency into a Setting for Team Training
- Integrated Health Care Systems
- Challenges of Rural Sites

1998   345pp   0-8261-1210-2   hard

536 Broadway, New York, NY 10012 • (212) 431-4370 • Fax (212) 941-7842
Order Toll-Free: 877-687-7476 • Order on-line: www.springerpub.com

Springer Publishing Company

Geriatric Nursing Research Digest

Joyce J. Fitzpatrick, PhD, RN, FAAN
Terry Fulmer, PhD, RN, FAAN

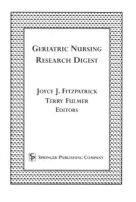

This unique synopsis of geriatric nursing research represents an important resource for the future care of the elderly. Written by leading experts in the forefront of the field, each entry describes the most significant research in a selected area and illuminates the relevance of this research to clinical practice.

Topics include: health promotion and risk reduction; normal aging through the lifespan; environments of care; emotional health; pathological conditions; and more.

For students of geriatric nursing to assist them in identifying significant research issues and questions. For geriatric nurses to apply the available research to practice.

Contents:
- **Section I:** Health Promotion & Risk Reduction
- **Section II:** Normalcy Throughout Lifespan
- **Section III:** Issues in Environments of Care
- **Section IV:** Geriatric Emotional Health
- **Section V:** Pathological Conditions
- **Section VI:** Neurobehavioral & Cognitive Changes of Aging
- References
- Index

2000   593pp   0-8261-1332-X   hard

536 Broadway, New York, NY 10012 • (212) 431-4370 • Fax (212) 941-7842
Order Toll-Free: 877-687-7476 • Order on-line: www.springerpub.com

Springer Publishing Company

Care of Arthritis in the Older Adult

Ann Schmidt Luggen, PhD, RN, ARNP, CNAA
Sue E. Meiner, EdD, RN, CS, GNP, Editors

"The editors' competence and compassion shine through...It is a pleasure to see this vital book come to fruition..." —from the Foreword by **Priscilla Ebersole,** PhD, RN, FAAN

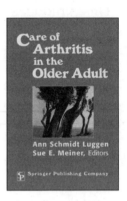

This concise guide provides nurses with the tools to help older adults with arthritis achieve the highest possible quality of life. Practical tips on nursing management, self care, and the importance of exercise are a focus throughout. Any nurse working with the elderly will find this a fundamental resource.

PARTIAL CONTENTS:

- Osteoarthritis, *P. Birchfield*
- Rheumatoid Arthritis, *A.S. Luggen*
- Gouty Arthritis, *S.E. Meiner*
- Polymyalgia Rheumatica and Giant Cell Arteritis, *L. Kennedy-Malone*
- Cervical and Lumbar Disk Problems, *S.E. Meiner*
- Osteoporosis, *P. Mezinskis*
- Assessing and Managing Pain,*A.S. Luggen*
- Exercise and Physical Therapy, *B. Resnick*
- Quality of Life Issues, *P.J. Atkinson*
- Alternative and Complementary Therapies, *M.R. Painter-Romanello*
- Participating in Sports with Arthritis, *C.A. Hill*

Springer Series on Geriatric Nursng
2002   232pp   0-8261-2362-7   hard

536 Broadway, New York, NY 10012 • (212) 431-4370 • Fax (212) 941-7842
Order Toll-Free: 877-687-7476 • Order on-line: www.springerpub.com